Orthopedic Physical Examination Tests

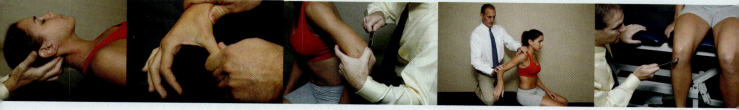

Orthopedic Physical Examination Tests
An Evidence-Based Approach

Chad E. Cook, PT, PhD, MBA, OCS, FAAOMPT
Assistant Professor
Duke University Medical Center
Durham, North Carolina

Eric J. Hegedus, PT, DPT, MHSc, OCS, CSCS
Assistant Professor
Duke University
Durham, North Carolina

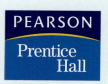

PEARSON

Prentice
Hall

Upper Saddle River, New Jersey 07458

Library of Congress Cataloging-in-Publication Data

Cook, Chad E.
  Orthopedic physical examination tests : a evidence-based approach / Chad E. Cook, Eric J. Hegedus.
    p. ; cm.
  Includes bibliographical references and index.
  ISBN-13 978-0-13-179100-8
  ISBN-10 0-13-179100-1
1. Manipulation (therapeutics) 2. Orthopedics. 3. Medicine, Physical. I. Title.
  [DLNM: 1. Manipulation, Orthopedic—methods—handbooks. WB 39 C771o 2008]
  RM724.C66 2008
  615.8'2—dc22
                                              2008015857

Publisher: Julie Levin Alexander
Executive Editor: Mark Cohen
Associate Editor: Melissa Kerian
Editorial Assistant: Nicole Ragonese
Media Editor: John J. Jordan
New Media Project Manager: Stephen Hartner
Managing Editor for Production: Patrick Walsh
Production Liaison: Christina Zingone
Production Editor: Jessica Balch, Pine Tree Composition
Manufacturing Manager: Ilene Sanford
Manufacturing Buyer: Pat Brown

Design Director: Maria Guglielmo
Cover Designer: Anthony Gemmellaro
Interior Design Coordinator: L.P. Zeidenstein, Pine Tree Composition
Director of Marketing: Karen Allman
Senior Marketing Manager: Harper Coles
Marketing Specialist: Michael Sirinides
Marketing Assistant: Wayne Celia
Composition: Pine Tree Composition, Inc.
Printer/Binder: Courier Kendallville
Cover Printer: Phoenix Color Corp.

Pearson Education Ltd., *London*
Pearson Education Australia Pty. Limited, *Sydney*
Pearson Education Singapore, Pte. Ltd.
Pearson Education North Asia Ltd., *Hong Kong*
Pearson Education Canada, Ltd., *Toronto*
Pearson Educación de Mexico, S.A. de C.V.
Pearson Education—Japan, *Tokyo*
Pearson Education Malaysia, Pte. Ltd.
Pearson Education, Upper Saddle River, New Jersey

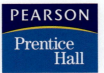

10 9 8 7 6 5

ISBN-13: 978-0-13-179100-8
ISBN-10:   0-13-179100-1

Contents

Contents

Foreword

"If you pour molten iron ore out on the ground you get 'pig iron' but if you beat it a lot you get steel."

Lenox D. Baker, MD, Chairman,
Orthopaedic Surgery, Duke University, 1937–1967

Such was the traditional philosophy of teaching residents at Duke during the Baker, Stead, and Sabiston (Chairman respectively of Orthopaedics, Medicine, and Surgery) era. The essence of this "beating" was a grounding in anatomy and physical examination which has been lost to a large extent and overshadowed by newer technologies. These technologies, while tremendous in sum, do not replace the foundation of a good history and physical examination. We would do well to return to these basics. In this light, it is my distinct pleasure to introduce the first edition of *Orthopedic Physical Examination Tests: An Evidence-Based Approach* by Chad E. Cook and Eric J. Hegedus, which forms a tremendous link between the ancient art of physical examination and current technology in statistical analysis and outcomes research. I believe that the authors have provided information in this text which will result in a paradigm shift in our understanding of physical findings.

There is no shortage of information on physical examination of the spine and extremities. The unusual and perhaps disappointing reality is that very little has been added to the armamentarium of the health care professional in this area since the work of Hoppenfeld,[1] originally published nearly 40 years ago. It is not surprising with the advent of the PET scan, 3D CT scan, functional MRI, MRA, and other advanced imaging studies that there has been a movement away from the basics. We currently operate in a high-tech, low-touch world where time constraints and financial issues occupy the mind of the busy practitioner. At Duke we have no shortage of decorum-laden tradition and the icons of the past— Baker, Stead, and Sabiston—call out to us to remain proficient in the most basic of the healing arts, the physical examination. Dr. Stead, addressing the house staff who had unsuccessfully attempted to diagnose a patient's disease, made his famous and acerbic comment, "What this patient needs is a doctor."[2] Perhaps in our day and time when we are facing a challenging clinical problem where specialized x-ray views, MRI, and neurologic studies have been unrevealing, we should suggest "maybe we should order a physical examination."

It is clear that the work presented in this text by Cook and Hegedus addresses this situation in spades. They have been tremendously thorough in covering the basic tests for all areas of the musculoskeletal system and have gone one step further in subjecting each of these tests to scientific scrutiny with modern statistical analysis and outcomes measures. This will allow for the appropriate placement of each of these tests in our armamentarium as we face a difficult diagnostic dilemma. I have no doubt that for years to come trainees, and ultimately patients, will thank the authors for this contribution to our knowledge base.

Claude T. Moorman III, MD
Director, Sports Medicine
Duke University Medical Center

References
1. Stanley Hoppenfeld, *Physical Examination of the Spine Extremities,* Upper Saddle River, NJ: Prentice Hall, 1976.
2. Eugene A. Stead, Jr., *What This Patient Needs is a Doctor,* Durham, NC: Carolina Academic Press, 1978.

Foreword

The key to finding a remedy to a problem is the accurate recognition of the problem. In medicine, the recognition of the problem is based on the examination process. One of the keys to a successful examination is the selection of appropriate tests. The question the clinician must ask him- or herself when examining a patient is, "Which test is best?" for identifying this specific patient's problem. The selected examination tests can assist the clinician in ruling out specific lesions and aid in ruling in others. The appropriate test should render true positive results, while minimizing false positive results. Thus, the selection of the best examination tests must exhibit a high degree of sensitivity and specificity.

Numerous textbooks and articles have been written describing the examination of specific body regions or anatomical structures. Often authors describe traditional tests or explain new tests or modification of existing ones. There are hundreds of examination tests available to the clinician, but which tests are the best for the specific patient's lesion? The question the practitioner must ask is whether the test is a "good test" for recognition of this patient's specific lesion.

This textbook is unique. Not only have the authors of this textbook described a plethora of examination tests, but they have also reviewed the literature extensively to analyze the foundation of the described tests. The authors have discussed the scientific evidence for all the tests described. In this era of evidence-based treatment, the authors have provided to the reader the reliability, validity, diagnostic values, and perhaps most importantly the clinical utility.

This textbook is a valuable tool to all practitioners (physicians, physical therapists, athletic trainers, etc.) when evaluating and treating musculoskeletal disorders. This textbook aides the clinician in selecting the "best available examination test" for their patients. Because, as the authors have stated in Chapter 1, "clearly all physical examination tests are not created equal."

Cook and Hegedus should be commended for their work. It appears to me that their efforts were a labor of love. The authors have put forth an enormous effort compiling this information from the current literature. Over 600 references have been utilized to write this textbook. This textbook is an excellent addition to any practitioner's library. Thank you to Cook and Hegedus for helping us practitioners in selecting the best available physical examination tests for our patients. Furthermore, thank you for guiding us through the often difficult and curvy road of the clinical examination.

Kevin E. Wilk, PT, DPT

Preface

Do orthopedic clinicians need another collection of special tests and measures? At first glance, one might think not. However, in the age of evidence-based practice, we believe that the previous methods of presenting physical examination tests are both incomplete and riddled with inaccuracies and bias. To truly demonstrate benefit, a test and measure for screening or for diagnostic confirmation must show appropriate diagnostic accuracy, be free from bias, and should be reproducible and effective for the condition and clinical environment at hand. To our knowledge no textbook has examined these aspects of tests and measures.

We have addressed four particular foci in this book. First, we provide a diagnostic value (Sensitivity, Specificity, Positive Likelihood Ratio [LR+], and Negative Likelihood Ratio [LR-]) for each of the tests (if they exist). Diagnostic accuracy scores for a given pathoanatomical diagnosis provide clinicians with quick information for appropriate test selection. Second, we have attempted to gather all studies that have examined the diagnostic value of teach test. By reviewing numerous studies for each test, we have reduced the chance that sampling bias, operator bias, or poor study design could significantly influence the findings. Third, we have scored each of the studies that have evaluated the tests using the Quality Assessment of Diagnostic Accuracy Studies (QUADAS) instrument; something no other text does. QUADAS assists the reader in appreciating the extent to which bias has influenced the estimates of diagnostic accuracy. When the QUADAS score is low, the statistics that estimate diagnostic accuracy should be viewed with a healthy skepticism by the reader. Finally, two summary scores are provided: (1) the diagnostic odds ratio (DOR) and (2) a "Utility Score." The DOR is a statistic that combines sensitivity, specificity, positive likelihood ratio, and negative likelihood ratio so that

a clinician can view one number that reflects diagnostic accuracy and allows quick comparison between articles. However, because the DOR lacks an easy translation to clinical practice, we provide a summary Utility Score for the body of research surrounding each test. Our Utility Score takes into account the reliability, the diagnostic accuracy, the study quality, and the usefulness of the test in clinical practice. The Utility Score is unabashedly homegrown and is based on our empirical and clinical expertise. The measure is our educated opinion as to the use of the test in the clinical environment. For ease of access, the tests are listed in each chapter according to pathoanatomical classification and ordered in a descending fashion, from best to worst, based on their Utility Score.

Chapter Overview

For some orthopedic clinicians, the statistical terminology may be as unfamiliar as viewing these physical examination measures in the light we have presented. Chapter 1 is essentially a user's guide for the textbook. Chapter 1 outlines the two primary purposes of a physical examination test and the required elements, including sensitivity, specificity, responsiveness, dedicated procedure, and referencing. The chapter also describes and discusses the use of a LR+ and LR-. Furthermore, the reader is introduced to the STARD and QUADAS scoring methods used for each study.

Chapter 2 outlines neurological testing methods, including reflex testing, sensibility testing, manual muscle testing, and selected procedures for upper motor neuron assessment. Structural differentiation testing is introduced to assist the clinician in differentiating between shoulder/cervical, lumbar/pelvis, and other difficult-to-isolate regions.

Chapter 3 outlines the physical examination tests for the cervical spine, and includes all case series and cohorts designs that have investigated the diagnostic values. Each test includes a utility score and a QUADAS score.

Chapter 4 reports the physical examination tests for the shoulder complex and includes all case series and cohorts designs that have investigated the diagnostic values. Each test includes a utility score and a QUADAS score.

Chapter 5 reports the physical examination tests of the elbow, wrist, and hand and includes all case series and cohorts designs that have investigated the diagnostic values. Each test includes a utility score and a QUADAS score.

Chapter 6 reports the physical examination tests of the thoracic spine and includes all case series and cohorts designs that have investigated the diagnostic values. Each test includes a utility score and a QUADAS score.

Chapter 7 includes the physical examination tests of the lumbar spine and includes all case series and cohorts designs that have investigated the diagnostic values. Each test includes a utility score and a QUADAS score.

Chapter 8 includes the physical examination tests of the sacroiliac joint and pelvis and includes all case series and cohorts designs that have investigated the diagnostic values. Each test includes a utility score and a QUADAS score.

Chapter 9 reports the physical examination tests of the hip and includes all case series and cohorts designs that have investigated the diagnostic values. Each test includes a utility score and a QUADAS score.

Chapter 10 reports the physical examination tests of the knee and includes all case series and cohorts designs that have investigated the diagnostic values. Each test includes a utility score and a QUADAS score.

Chapter 11 reports the special clinical tests of the lower leg, ankle, and foot and includes all case series and cohorts designs that have investigated the diagnostic values. Each test includes a utility score and a QUADAS score.

We hope that the information presented in this book adds to a growing pool of evidence for orthopedic testing and stimulates meaningful thought and discussion.

Chad E. Cook PT, PhD, MBA, OCS, FAAOMPT
Duke University

Eric J. Hegedus PT, DPT, MHSc, OCS, CSCS
Duke University

Contributors

Dawn Driesner PT, DPT
Physical Therapist
Dunn Physical Therapy
Cary, North Carolina
Chapter 10: Physical Examination Tests for the Knee

Adam Goode PT, DPT, CSCS
Clinical Instructor
Division of Physical Therapy
Department of Community and Family Medicine
School of Medicine
Duke University
Durham, North Carolina
Chapter 5: Physical Examination Tests for the Elbow, Wrist, and Hand

Alexis Wright, PT, DPT
Physical Therapist
Department of Physical and Occupational Therapy
Duke University Medical Center
Durham, North Carolina
Chapter 10: Physical Examination for the Knee

Reviewers

Aimie F. Kachingwe, PT, EdD, OCS, MTC
Assistant Professor, Physical Therapy
California State University–Northridge
Northridge, California

Morey J. Kolber, PT, PhD(c), MDT, CSCS
Assistant Professor, Physical Therapy
Nova Southeastern University
Fort Lauderdale, Florida

Eric R. Miller, PT, DSc, OCS
Associate Professor, Physical Therapy
D'Youville College
Buffalo, New York

David M. Selowitz, PT, PhD, OCS, DAAPM
Professor, Physical Therapy Education
Western University of Health Sciences
Pomona, California

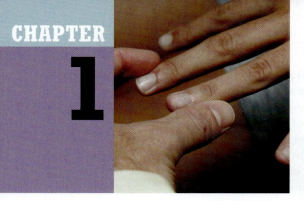

Introduction to Diagnostic Accuracy

Introduction

Diagnosis of patients with orthopedic problems is a complex cognitive and psychomotor task that primarily consists of a patient interview and physical examination. A well-performed patient interview produces the patient history and the range of possible diagnoses and begins to narrow the range of possible diagnoses.[3,19,32] The physical examination of patients with orthopedic problems is the next step in the patient encounter and a cornerstone of the diagnostic process. During the physical examination, the clinician uses findings to further modify the probability of the range of diagnoses,[1,3,27,39] ruling in some, ruling out others, and creating a list of impairments ultimately arriving at a hypothesis as to the pathology that produced functional limitation and disability. We have used the term "Physical Examination Tests" to capture diagnostic elements of observation, motion testing, strength testing, accessory motions, palpations, and special tests.

Physical Examination Tests have historically been an integral part of the clinical examination and have great allure to the clinician who may want to simplify the complex diagnostic process or save the patient from expensive and often painful imaging and lab tests. Evidence as to the allure of Physical Examination Tests is obvious in that the rate of publication of these tests continues to accelerate and musculoskeletal textbooks are rife with descriptions of tests.[9,22,23,30] Unfortunately, many published articles lack sound methodology.[11,20,29] Furthermore, many of the current textbooks[23,30] offer no guidance as to the clinical utility of the test, the reliability with which the test is performed, or the quality of the research evaluating the test, leading the reader to the conclusion that "all Physical Examination Tests are created equal." Clearly, all Physical Examination Tests are not created equal.[28]

The Purpose of Physical Examination Tests

Physical Examination Tests exist as part of the overall physical examination scheme of the patient. These tests are typically performed at two different time periods: (1) at the beginning of the physical examination as a screening test and (2) toward the end of an orderly examination as a diagnostic test.[39] The purpose of the Physical Examination Test as a screen is to help the clinician rule out some of the many possible diagnoses.[31] As a diagnostic test, the purpose of the Physical Examination Test is to validly differentiate among the few remaining competing diagnoses. These diagnoses are close to each other with regard to nature and severity and therefore the clinician uses the Physical Examination Test to ease any remaining confusion with regard to the condition or disorder.[16]

Regardless of whether the Physical Examination Test is used for screening or diagnostic purposes, the test must be performed reliably by the practitioner or practitioners in order for that test to be a valuable guide during the clinical diagnostic process.[9,37,38] Reliability captures the extent to which a test or measurement is free from error. In reference to Physical Examination Tests, reliability is often used to capture agreement and is subdivided into intrarater reliability and interrater reliability.[35] Intrarater reliability examines whether the same single examiner can repeat the test consistently whereas interrater reliability captures whether two or more examiners can repeat the test. Both intra- and interrater reliability can be represented by a statistic called the intraclass correlation coefficient (ICC). Many Physical Examination Tests have a dichotomous outcome, meaning that the result of the test is either positive (the patient has the pathol-

TABLE 1-1 Agreement Guidelines of Kappa (κ) (Adapted from Landis and Koch[21])

Kappa (κ) Value	Explanation
0	Poor/less than chance agreement
.01 to .20	Slight agreement
.21 to .40	Fair agreement
.41 to .60	Moderate agreement
.61 to .80	Substantial agreement
.81 to .99	Almost perfect agreement

ogy) or negative (the patient does not have the pathology). When the Physical Examination Test has a dichotomous outcome, there is a high possibility that two or more examiners will agree with each other by chance alone. The statistic used frequently to adjust for this chance agreement in dichotomous outcome tests is called kappa (κ). Kappa measures the amount of agreement beyond what would be expected by chance alone. Values for κ were categorized and value-labeled in 1976 by Landis and Koch[21] and this categorization remains prevalent today despite its arbitrary nature (Table 1-1). In order to determine if the Physical Examination Test is both reliable and valid as a screening or diagnostic tool, the test must be examined in a research study and, preferably, multiple studies.

Research Studies Assessing Physical Examination Tests

Research examining the reliability and diagnostic accuracy of a Physical Examination Test should be of high quality. Unfortunately, the quality of research is an issue that has plagued studies on Physical Examination Tests.[11,20,22,29,37] In an effort to improve the quality of research design in the area of Physical Examination Tests, the quality of publication of Physical Examination Tests research, and the critique of that research, the scientific community has produced tools to aide the clinician on all counts.[5,6,24,37] Tables 1-2 and 1-3 show tools developed by the Cochrane Diagnostic and

Screening Test Methods Group through their Standards for Reporting of Diagnostic Accuracy (STARD) initiative[5,6] and by Whiting et al.[37] with their Quality Assessment of Diagnostic Accuracy Studies (QUADAS) initiative, respectively. While both the STARD and the QUADAS tools help the evidence-based researcher detect error and bias in diagnostic accuracy studies, the tools do differ. The STARD checklist is used as a guide for reporting diagnostic research[5,6] and is presented here for the convenience of the reader who may one day design his or her own diagnostic accuracy study and attempt to submit the results to a peer-reviewed journal for publication (Table 1-2). The QUADAS tool was developed to assess the quality of primary research studies of diagnostic accuracy.[37] In research terms, the QUADAS tool provides an organized format in which a reader can examine the internal validity and external validity of a study. Internal validity is improved when the research design minimizes bias. External validity is judged by whether the estimates of diagnostic accuracy can be applied to the clinical practice setting. QUADAS involves individualized scoring of 14 components. Each of the 14 steps is scored as "yes," "no," or "unclear." Individual procedures for scoring each of the 14 items, including operational standards for each question, have been published, although a cumulative methodological score is not advocated.[36] Past studies[10,33,34] have used a score of 7 of 14 or greater "yes's" to indicate a high-quality diagnostic accuracy study, whereas scores below 7 were indicative of low quality. Based on our experience in the use of the QUADAS tool, the consensus is that higher-quality articles are associated with 10 or greater unequivocal "yes's," whereas those articles with less than 10 unequivocal "yes's" are associated with poorly designed studies (Table 1-3).

Estimates of diagnostic accuracy are captured using various statistical terms. The simplest way to examine these statistical terms is via the 2 × 2 table. The 2 × 2 table in Figure 1-1 is an epidemiologist's way to show the results of the performance of the special test when that special test is compared to a "gold" standard or a criterion standard. The criterion standard can be a laboratory test or an imaging test but in the area of musculoskeletal practice, the criterion standard is often confirmation of the pathology via surgery.[7,8,12,25,26] Regardless of which criterion standard is chosen, the assumption in a 2 × 2 table is that the

(text continues on p. 6)

TABLE 1-2   STARD Checklist for the Reporting of Studies of Diagnostic Accuracy
(*First official version, January 2003*)

Section and Topic	Item #		On Page #
Title/Abstract/ Keywords	1	Identify the article as a study of diagnostic accuracy (recommend MeSH heading "sensitivity and specificity").	
Introduction	2	State the research questions or study aims, such as estimating diagnostic accuracy or comparing accuracy between tests or across participant groups.	
Methods *Participants*	3	Describe the study population: the inclusion and exclusion criteria, setting, and locations where the data were collected.	
	4	Participant recruitment: was recruitment based on presenting symptoms, results from previous tests, or the fact that the participants had received the index tests or the reference standard?	
	5	Participant sampling: was the study population a consecutive series of participants defined by the selection criteria in items 3 and 4? If not, specify how participants were further selected.	
	6	Data collection: Was data collection planned before the index test and reference standard performed before (prospective study) or after (retrospective study)?	
Test methods	7	The reference standard and its rationale	
	8	Technical specifications of material and methods involved including how and when measurements were taken, and/or cite references for index tests and reference standard	
	9	Definition of and rationale for the units, cutoffs, and/or categories of the results of the index tests and the reference standard	
	10	The number, training, and expertise of the persons executing and reading the index tests and the reference standard	
	11	Whether or not the readers of the index tests and reference standard were blinded (masked) to the results of the other test and describe any other clinical information available to the readers	
Statistical methods	12	Methods for calculating or comparing measures of diagnostic accuracy, and the statistical methods used to quantify uncertainty (e.g., 95% confidence intervals)	
	13	Methods for calculating test reproducibility, if done	

(*continued*)

TABLE 1-2 (*cont.*) STARD Checklist for the Reporting of Studies of Diagnostic Accuracy (*First official version, January 2003*)

Section and Topic	Item #		On Page #
Results		Report	
Participants	14	When study was done, including beginning and ending dates of recruitment	
	15	Clinical and demographic characteristics of the study population (e.g., age, sex, spectrum of presenting symptoms, comorbidity, current treatments, recruitment centers)	
	16	The number of participants satisfying the criteria for inclusion that did or did not undergo the index tests and/or the reference standard; describe why participants failed to receive either test (a flow diagram is strongly recommended)	
	17	Time interval from the index tests to the reference standard, and any treatment administered between	
	18	Distribution of severity of disease (define criteria) in those with the target condition; other diagnoses in participants without the target condition	
	19	A cross-tabulation of the results of the index tests (including indeterminate and missing results) by the results of the reference standard; for continuous results, the distribution of the test results by the results of the reference standard	
	20	Any adverse events from performing the index tests or the reference standard	
	21	Estimates of diagnostic accuracy and measures of statistical uncertainty (e.g., 95% confidence intervals)	
	22	How indeterminate results, missing responses, and outliers of the index tests were handled	
	23	Estimates of variability of diagnostic accuracy between subgroups of participants, readers, or centers, if done	
	24	Estimates of test reproducibility, if done	
Discussion	25	Discuss the clinical applicability of the study findings	

TABLE 1-3   Quality Assessment of Diagnostic Accuracy Studies (QUADAS) Tool

Item #		Yes	No	Unclear
1	Was the spectrum of patients representative of the patients who will receive the test in practice?			
2	Were selection criteria clearly described?			
3	Is the reference standard likely to classify the target condition correctly?			
4	Is the period between reference standard and index test short enough to be reasonably sure that the target condition did not change between the two tests?			
5	Did the whole sample or a random selection of the sample receive verification using a reference standard of diagnosis?			
6	Did patients receive the same reference standard regardless of the index test result?			
7	Was the reference standard independent of the index test (i.e., the index test did not form part of the reference standard)?			
8	Was the execution of the index test described in sufficient detail to permit replication of the test?			
9	Was the execution of the reference standard described in sufficient detail to permit replication of the test?			
10	Were the index test results interpreted without knowledge of the results of the reference standard?			
11	Were the reference standard results interpreted without knowledge of the results of the index test?			
12	Were the same clinical data available when test results were interpreted as would be available when the test is used in practice?			
13	Were uninterpretable/intermediate test results reported?			
14	Were withdrawals from the study explained?			

<u>Truth about the Pathology</u>

	Present	Absent
Test Result +	True Positives (TP) *a*	False Positives (FP) *b*
—	False Negatives (FN) *c*	True Negatives (TN) *d*

FIGURE 1-1   A 2 × 2 contingency table.

truth about the presence or absence of the pathology under investigation is known. Common information gleaned from the 2 × 2 table is as follows:

True positive (TP)—The special test is positive and the patient truly has the pathology. Traditionally represented by *a*.

False positive (FP)—The special test is positive but the patient does not have the pathology. Traditionally represented by *b*.

False negative (FN)—The special test is negative but the patient truly has the pathology. Traditionally represented by *c*.

True negative (TN)—The special test was negative and the patient truly does not have the pathology. Traditionally represented by *d*.

Sensitivity (SN)—The probability of a positive test result in someone with the pathology. Formula: $a/(a+c)$

Specificity (SP)—The probability of a negative test result in someone without the pathology. Formula: $b/(b+d)$

Positive Likelihood Ratio (LR+)—The ratio of a positive test result in people with the pathology to a positive test result in people without the pathology. The LR+ is a multiplier in Bayes' Theorem and is used to modify the posttest probability. Formula: $SN/(1-SP)$

Negative Likelihood Ratio (LR−)—The ratio of a negative test result in people with the pathology to a negative test result in people without the pathology. Formula: $(1-SN/SP)$

Bayes' Theorem—Pretest probability of a pathology × LR+ = Posttest probability of a pathology. See Fagan's nomogram[13] (Figure 1-2) for an example of the clinical application of likelihood ratios and Bayes' Theorem.

Diagnostic Odds Ratio (DOR)—A single measure of diagnostic test accuracy combining LR+ and LR−. Formula: $(LR+)/(LR-)$

Positive Predictive Value (PPV)—The proportion of people with the disease of those with a positive test result. Formula: $a/(a+b)$

Negative Predictive Value (NPV)—The proportion of people without the disease who had a negative test result. Formula: $c/(c+d)$

Accuracy—The proportion of subjects correctly identified by the test results. Formula: $(a+d)/(a+b+c+d)$

FIGURE 1-2   Fagan's nomogram for using a likelihood ratio (LR) to modify pretest probability into an estimate of posttest probability accuracy.[13]

TABLE 1-4   Guidelines for the Use of Likelihood Ratios (Adapted from Jaeschke et al.[17])

+LR	Explanation	LR−
1 to 2	Alters posttest probability of a diagnosis to a minimal degree	.5 to 1
2 to 5	Alters posttest probability of a diagnosis to a small degree	.2 to .5
5 to 10	Alters posttest probability of a diagnosis to a moderate degree	.1 to .2
More than 10	Alters posttest probability of a diagnosis significantly and almost conclusively	Less than .1

True positives, true negatives, false positives, and false negatives are terms to capture the raw data from a study examining the accuracy of special tests. All four of these measures contribute to sensitivity (SN) and specificity (SP). Tests with a high SN are valued as screening tests to rule out pathology when they are negative.[31,39] In studies that examine the diagnostic ability of a test, SN and SP are arguably the most popular measures of test performance. While SN and SP are popular, they are nonetheless incomplete measures of test performance. As SN increases, SP often decreases.[14] Furthermore, paired indicators like SN/SP, PPV/NPV, and LR+/LR− cannot be used to easily rank special tests so that a clinician may easily pick the best test,[14] despite the fact that in 1994, Jaeschke et al.[17] attempted to make likelihood ratios more clinician-friendly by producing an outline of acceptable likelihood ratios (Table 1-4).

Accuracy is a single easily understood measure of test performance but accuracy is greatly affected by the prevalence of a pathology.[14] The prevalence of a pathology can change from clinic to clinic. For example, a sports clinic is more likely to see patients with a torn anterior cruciate ligament than a primary care practice and thus, a special test that detects a torn anterior cruciate ligament is likely to appear to have greater accuracy when used in the sports clinic. The diagnostic odds ratio (DOR) is a single indicator of test performance that is somewhat resistant to changes in prevalence, which is why we included this measure in our tables throughout the book. The DOR ranges from 0 to infinity with the higher value being better, but its interpretation and therefore, application back to the clinical environment is somewhat limited.[14] The reader should view the DOR as another measure of the diagnostic strength of the individual Physical Examination Test. Finally, all of these measures, while capturing the performance of a special test in a research study, lack the ability to comment on the consistency/reliability with which the diagnostic test was performed and the overall quality of that study. If examiners are performing the same special test in a different fashion, then they will have difficulty making valid decisions about patients.[2] Moreover, if the overall quality of a study is poor and full of bias, the accuracy of the special test will be overestimated in that study and the measures from that study should be used with caution.[28,38]

How to Use This Book

The purposes of this textbook are to (1) produce a comprehensive current list of Physical Examination Tests and, when possible, their original descriptions and (2) aid the musculoskeletal practitioner in choosing the best available Physical Examination Tests for his or her practice. With these goals in mind, we have attempted to make this book as clinician-friendly as possible. The book is divided into broad anatomical areas and subdivided into Physical Examination Tests that detect pathologies within those anatomical areas. Within each pathoanatomical category, the studies are ordered so that the clinician will find the best tests first and the tests with little or no research to back them last. We do realize that this will cause some consternation when selected favorite clinical Physical Examination Tests are not listed first. A detailed description, original if possible, and photographs accompany each Physical Examination Test. All relevant literature studying the test's discriminatory ability and reliability are summarized in a table format along with the epidemiological statistics gathered from that article (see p. 9). Finally, the number of "yes's" on the QUADAS tool is recorded for each article and we will give the test a summary "Utility Score," which is our opinion of the clinical use of that special test after gathering and critically evaluating all of the literature. Please see p. 9 for an example of the textbook's format. We feel it is important for the reader to know that because the quality of research literature in the area of special tests is mediocre, some would say that providing a quality score for Physical Examination Tests is unwise.[36] Be that as it may, we endeavored to create a handbook that is as clinician-friendly as possible and the "Utility Score" is our expert opinion, as clinicians, teachers, and researchers, as to the clinical import of each Physical Examination Test. Our scale for the "Utility Score" is as follows:

1   Evidence strongly supports the use of this test

2   Evidence moderately supports the use of this test

3   Evidence minimally supports or does not support the use of this test

?   The test has not been researched sufficiently so we are unsure of its value

We hope that you find this textbook of use and that we contribute, in some small way, to the value of your clinical practice.

TESTS FOR ANTERIOR CRUCIATE LIGAMENT (ACL) TEAR

Anterior Drawer Test

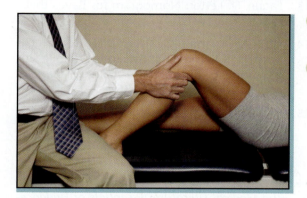

1. The patient is supine with the knee flexed to 90 degrees so that the foot is flat.

2. The examiner sits on the patient's foot and grasps behind the proximal tibia with thumbs palpating the tibial plateau and index fingers palpating the tendons of the hamstring muscle group medially and laterally.

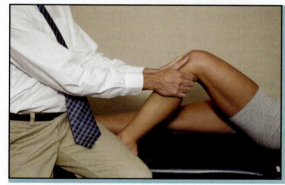

3. An anterior tibial force is applied by the examiner.

4. A positive test for a torn ACL is indicated by greater anterior tibial displacement on the affected side when compared to the unaffected side.

UTILITY SCORE 2

Study	Reliability	Sensitivity	Specificity	LR+	LR−	DOR	QUADAS Score (0–14)
Hardaker[15]	NT	18	NT	NA	NA	NA	8
Bomberg[4]	NT	41	100	NA	NA	NA	9
Jonsson[18] Acute (A)	NT	33	NT	NA	NA	NA	8
Chronic (C)	NT	95	NT	NA	NA	NA	8

Comments: The Anterior Drawer Test appears to be a specific test helpful at ruling in a torn ACL when the test is positive. The Anterior Drawer Test may become more sensitive in nonacute patients.
NT = Not tested. This designation is used when the statistic was not reported in the study for whatever reason. Also, if a study reported only one of either sensitivity or specificity, then the rest of the statistics for that study are reported as NA.
NA = Not applicable. This designation, in addition to being used when only one of either sensitivity or specificity are reported, is used for the likelihood ratios (LR+/LR−) and diagnostic odds ratio (DOR) when either sensitivity or specificity is reported as perfect (100) for a study. Also, if the study was not one of diagnostic accuracy, then NA was used to indicate that QUADAS cannot be used to critique study quality.

References

1. Guide to Physical Therapist Practice. Second Edition. American Physical Therapy Association. *Phys Ther.* 2001;81:9–746.

2. Bartko JJ, Carpenter WT, Jr. On the methods and theory of reliability. *J Nerv Ment Dis.* 1976;163:307–317.

3. Benbassat J, Baumal R, Heyman SN, Brezis M. Viewpoint: suggestions for a shift in teaching clinical skills to medical students: the reflective clinical examination. *Acad Med.* 2005;80:1121–1126.

4. Bomberg BC, McGinty JB. Acute hemarthrosis of the knee: indications for diagnostic arthroscopy. *Arthroscopy.* 1990;6:221–225.

5. Bossuyt PM, Reitsma JB, Bruns DE, et al. Towards complete and accurate reporting of studies of diagnostic accuracy: The STARD Initiative. *Ann Intern Med.* 2003;138:40–44.

6. Bossuyt PM, Reitsma JB, Bruns DE, et al. The STARD statement for reporting studies of diagnostic accuracy: explanation and elaboration. *Ann Intern Med.* 2003;138:W1–12.

7. Chan YS, Lien LC, Hsu HL, et al. Evaluating hip labral tears using magnetic resonance arthrography: a prospective study comparing hip arthroscopy and magnetic resonance arthrography diagnosis. *Arthroscopy.* 2005;21:1250.

8. Charnley J. Orthopaedic signs in the diagnosis of disc protrusion. With special reference to the straight-leg-raising test. *Lancet.* 1951;1:186–192.

9. Cleland J. *Orthopaedic Clinical Examination: An Evidence-Based Approach for Physical Therapists.* First ed. Carlstadt, NJ: Icon Learning Systems; 2005.

10. de Graaf I, Prak A, Bierma-Zeinstra S, Thomas S, Peul W, Koes B. Diagnosis of lumbar spinal stenosis: a systematic review of the accuracy of diagnostic tests. *Spine.* 2006;31:1168–1176.

11. Deeks JJ. Systematic reviews in health care: systematic reviews of evaluations of diagnostic and screening tests. *Bmj.* 2001;323:157–162.

12. Eren OT. The accuracy of joint line tenderness by physical examination in the diagnosis of meniscal tears. *Arthroscopy.* 2003;19:850–854.

13. Fagan TJ. Letter: Nomogram for Bayes theorem. *N Engl J Med.* 1975;293:257.

14. Glas AS, Lijmer JG, Prins MH, Bonsel GJ, Bossuyt PM. The diagnostic odds ratio: a single indicator of test performance. *J Clin Epidemiol.* 2003;56:1129–1135.

15. Hardaker WT, Jr., Garrett WE, Jr., Bassett FH, 3rd. Evaluation of acute traumatic hemarthrosis of the knee joint. *South Med J.* 1990;83:640–644.

16. Jaeschke R, Guyatt G, Lijmer JG. *User's Guide to the Medical Literature: Essentials of Evidence-Based Practice.* Chicago: AMA Press; 2002.

17. Jaeschke R, Guyatt GH, Sackett DL. Users' guides to the medical literature. III. How to use an article about a diagnostic test. B. What are the results and will they help me in caring for my patients? The Evidence-Based Medicine Working Group. *JAMA.* 1994;271:703–707.

18. Jonsson T, Althoff B, Peterson L, Renstrom P. Clinical diagnosis of ruptures of the anterior cruciate ligament: a comparative study of the Lachman test and the anterior drawer sign. *Am J Sports Med.* 1982;10:100–102.

19. Kassirer JP. Teaching clinical medicine by iterative hypothesis testing. Let's preach what we practice. *N Engl J Med.* 1983;309:921–923.

20. Knottnerus JA, van Weel C, Muris JW. Evaluation of diagnostic procedures. *BMJ.* 2002;324:477–480.

21. Landis JR, Koch GG. The measurement of observer agreement for categorical data. *Biometrics.* 1977;33:159–174.

22. Lijmer JG, Mol BW, Heisterkamp S, et al. Empirical evidence of design-related bias in studies of diagnostic tests. *JAMA.* 1999;282:1061–1066.

23. Magee DJ. *Orthopedic Physical Assessment.* Third ed. Philadelphia: W.B. Saunders Company; 1997.

24. Mulrow CD, Linn WD, Gaul MK, Pugh JA. Assessing quality of a diagnostic test evaluation. *J Gen Intern Med.* 1989;4:288–295.

25. Murrell GA, Walton JR. Diagnosis of rotator cuff tears. *Lancet.* 2001;357:769–770.

26. Park HB, Yokota A, Gill HS, El Rassi G, McFarland EG. Diagnostic accuracy of clinical tests for the different degrees of subacromial impingement syndrome. *J Bone Joint Surg Am.* 2005;87:1446–1455.

27. Pauker SG, Kassirer JP. The threshold approach to clinical decision making. *N Engl J Med.* 1980;302:1109–1117.

28. Pewsner D, Battaglia M, Minder C, Marx A, Bucher HC, Egger M. Ruling a diagnosis in or out with "SpPIn" and "SnNOut": a note of caution. *BMJ.* 2004;329:209–213.

29. Reid MC, Lachs MS, Feinstein AR. Use of methodological standards in diagnostic test research. Getting better but still not good. *JAMA.* 1995;274:645–651.

30. Richardson J, Iglarsh Z. *Clinical Orthopaedic Physical Therapy.* Philadelphia: W.B. Saunders Company; 1994.

31. Sackett D, Strauss S, Richardson W, Rosenberg W, Haynes R. *Evidence-Based Medicine: How to Practice and Teach EBM.* Second ed. Churchill Livingstone; 2000.

32. Schmitt BP, Kushner MS, Wiener SL. The diagnostic usefulness of the history of the patient with dyspnea. *J Gen Intern Med.* 1986;1:386–393.

33. Sehgal N, Shah RV, McKenzie-Brown AM, Everett CR. Diagnostic utility of facet (zygapophysial) joint injections in chronic spinal pain: a systematic review of evidence. *Pain Physician.* 2005;8:211–224.

34. Shah RV, Everett CR, McKenzie-Brown AM, Sehgal N. Discography as a diagnostic test for spinal pain: a systematic and narrative review. *Pain Physician.* 2005;8:187–209.

35. Sim J, Wright CC. The kappa statistic in reliability studies: use, interpretation, and sample size requirements. *Phys Ther.* 2005;85:257–268.

36. Whiting P, Harbord R, Kleijnen J. No role for quality scores in systematic reviews of diagnostic accuracy studies. *BMC Med Res Methodol.* 2005;5:19.

37. Whiting P, Rutjes AW, Dinnes J, Reitsma J, Bossuyt PM, Kleijnen J. Development and validation of methods for assessing the quality of diagnostic accuracy studies. *Health Technol Assess.* 2004;8:iii, 1–234.

38. Whiting P, Rutjes AW, Reitsma JB, Glas AS, Bossuyt PM, Kleijnen J. Sources of variation and bias in studies of diagnostic accuracy: a systematic review. *Ann Intern Med.* 2004; 140:189–202.

39. Woolf AD. How to assess musculoskeletal conditions: history and physical examination. *Best Pract Res Clin Rheumatol.* 2003;17:381–402.

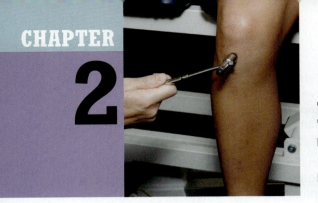

Physical Examination Tests for Neurological Testing and Screening

TESTS FOR PATHOLOGICAL UPPER MOTOR NEURON REFLEX OR SPINAL CORD COMPRESSION

Hoffmann's Reflex

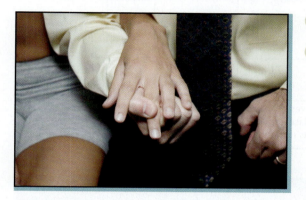

1 The patient is placed in sitting or standing.

2 The examiner stabilizes the middle finger proximally to the distal interphalangeal joint and cradles the hand of the patient.

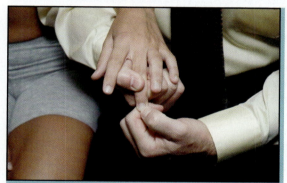

3 The examiner applies a stimulus to the middle finger by nipping the fingernail of the patient between his or her thumb and index finger or by flicking the middle finger with the examiner's fingernail.

4 A positive test is adduction and opposition of thumb and slight flexion of the fingers.

UTILITY SCORE 2

Study	Reliability	Sensitivity	Specificity	LR+	LR−	DOR	QUADAS Score (0–14)
Denno & Meadows[7] (sample was biased, negative Hoffmann's was selected)	NT	0	0	0	0	0	6
Sung & Wang[32] (sample consisted of those with positive tests only)	NT	94	NT	NA	NA	NA	7

(continued)

TESTS FOR PATHOLOGICAL UPPER MOTOR NEURON REFLEX OR SPINAL CORD COMPRESSION

Study	Reliability	Sensitivity	Specificity	LR+	LR−	DOR	QUADAS Score (0–14)
Wong et al.[37] (sample consisted of patients with cervical myelopathy)	NT	82	NT	NA	NA	NA	3
Glaser et al.[10] (Unblinded Tester)	NT	58	74	2.23	0.57	3.93	8
Glaser et al.[10] (Blinded Tester)	NT	28	71	0.96	1.01	0.95	8
Comments: Positive findings are typically very subtle. False positives may occur in patients with a history of head injury or concussion. Note that the only blinded reference involves the Glaser et al.[10] study. The values associated with blinding and unblinding are significantly affected. We feel that the Hoffmann's is not a good screening test.							

Babinski Sign

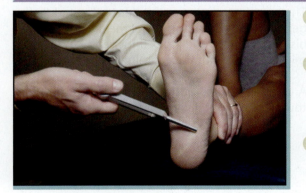

1 The patient is placed in supine. The foot is held in relative neutral by the examiner.

2 The examiner applies stimulation with the blunt end of a reflex hammer to the plantar aspect of the foot (typically laterally to medial from heel to metatarsal)

3 A negative finding is slight toe flexion, smaller digits greater than great toe.

UTILITY SCORE 2

Study	Reliability	Sensitivity	Specificity	LR+	LR−	DOR	QUADAS Score (0–14)
Bertilson et al.[4]	98% agreement	NT	NT	NA	NA	NA	NA
De Freitas & Andre[6] (tested to determine brain death)	NT	0	NT	NA	NA	NA	6
Berger et al.[2] (tested concurrently with sock off and sheet removal)	NT	80	90	8	0.05	156	7

TESTS FOR PATHOLOGICAL UPPER MOTOR NEURON REFLEX OR SPINAL CORD COMPRESSION

Study	Reliability	Sensitivity	Specificity	LR+	LR−	DOR	QUADAS Score (0–14)
Ghosh et al.[9]	NT	76	NT	NA	NA	NA	11
Hindfelt et al.[14]	NT	18	NT	NA	NA	NA	6
Miller & Johnston[24]	.73 Kappa	35	77	1.5	0.8	1.8	9
Comments: A positive finding is generally associated with a pyramidal defect. Response changes after 1 year of birth. There are a number of ways to perform the stroking of the foot, and it is doubtful if technique or location affects findings.							

Lhermitte's Sign

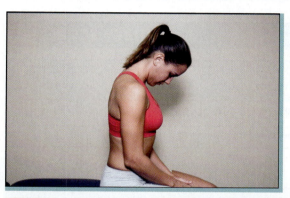

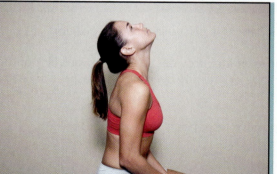

1. The patient is placed in sitting or supine.

2. The patient is instructed to flex the neck with emphasis in lower cervical flexion.

3. Some examiners have advocated use of hyperextension to produce a Lhermitte's response.

4. The patient is queried for "electrical-type" responses during the flexion or if used, extension. A positive test is an "electrical-type" sensation in the midline and occasionally to the extremities during flexion.

UTILITY SCORE 2

Study	Reliability	Sensitivity	Specificity	LR+	LR−	DOR	QUADAS Score (0–14)
Uchihara et al.[34]	NT	3	97	1	1	1	8
Comments: A positive finding is associated with focal lesions of the spinal cord, multiple sclerosis, or other degenerative processes causing stenosis (cord compression).							

TESTS FOR PATHOLOGICAL UPPER MOTOR NEURON REFLEX OR SPINAL CORD COMPRESSION

Gonda-Allen Sign

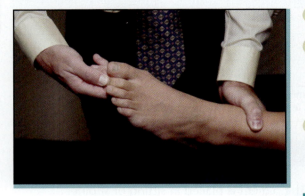

1. The patient is placed in a supine position.

2. The examiner provides a forceful downward stretch or snaps the distal phalanx of the 2nd or 4th toe. The examiner may also press on the toe nail, twist the toe, and hold for a few seconds.

3. A positive response is the extensor toe sign (great toe extension), a similar response to a positive Babinski test.

UTILITY SCORE 2

Study	Reliability	Sensitivity	Specificity	LR+	LR−	DOR	QUADAS Score (0–14)
Denno & Meadows[7]	NT	90	NT	NA	NA	NA	11

Comments: The sample was biased because only patients with a negative Hoffmann's were selected.

Allen-Cleckley Sign

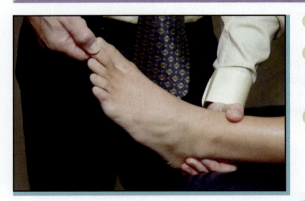

1. The patient is placed in a supine position.

2. The examiner provides a sharp upward flick of the 2nd toe or pressure over the distal aspect or ball of the toe.

3. A positive response is the extensor toe sign.

UTILITY SCORE 2

Study	Reliability	Sensitivity	Specificity	LR+	LR−	DOR	QUADAS Score (0–14)
Denno & Meadows[7]	NT	82	NT	NA	NA	NA	11

Comments: The diagnostic value of this test suggests high sensitivity but caution must be taken. The sample was biased, only patients with a negative Hoffmann's were selected.

TESTS FOR PATHOLOGICAL UPPER MOTOR NEURON REFLEX OR SPINAL CORD COMPRESSION

Inverted Supinator Sign

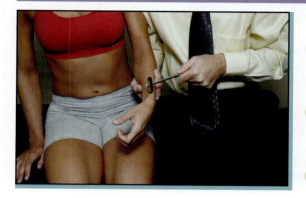

1. The patient assumes a sitting position.

2. The examiner places the patient's forearm on his or her forearm to ensure relaxation. The patient's forearm is held in slight pronation.

3. The examiner applies a series of quick strikes near the styloid process of the radius at the attachment of the brachioradialis and the tendon.

4. A positive test is finger flexion or slight elbow extension.

UTILITY SCORE ?

Study	Reliability	Sensitivity	Specificity	LR+	LR−	DOR	QUADAS Score (0–14)
Estanol & Marin[8]	NT	NT	NT	NA	NA	NA	NA

Comments: Although not studied, this test is commonly used during screening. A positive finding is likely related to increased alpha motor neuron below the level of the lesion.

TESTS FOR PATHOLOGICAL UPPER MOTOR NEURON REFLEX OR SPINAL CORD COMPRESSION

Crossed Upgoing Toe Sign (Cut)

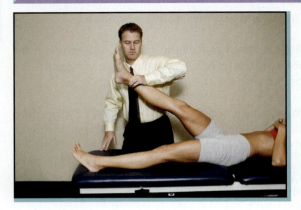

1 The patient is placed in a supine position.

2 The examiner passively raises the opposite limb into hip flexion. The examiner then instructs the patient to hold the leg in flexion.

3 The examiner applies a downward force against the leg.

4 Visual inspection of the opposite great toe is required to observe great toe extension.

5 A positive test is associated with great toe extension of the opposite leg during resistance of hip flexion.

UTILITY SCORE ?

Study	Reliability	Sensitivity	Specificity	LR+	LR−	DOR	QUADAS Score (0–14)
Hindfelt et al.[14]	NT	31	96	7.8	0.72	10.8	6
Comments: Bias limits the true assessment of diagnostic value.							

Mendal Bechtrew Sign

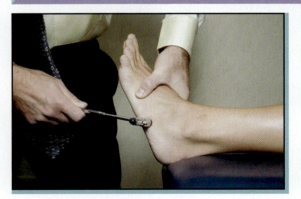

1 The patient is placed in a supine or sitting position.

2 The examiner taps on the cuboid bone (on the dorsal aspect) using the sharp end of the reflex hammer.

3 A positive response is flexion of the four lateral toes.

TESTS FOR PATHOLOGICAL UPPER MOTOR NEURON REFLEX OR SPINAL CORD COMPRESSION

UTILITY SCORE ?

Study	Reliability	Sensitivity	Specificity	LR+	LR−	DOR	QUADAS Score (0–14)
Kumar & Ramasubramanian[19]	NT	NT	NT	NA	NA	NA	NT

Comments: The diagnostic value of this test is unknown.

▶ Schaefer's Sign

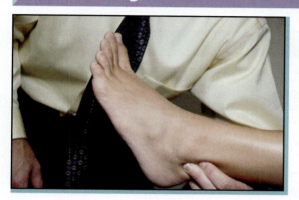

1 The patient is placed in a supine or sitting position.

2 The examiner provides a sharp, quick squeeze of the Achilles tendon.

3 A positive response is the extensor toe sign.

UTILITY SCORE ?

Study	Reliability	Sensitivity	Specificity	LR+	LR−	DOR	QUADAS Score (0–14)
Kumar & Ramasubramanian[19]	NT	NT	NT	NA	NA	NA	NT

Comments: The diagnostic value of this test is unknown.

TESTS FOR PATHOLOGICAL UPPER MOTOR NEURON REFLEX OR SPINAL CORD COMPRESSION

Oppenheim Sign

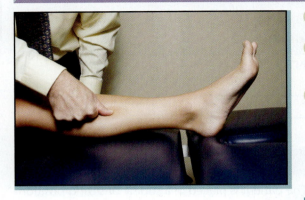

1. The patient is placed in a supine or sitting position.

2. The examiner provides pressure along the shin of the tibia, while sliding downward toward the foot.

3. A positive response is the extensor toe sign.

UTILITY SCORE ?

Study	Reliability	Sensitivity	Specificity	LR+	LR−	DOR	QUADAS Score (0–14)
Kumar & Ramasubramanian[19]	NT	NT	NT	NA	NA	NA	NT
Comments: The diagnostic value of this test is unknown.							

Chaddock's Sign

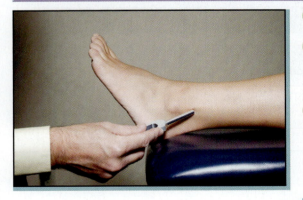

1. The patient is placed in a supine or sitting position.

2. The examiner strokes the lateral malleolus from proximal to distal with a solid, relatively sharp object.

3. A positive response is the extensor toe sign.

UTILITY SCORE ?

Study	Reliability	Sensitivity	Specificity	LR+	LR−	DOR	QUADAS Score (0–14)
Kumar & Ramasubramanian[19]	NT	NT	NT	NA	NA	NA	NT
Comments: The diagnostic value of this test is unknown.							

TESTS FOR PATHOLOGICAL UPPER MOTOR NEURON REFLEX OR SPINAL CORD COMPRESSION

Clonus

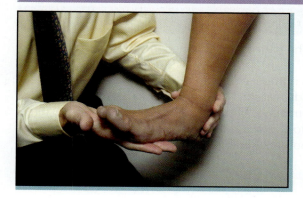

1 The patient is placed in a supine or sitting position.

2 The technique can be applied to the wrist or to the ankle.

3 The examiner takes up the slack of the wrist (into extension; not pictured). The examiner then applies a quick overpressure with maintained pressure to the wrist.

4 The examiner takes up the slack of the ankle (into dorsiflexion; pictured). The examiner then applies a quick overpressure with maintained pressure to the ankle.

5 A positive response is more than three involuntary beats of the ankle or wrist.

UTILITY SCORE   ?

Study	Reliability	Sensitivity	Specificity	LR+	LR−	DOR	QUADAS Score (0–14)
Not tested	NT	NT	NT	NA	NA	NA	NT

Comments: One or two beats is relatively normal and is not indicative of pathology. Three beats or more is considered abnormal. One may see a positive for patients with a history of concussion.

TEST FOR PATHOLOGICAL UPPER MOTOR NEURON REFLEX

Palmomental Reflex

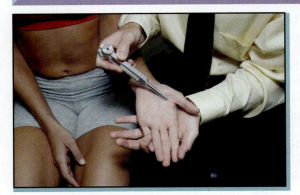

1 The patient is positioned in sitting or supine.

2 A number of methods to elicit this reflex have been advocated. The examiner may stroke the thenar eminence of the hand in a proximal to distal direction with a reflex hammer or may stroke the hypothenar eminence in a similar fashion.

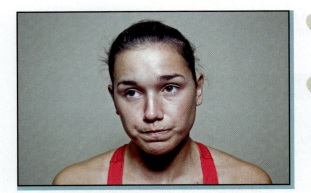

3 The process can be repeated up to five times to detect a continuous response. If the response diminishes the test is considered negative.

4 A positive test is contraction of the mentalis and orbicularis oris muscles causing wrinkling of the skin of the chin and slight retraction (and occasionally elevation of the mouth).

UTILITY SCORE 2

Study	Reliability	Sensitivity	Specificity	LR+	LR−	DOR	QUADAS Score (0–14)
Gotkine et al.[11]	98.9% agreement	24	NT	NA	NA	NA	9
August & Miller[1]	NT	95	98	38	.21	181.5	4
Isakov et al.[15]	NT	78	58	1.8	.22	8.3	11

Comments: This test is associated with a high degree of false positives. There is a higher prevalence of positive findings in Parkinson's and other neurological diseases.

TESTS FOR PERIPHERAL NEUROPATHY

Superficial Pain

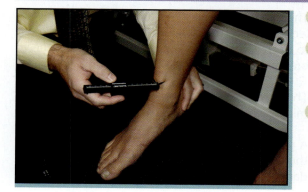

1 The patient is placed in sitting or standing.

2 The examiner applies a superficial painful stimuli and queries the patient regarding pain level. The patient's eyes are closed during the testing.

3 A positive response is a lack of report of pain during application of painful stimuli.

UTILITY SCORE   1

Study	Reliability	Sensitivity	Specificity	LR+	LR−	DOR	QUADAS Score (0–14)
Olaleye et al.[25] (2 correct responses)	NT	47	89	4.27	0.59	7.17	7
Olaleye et al.[25] (3 correct responses)	NT	42	90	4.2	0.64	6.51	7
Olaleye et al.[25] (4 correct responses)	NT	25	97	8.33	0.77	10.8	7
Olaleye et al.[25] (5 correct responses)	NT	23	98	11.5	0.78	14.6	7
Perkins et al.[27] (>5 out of 8 attempts)	NT	59	97	19.7	0.42	46.5	9

Comments: To stimulate superficial pain, a sharp–dull response was used. Anesthesia is considered a positive finding.

TESTS FOR PERIPHERAL NEUROPATHY

Vibration Testing

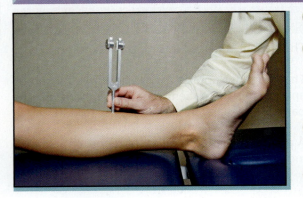

1 The patient is placed in sitting or supine position.

2 The examiner applies the tuning fork over the selected bony prominence. The patient is instructed to close his or her eyes and to indicate when the vibration begins and when the vibration is complete.

3 The examiner applies a series of five trials to determine the cumulative ability of correct responses.

4 A positive test is decreased ability to report when the vibration was applied and when the vibration dampened while still applied.

UTILITY SCORE 1

Study	Reliability	Sensitivity	Specificity	LR+	LR−	DOR	QUADAS Score (0–14)
Olaleye et al.[25] (2 correct responses)	NT	46	94	7.66	0.57	13.3	7
Olaleye et al.[25] (3 correct responses)	NT	42	97	14	0.59	23.4	7
Olaleye et al.[25] (4 correct responses)	NT	25	99	25	0.75	33	7
Olaleye et al.[25] (5 correct responses)	NT	22	99	22	0.78	27.9	7
Perkins et al.[27] (>5 out of 8 attempts) (On–Off method)	NT	53	99	53	0.47	111.6	9
Perkins et al.[27] (>5 out of 8 attempts) (Timed Method)	NT	80	98	40	0.20	196	9
Jepsen et al.[16] (Median Nerve)	.70 Kappa	NT	NT	NA	NA	NA	NA
Jepsen et al.[16] (Ulnar Nerve)	.45 Kappa	NT	NT	NA	NA	NA	NA

Comments: Although primarily tested in this population, the test is not specific for peripheral neuropathy.

TESTS FOR PERIPHERAL NEUROPATHY

Monofilament Testing

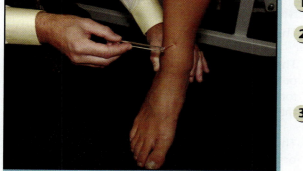

1. The patient is placed in sitting.

2. The examiner applies a Semmes-Weinstein 10-g monofilament to the selected noncalloused areas of the body. With eyes closed, the patient is queried to whether he or she feels the application.

3. A positive response is the inability to feel the applied stimulus. If no stimulus is felt at the palmar aspect of the foot, this reflects the lack of a protective sensation from the patient.

UTILITY SCORE 2

Study	Reliability	Sensitivity	Specificity	LR+	LR−	DOR	QUADAS Score (0–14)
Olaleye et al.[25] (2 correct responses)	NT	70	75	2.8	0.4	7	7
Olaleye et al.[25] (3 correct responses)	NT	63	82	3.5	0.45	7.8	7
Olaleye et al.[25] (4 correct responses)	NT	39	96	9.8	0.63	15.3	7
Olaleye et al.[25] (5 correct responses)	NT	31	97	10.3	0.71	14.5	7
Perkins et al.[27] (>5 out of 8 attempts)	NT	77	96	19.3	0.24	80.3	9

Comments: The articles addressed the protective sensation secondary to peripheral neuropathy of the diabetic foot. Each article used a 10-g monofilament to test protective sensation. This procedure is different from a standard assessment of monofilament testing, which has not undergone diagnostic accuracy analysis. The test is frequently performed as a component of the upper quarter screen.

TESTS FOR CERVICAL RADICULOPATHY

▶ Biceps Deep Tendon Reflex

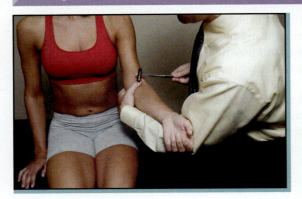

1 The patient assumes a sitting position.

2 The examiner places the patient's forearm on his or her forearm to ensure relaxation. The patient's forearm is held in slight supination. The examiner's thumb is placed on the biceps tendon of the patient.

3 The examiner applies a series of quick strikes to his or her own thumb. The quick strikes should elicit a reflex response of elbow flexion.

4 A positive test is a depression of reflex when compared to the opposite side or "normal."

5 The patient may be instructed to perform the lower extremity Jendrassik maneuver to improve the response of the reflex.

UTILITY SCORE 2

Study	Reliability	Sensitivity	Specificity	LR+	LR−	DOR	QUADAS Score (0–14)
Bertilson et al.[4]	94% agreement	NT	NT	NA	NA	NA	NA
Wainner et al.[36]	.73 kappa	24	95	4.8	0.8	6	10
Matsumoto et al.[22] (C4-5)	NT	65	95	13	0.37	35.3	6
Matsumoto et al.[22] (C5-6)	NT	65	94	10.8	0.37	29.1	6
Lauder et al.[20] (C5-6)	NT	14	90	1.4	0.95	1.47	9

Comments: Reflex testing is commonly scored as 0+ = absent (no visible or palpable muscle contraction with reinforcement), 1+ = tone change (slight, transitory impulse, with no movement of the extremities), 2+ = normal (visual, brief movement of the extremity), 3+ = exaggerated (full movement of the extremities), 4+ = abnormal (compulsory and sustained movement, lasting for more than 30 seconds). The test is frequently performed as a component of the upper quarter screen. The test is purported to target C6.

Triceps Deep Tendon Reflex

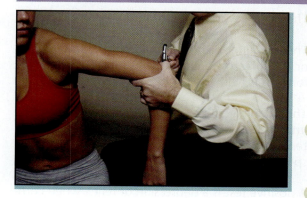

(1) The patient assumes a sitting position.

(2) The examiner flexes the patient's elbow and lifts the shoulder to 90 degrees. The examiner places his or her thumb over the distal aspect of the triceps tendon.

(3) The examiner applies a series of strikes to his or her thumb. The strikes should elicit a reflex response of elbow extension.

(4) A positive test is a depression of reflex when compared to the opposite side or "normal."

UTILITY SCORE   2

Study	Reliability	Sensitivity	Specificity	LR+	LR−	DOR	QUADAS Score (0–14)
Bertilson et al.[4]	88% agreement	NT	NT	NA	NA	NA	NA
Wainner et al.[36]	NT	3	93	0.42	1.04	0.4	10
Matsumoto et al.[22]	NT	38	98	19	0.63	30.03	6
Lauder et al.[20] (C7)	NT	14	92	1.75	0.93	1.87	9

Comments: Reflex testing is commonly scored as 0+ = absent (no visible or palpable muscle contraction with reinforcement), 1+ = tone change (slight, transitory impulse, with no movement of the extremities), 2+ = normal (visual, brief movement of the extremity), 3+ = exaggerated (full movement of the extremities), 4+ = abnormal (compulsory and sustained movement, lasting for more than 30 seconds). The test is frequently performed as a component of the upper quarter screen. The test is purported to target C7.

TESTS FOR CERVICAL RADICULOPATHY

Brachioradialis Deep Tendon Reflex

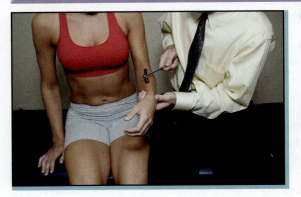

1. The patient assumes a sitting position.

2. The examiner places the patient's forearm on his or her forearm to ensure relaxation. The patient's forearm is held in slight pronation.

3. The examiner applies a series of quick strikes to the intersection point of the brachioradialis and the tendon. The quick strikes should elicit a reflex response of pronation and elbow flexion.

4. A positive test is a depression of reflex when compared to the opposite side or "normal."

UTILITY SCORE 3

Study	Reliability	Sensitivity	Specificity	LR+	LR−	DOR	QUADAS Score (0–14)
Bertilson et al.[4]	92% agreement	NT	NT	NA	NA	NA	NA
Wainner et al.[36]	NT	6	95	1.2	0.98	1.21	10
Lauder et al.[20] (C6-7)	NT	17	94	2.8	0.88	3.2	9

Comments: Reflex testing is commonly scored as 0+ = absent (no visible or palpable muscle contraction with reinforcement), 1+ = tone change (slight, transitory impulse, with no movement of the extremities), 2+ = normal (visual, brief movement of the extremity), 3+ = exaggerated (full movement of the extremities), 4+ = abnormal (compulsory and sustained movement, lasting for more than 30 seconds). The test is frequently performed as a component of the upper quarter screen. The test is purported to target C6.

Muscle Power Testing

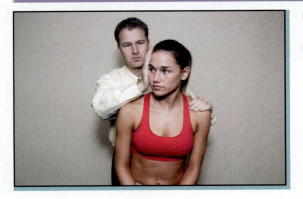

1. The patient is placed in sitting.

2. To test C1-3, cervical rotation is resisted.

TESTS FOR CERVICAL RADICULOPATHY

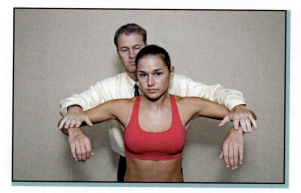

1. The patient is placed in sitting.

2. To test C4, shoulder shrug is resisted.

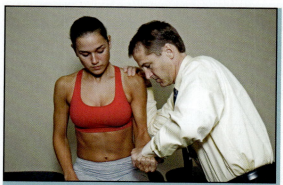

1. The patient is placed in sitting.

2. To test C5, shoulder abduction is resisted.

1. The patient is placed in sitting.

2. To test C6, the biceps are resisted.

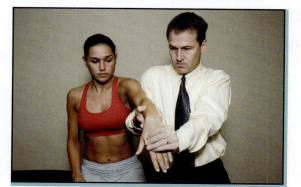

1. The patient is placed in sitting.

2. To test C7, resist wrist flexion.

(continued)

TESTS FOR CERVICAL RADICULOPATHY

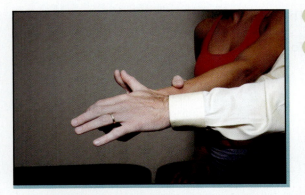

1 The patient is placed in sitting.

2 To test C8, thumb extension is resisted.

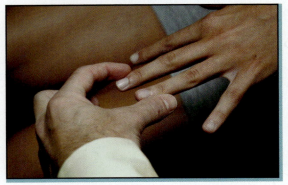

1 The patient is placed in sitting.

2 To test T1, finger abduction is resisted.

3 With all areas, a positive test is noticeable weakness when compared to the opposite side or versus expectations if bilateral symptoms are present.

UTILITY SCORE | **2**

Study	Reliability	Sensitivity	Specificity	LR+	LR−	DOR	QUADAS Score (0–14)
Wainner et al.[36] (Deltoid)	.62 kappa	24	89	2.18	0.85	2.55	10
Wainner et al.[36] (Biceps)	.69 kappa	24	94	4	0.8	4.84	10
Wainner et al.[36] (Extensor Carpi Radialis)	.63 kappa	12	90	1.2	0.97	1.23	10
Wainner et al.[36] (Triceps Brachii)	.29 kappa	12	94	2	0.93	2.13	10
Wainner et al.[36] (Flexor Carpi Radialis)	.23 kappa	6	89	0.54	1.05	0.51	10
Wainner et al.[36] (Abductor Pollicis Brevis)	.39 kappa	6	84	0.37	1.12	0.33	10

TESTS FOR CERVICAL RADICULOPATHY

Study	Reliability	Sensitivity	Specificity	LR+	LR−	DOR	QUADAS Score (0–14)
Wainner et al.[36] (First Dorsal Interosseus)	.37 kappa	3	93	0.42	1.04	0.41	10
Matsumoto et al.[22] (C4-5) (Deltoid Weakness)	NT	35	98	17.5	0.66	26.4	6
Matsumoto et al.[22] (C7 or below) (Wrist Extensor Weakness)	NT	28	74	1.07	0.97	1.10	6
Comments: Note that the test tends to exhibit strong specificity and low sensitivity, suggesting it may lack practicality as a screen. The test is frequently performed as a component of the upper quarter screen.							

Sensibility Testing

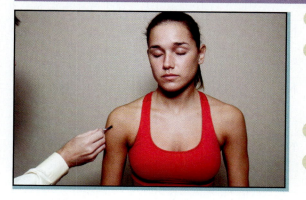

1 The patient is placed in sitting or supine.

2 The examiner applies a series of concurrent sensibility tests to both sides (light touch, sharp/dull). The examiner makes careful effort to apply sensation testing along known dermatomes.

3 Sharp/dull is assessed using pin prick.

4 A positive test is considered impaired sensation when tested against the opposite side.

UTILITY SCORE   2

Study	Reliability	Sensitivity	Specificity	LR+	LR−	DOR	QUADAS Score (0–14)
Jepsen et al.[16] (Axillary Nerve) (Light Touch)	.69 kappa	NT	NT	NA	NA	NA	NA
Jepsen et al.[16] (Medial Cutaneous of Arm) (Light Touch)	.90 kappa	NT	NT	NA	NA	NA	NA

(continued)

TESTS FOR CERVICAL RADICULOPATHY

Study	Reliability	Sensitivity	Specificity	LR+	LR−	DOR	QUADAS Score (0–14)
Jepsen et al.[16] (Medial Cutaneous of Forearm) (Light Touch)	.75 kappa	NT	NT	NA	NA	NA	NA
Jepsen et al.[16] (Musculocutaneous) (Light Touch)	.67 kappa	NT	NT	NA	NA	NA	NA
Jepsen et al.[16] (Radial Nerve) (Light Touch)	.31 kappa	NT	NT	NA	NA	NA	NA
Jepsen et al.[16] (Median Nerve) (Light Touch)	.73 kappa	NT	NT	NA	NA	NA	NA
Jepsen et al.[16] (Ulnar Nerve) (Light Touch)	.59 kappa	NT	NT	NA	NA	NA	NA
Jepsen et al.[16] (Axillary Nerve) (Pain)	.54 kappa	NT	NT	NA	NA	NA	NA
Jepsen et al.[16] (Medial Cutaneous of Arm) (Pain)	.42 kappa	NT	NT	NA	NA	NA	NA
Jepsen et al.[16] (Medial Cutaneous of Forearm) (Pain)	.69 kappa	NT	NT	NA	NA	NA	NA
Jepsen et al.[16] (Musculocutaneous) (Pain)	.48 kappa	NT	NT	NA	NA	NA	NA
Jepsen et al.[16] (Radial Nerve) (Pain)	.48 kappa	NT	NT	NA	NA	NA	NA
Jepsen et al.[16] (Median Nerve) (Pain)	.43 kappa	NT	NT	NA	NA	NA	NA
Jepsen et al.[16] (Ulnar Nerve) (Pain)	.48 kappa	NT	NT	NA	NA	NA	NA

TESTS FOR CERVICAL RADICULOPATHY

Study	Reliability	Sensitivity	Specificity	LR+	LR−	DOR	QUADAS Score (0–14)
Wainner et al.[36] (C5) (Pin Prick)	.67 kappa	29	86	2.07	0.82	2.51	10
Wainner et al.[36] (C6) (Pin Prick)	.28 kappa	24	66	0.70	1.15	0.61	10
Wainner et al.[36] (C7) (Pin Prick)	.40 kappa	28	77	1.21	0.93	1.30	10
Wainner et al.[36] (C8) (Pin Prick)	.16 kappa	12	81	0.63	1.08	0.58	10
Wainner et al.[36] (T1) (Pin Prick)	.46 kappa	18	79	0.85	1.03	0.82	10
Matsumoto et al.[22] (C3,4,5)	NT	56	82	3.11	0.53	5.79	6
Matsumoto et al.[22] (6 and below)	NT	45	81	2.36	0.68	3.49	6

Comments: Results suggest that bilateral stimulus with the patient's eyes closed generates the most valid findings. Unless indicated, results were associated with light touch sensibility testing. The test is frequently performed as a component of the upper quarter screen.

Combined Tests Upper Extremity

UTILITY SCORE 2

Study	Reliability	Sensitivity	Specificity	LR+	LR−	DOR	QUADAS Score (0–14)
Matsumoto et al.[23] (All Deep Tendon Reflexes)	63% agreement	52	NT	NA	NA	NA	7
Matsumoto et al.[23] (All Muscle Weakness)	63% agreement	23	NT	NA	NA	NA	7
Matsumoto et al.[23] (All Dermatomes)	63% agreement	62	NT	NA	NA	NA	7
Lauder et al.[20] (Weakness Any Muscle)	NT	73	61	1.87	0.44	4.22	9
Lauder et al.[20] (Sensory and Reflexes)	NT	9	97	3	0.93	1.87	9

(continued)

TESTS FOR CERVICAL RADICULOPATHY

Study	Reliability	Sensitivity	Specificity	LR+	LR−	DOR	QUADAS Score (0–14)
Lauder et al.[20] (Sensory and Weakness)	NT	27	74	1.04	0.98	1.1	9
Lauder et al.[20] (Weakness and Reflexes)	NT	18	98	9	0.83	10.7	9
Lauder et al.[20] (Weakness, Sensory, and Reflex Abnormalities)	NT	7	98	3.5	0.94	3.68	9
Lauder et al.[20] (Any Component-Weakness or Sensory or Reflex Abnormalities)	NT	84	31	1.2	0.51	2.35	9
Lauder et al.[20] (Sensation Loss-Vibration or Pin Prick)	NT	38	46	0.70	1.35	0.522	9
Davidson et al.[5] (Loss or Depression of Reflexes)	NT	50	NT	NA	NA	NA	8
Davidson et al.[5] (Any Muscle Strength Loss)	NT	91	NT	NA	NA	NA	8
Spurling & Scoville[31] (Any Muscle Strength Loss)	NT	58	NT	NA	NA	NA	4
Spurling & Scoville[31] (Any Loss or Depression of Reflexes)	NT	33	NT	NA	NA	NA	4

Comments: For diagnostic purposes, combined values exceeded the findings of single neurological screening testing.

TESTS FOR LUMBAR RADICULOPATHY

Quadriceps Deep Tendon Reflex

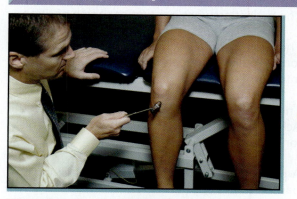

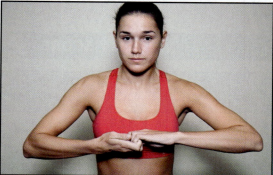

1 The patient assumes a sitting position.

2 The examiner strikes the infrapatellar tendon just above the tibial tuberosity. Three to 5 strikes are necessary to examine fatigue.

3 A positive test is a depression of knee extension directly after the tendon strike in comparison to the opposite side.

4 The Jendrassik maneuver is often used to improve reflex response.

UTILITY SCORE 2

Study	Reliability	Sensitivity	Specificity	LR+	LR−	DOR	QUADAS Score (0–14)
Knuttson[18] (L3-L4)	NT	100	65	NA	NA	NA	3
Knuttson[18] (L5-S1)	NT	14	65	0.41	1.32	0.31	3
Knuttson[18] (L4-L5)	NT	12	65	0.34	1.36	0.25	3
Hakelius & Hindmarsh[13] (All Levels Included)	NT	75	NT	NA	NA	NA	3
Lauder et al.[20] (All Levels Included)	NT	12	96	3	0.92	3.27	6

Comments: Reflex testing is commonly scored as 0 + = absent (no visible or palpable muscle contraction with reinforcement), 1 + = tone change (slight, transitory impulse, with no movement of the extremities), 2 + = normal (visual, brief movement of the extremity), 3 + = exaggerated (full movement of the extremities), 4 + = abnormal (compulsory and sustained movement, lasting for more than 30 seconds). Please note that the majority of the studies were very poorly performed and this predicament likely biases findings. The test is frequently performed as a component of the lower quarter screen. The test is purported to target L2–3.

TESTS FOR LUMBAR RADICULOPATHY

Achilles Deep Tendon Reflex (Lumbar Radiculopathy Secondary to Disk Herniation or Protrusion)

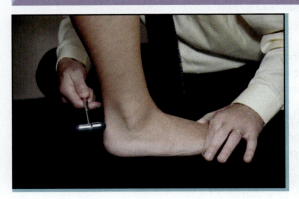

1. The patient assumes a sitting or supine position.

2. The examiner places the ankle in slight dorsiflexion by pulling the palmar aspect of the forefoot into dorsiflexion.

3. The examiner applies 3 to 5 quick strikes to the Achilles tendon. The examiner observes plantarflexion immediately after each strike.

4. A positive test is depression of the reflex in comparison to the opposite side.

UTILITY SCORE **2**

Study	Reliability	Sensitivity	Specificity	LR+	LR−	DOR	QUADAS Score (0–14)
Knuttson[18] (L5-S1)	NT	80	76	3.36	0.26	12.8	3
Knuttson[18] (L4-L5)	NT	36.5	76	1.53	0.83	1.84	3
Kerr et al.[17] (L5-S1)	NT	87	89	7.91	0.15	54.2	7
Kerr et al.[17] (L4-L5)	NT	12	89	1.1	0.99	1.1	7
Hakelius & Hindmarsh[13] (All Levels Included)	NT	80	NT	NA	NA	NA	3
Lauder et al.[20] (All Levels Included)	NT	15	92	1.88	0.9	2.03	6
Rico & Jonkman[2930] (S1)	NT	85	89	7.9	0.2	48.4	6

Comments: Reflex testing is commonly scored as 0+ = absent (no visible or palpable muscle contraction with reinforcement), 1+ = tone change (slight, transitory impulse, with no movement of the extremities), 2+ = normal (visual, brief movement of the extremity), 3+ = exaggerated (full movement of the extremities), 4+ = abnormal (compulsory and sustained movement, lasting for more than 30 seconds). Studies were poorly done. The test is frequently performed as a component of the lower quarter screen. The test is purported to target L5–S1.

TESTS FOR LUMBAR RADICULOPATHY

Extensor Digitorum Brevis Deep Tendon Reflex Test (Radiculopathy of L5–S1)

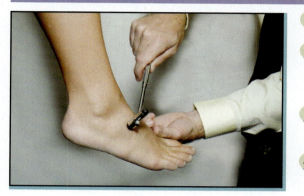

1 The patient assumes a sitting position.

2 The examiner prepositions the foot into slight inversion and plantarflexion. The great toe is placed in plantarflexion.

3 The examiner taps the EDB tendons distal to the muscle belly near the metatarsalphalangeal joints.

4 The examiner repeats the process six times in an effort to elicit a reflex response.

5 A positive test is absence of a reflex (L5 with small contribution of S1) and is indicative of radiculopathy.

UTILITY SCORE 3

Study	Reliability	Sensitivity	Specificity	LR+	LR−	DOR	QUADAS Score (0–14)
Marin et al.[21] (L5)	NT	18	91	2	.90	2.22	8
Marin et al.[21] (S1)	NT	11	91	1.22	.98	1.25	8
Marin et al.[21] (L5 and S1)	NT	14	91	1.56	.95	1.64	8

Comments: Although not acknowledged by Marin et al., eliciting any reflex response with this test has shown to be very difficult. The test is purported to target L4–L5.

Muscle Power Testing (Lumbar Radiculopathy Secondary to Disk Herniation or Protrusion)

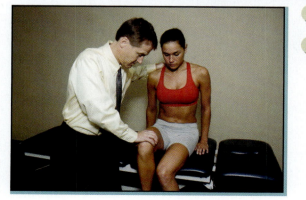

1 The patient is placed in sitting.

2 To test L1–2, hip flexion is resisted.

(continued)

TESTS FOR LUMBAR RADICULOPATHY

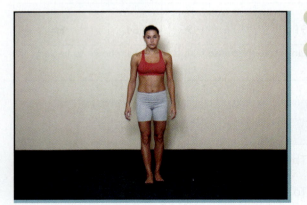

1 The patient is placed in sitting.

2 To test L3–4, knee extension is resisted.

1 The patient is placed in sitting.

2 To test L5, great toe extension is resisted.

1 The patient is placed in standing.

2 To test L4–5 (dorsiflexion), the patient is requested to walk on his or her heels.

TESTS FOR LUMBAR RADICULOPATHY

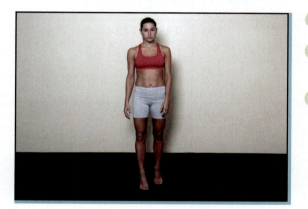

1 The patient is placed in standing.

2 To test L5–S1, the patient is requested to unilaterally stand.

3 The examiner observes pelvic drop on the opposite side for weakness in the hip abductors.

1 The patient is placed in standing.

2 To test S1, the patient is requested to walk on his or her toes.

3 With all areas, a positive test is noticeable weakness when compared to the opposite side or versus expectations if bilateral symptoms are present.

UTILITY SCORE 2

Study	Reliability	Sensitivity	Specificity	LR+	LR−	DOR	QUADAS Score (0–14)
Knuttson[18] (L5-S1) (Great Toe Weakness)	NT	48	50	0.95	1.1	0.9	3
Knuttson[18] (L4-L5) (Great Toe Weakness)	NT	74	50	1.5	0.52	2.9	3
Knuttson[18] (L3-L4) (Great Toe Weakness)	NT	100	50	NA	NA	NA	3
Knuttson[18] (L4-L5) (Great Toe Weakness)	NT	36	50	0.72	1.3	0.56	3
Gurdjian et al.[12] (Great Toe Weakness)	NT	16	50	0.32	1.7	0.19	4

(continued)

TESTS FOR LUMBAR RADICULOPATHY

Study	Reliability	Sensitivity	Specificity	LR+	LR−	DOR	QUADAS Score (0–14)
Gurdjian et al.[12] (Foot Drop-Dorsiflexion)	NT	1	50	0.02	1.98	0.01	4
Kerr et al.[17] (L4-L5) (Hip Extension Weakness)	NT	12	96	3	0.92	3.3	7
Kerr et al.[17] (L5-S1) (Hip Extension Weakness)	NT	9	89	0.77	1.03	0.75	7
Kerr et al.[17] (L3-L4) (Ankle Dorsiflexion)	NT	33	89	3.03	0.75	4.04	7
Kerr et al.[17] (L4-5) (Ankle Dorsiflexion)	NT	60	89	5.45	0.45	12.1	7
Kerr et al.[17] (L5-S1) (Ankle Dorsiflexion)	NT	49	89	4.45	0.6	7.7	7
Kerr et al.[17] (L3-L4) (Ankle Plantarflexion)	NT	0	100	NA	NA	NA	7
Kerr et al.[17] (L4-5) (Ankle Plantarflexion)	NT	0	100	NA	NA	NA	7
Kerr et al.[17] (L5-S1) (Ankle Plantarflexion)	NT	28	100	NA	NA	NA	7
Hakelius & Hindmarsh[13] (Great Toe Extension, All Levels)	NT	79	NT	NA	NA	NA	3
Hakelius & Hindmarsh[13] (Dorsiflexion, All Levels)	NT	75	NT	NA	NA	NA	3
Hakelius & Hindmarsh[13] (Quadriceps, All Levels)	NT	79	NT	NA	NA	NA	3

Comments: Note that the study results are highly variable and depend on the population examined. In addition, positive findings are affected by the prevalence of conditions represented in the study. Most patients in the studies demonstrated L4–5 or L5–S1 disorders, thus it's expected to see better diagnostic value with muscle groups that reflect this innervation pattern. The test is frequently performed as a component of the lower quarter screen.

Sensibility Testing (Lumbar Radiculopathy from Disk Herniation or Protrusion)

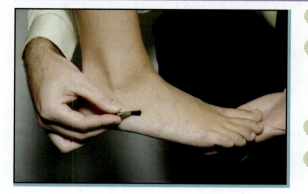

1 The patient is placed in sitting or supine.

2 The examiner applies a series of concurrent sensibility tests (light touch) to both sides. The examiner makes careful effort to apply sensation testing along known dermatomes.

3 Sharp/dull is assessed using pin prick.

4 A positive test is considered impaired sensation when tested against the opposite side.

UTILITY SCORE 2

Study	Reliability	Sensitivity	Specificity	LR+	LR−	DOR	QUADAS Score (0–14)
Porchet et al.[28]	NT	57	NT	NA	NA	NA	5
Kerr et al.[17] (L5 Dermatome)	NT	16	86	1.14	0.98	1.17	7
Kerr et al.[17] (S1 Dermatome)	NT	28	86	2	0.84	2.4	7
Lauder et al.[20] (Any Level, Vibration and Pinprick)	NT	55	77	2.4	0.6	4.1	6
Vroomen et al.[35] (Any Form, Any Level—Sensory Loss)	NT	45	50	0.9	1.1	0.8	10
Knuttson[18] (L3-L4)	NT	67	65	1.9	0.5	3.7	3
Knuttson[18] (L4-L5)	NT	30	65	0.87	1.1	0.81	3
Knuttson[18] (L5-S1)	NT	27	65	.8	1.1	0.69	3
Gurdjian et al.[12] (Hyperesthesia, Anesthesia, or Paresthesia)	NT	40	NT	NA	NA	NA	4

(continued)

TESTS FOR LUMBAR RADICULOPATHY

Study	Reliability	Sensitivity	Specificity	LR+	LR−	DOR	QUADAS Score (0–14)
Peeters et al.[26] (L4) (L3-L4 Disc Herniation)	NT	50	87.5	4	0.6	7	8
Peeters et al.[26] (L5) (L3-L4 Disc Herniation)	NT	50	100	NA	NA	NA	8
Peeters et al.[26] (S1) (L3-L4 Disc Herniation)	NT	0	87.5	0	0	0	8
Peeters et al.[26] (L4) (L4-L5 Disc Herniation)	NT	59	87.5	4.7	0.5	10.1	8
Peeters et al.[26] (L5) (L4-L5 Disc Herniation)	NT	50	100	NA	NA	NA	8
Peeters et al.[26] (S1) (L4-L5 Disc Herniation)	NT	23	87.5	1.8	0.9	2.1	8
Peeters et al.[26] (L4) (L5-S1 Disc Herniation)	NT	16	87.5	1.3	0.96	1.3	8
Peeters et al.[26] (L5) (L5-S1 Disc Herniation)	NT	42	100	NA	NA	NA	8
Peeters et al.[26] (S1) (L5-S1 Disc Herniation)	NT	74	87.5	5.9	0.3	19.6	8
Tokuhashi et al.[33] (L4,5,S1) (Light Touch)	NT	62	NT	NA	NA	NA	4
Tokuhashi et al.[33] (L4,5,S1) (Tuning Fork)	NT	53	NT	NA	NA	NA	4
Tokuhashi et al.[33] (L4,5,S1) (Pressure)	NT	52	NT	NA	NA	NA	4
Bertilson et al.[3] (L4)	.50 Kappa	NT	NT	NA	NA	NA	NA
Bertilson et al.[3] (L5)	.71 Kappa	NT	NT	NA	NA	NA	NA
Bertilson et al.[3] (S1)	.68 Kappa	NT	NT	NA	NA	NA	NA

Comments: Results suggest that bilateral stimulus with the patient's eyes closed generates the most valid findings. Unless indicated, results were associated with light touch sensibility testing. The test is frequently performed as a component of the lower quarter screen.

TESTS FOR LUMBAR RADICULOPATHY

Combined Tests Lower Extremity

UTILITY SCORE 2

Study	Reliability	Sensitivity	Specificity	LR+	LR−	DOR	QUADAS Score (0–14)
Porchet et al.[28] (All LE Reflexes, Lateral Disc Herniation)	NT	82	NT	NA	NA	NA	5
Porchet et al.[28] (Any Sensory Deficit, Lateral Disc Herniation)	NT	57	NT	NA	NA	NA	5
Porchet et al.[28] (Any Strength Loss, Lateral Disc Herniation)	NT	79	NT	NT	NT	NT	5
Lauder et al.[20] (Weakness, Any Muscle)	NT	69	61	1.77	0.51	3.48	6
Lauder et al.[20] (Sensory Loss and Weakness)	NT	41	88	3.41	0.67	5.1	6
Lauder et al.[20] (Sensory Loss and Reflexes)	NT	14	96	3.5	8.9	3.9	6
Lauder et al.[20] (Weakness and Reflexes)	NT	19	96	4.75	0.84	5.6	6
Lauder et al.[20] (Sensory, Reflexes and Weakness)	NT	12	100	NA	NA	NA	6
Vroomen et al.[35] (Ankle and Knee Loss)	NT	14	93	2.2	0.92	2.38	10

Comments: For diagnostic purposes, combined values exceed the findings of single neurological screening testing.

Key Points

1. Nearly all of the neurological clinical special tests exhibit high levels of procedural bias.

2. Despite the fact that many of the neurological clinical special tests are purported to function as screens, the majority demonstrate poor sensitivity and fair to strong specificity, the opposite diagnostic values expected in a screening examination.

3. Hoffmann's test, a test for upper motor neuron assessment, is frequently included as a gold standard in most studies, but demonstrates only poor to fair diagnostic value when examined independently.

4. Those studies with higher QUADAS values routinely demonstrate that many of the neurological screen tests have less accuracy than studies with lower QUADAS scores.

5. The Babinski sign and offshoots of this test (Allen-Cleckley and Gonda-Allen) demonstrate good sensitivity for testing UMN disorders.

6. The sensibility tests for peripheral neuropathy demonstrate very good diagnostic value but the sensibility tests for radiculopathy demonstrate poor value for lower extremities and poor to moderate value for upper extremities.

7. Only the biceps reflex test demonstrates fair diagnostic value. The brachioradialis and triceps reflex test demonstrates poor diagnostic value and do not function well as screens.

8. Nearly all the lower extremity reflex studies are riddled with bias.

9. As a whole, muscle power testing yields poor diagnostic value in lower and upper extremities.

10. Combined tests only marginally improve the diagnostic value of tests and when tests are combined but are required all present, sensitivity declines.

References

1. August B, Miller FB. Clinical value of the palmomental reflex. *J Am Med Assoc.* 1952; 148(2):120–121.

2. Berger JR, Fannin M. The "bedsheet" Babinski. *South Med J.* 2002;95(10):1178–1179.

3. Bertilson B, Bring J, Sjoblom A, Sundell K, Strender LE. Inter-examiner reliability in the assessment of low back pain (LBP) using the Kirkaldy-Willis classification (KWC). *Eur Spine J.* 2006;E-pub.

4. Bertilson B, Grunnesjo M, Strender LE. Reliability of clinical tests in the assessment of patient with neck/shoulder problems—impact of history. *Spine.* 2003;19:2222–2231.

5. Davidson R, Dunn E, Metzmaker J. The shoulder abduction test in the diagnosis of radicular pain in cervical extradural compression monoradiculopathies. *Spine.* 1981;6:441–445.

6. De Freitas G, Andre C. Absence of the Babinski sign in brain death. *J Neurol.* 2005;252: 106–107.

7. Denno JJ, Meadows GR. Early diagnosis of cervical spondylotic myelopathy. A useful clinical sign. *Spine.* 1991;16(12):1353–1355.

8. Estanol BV, Marin OS. Mechanism of the inverted supinator reflex. A clinical and neurophysiological study. *J Neurol Neurosurg Psychiatry.* 1976;39:905–908.

9. Ghosh D, Pradhan S. Extensor toe sign: by various methods in spastic children with cerebral palsy. *J Child Neurol.* 1998;13(5):216–220.

10. Glaser J, Cure J, Bailey K, Morrow D. Cervical spinal cord compression and the Hoffmann sign. *Iowa Orthop J.* 2001;21:49–52.

11. Gotkine M, Haggiag S, Abramsky O, Biran I. Lack of hemispheric localizing value of the palmomental reflex. *Neurology.* 2005;64(9):1656.

12. Gurdijan E, Webster J, Ostrowski AZ, Hardy W, Lindner D, Thomas L. Herniated lumbar intervertebral discs: an analysis of 1176 operated cases. *J Trauma.* 1961;1:158–176.

13. Hakelius A, Hindmarsh J. The comparative reliability of preoperative diagnostic methods in lumbar disc surgery. *Acta Orthop Scand.* 1972; 43:234–238.

14. Hindfelt B, Rosen I, Hanko J. The significance of a crossed extensor hallucis response in neurological disorders: a comparison with the Babinski sign. *Acta Neurol Scandinav.* 1976; 53:241–250.

15. Isakov E, Sazbon L, Costeff H, Luz Y, Najenson T. The diagnostic value of three common primitive reflexes. *Eur Neurol.* 1984;23(1):17–21.

16. Jepsen JR, Laursen LH, Hagert CG, Kreiner S, Larsen A. Diagnostic accuracy of the neurological upper limb examination I: inter-rater reproducibility of selected findings and patterns. *BMC Neurology.* 2006;6:8.

17. Kerr RSC, Cadoux-Hudson TA, Adams CBT. The value of accurate clinical assessment in the surgical management of the lumbar disc protrusion. *J Neurol Neurosurg Psychiatr.* 1988;51: 169–173.

18. Knuttson B. Comparative value of electromyographic, myelographic, and clinical-neurological examinations in diagnosis of lumbar root compression syndrome. *Acta Ortho Scand.* 1961;(Suppl 49):19–49.

19. Kumar SP, Ramasubramanian D. The Babinski sign—a reappraisal. *Neurology India.* 2000;48: 314–318.

20. Lauder T, Dillingham T, Andary M, Kumar S, Pezzin L, Stephens R. Predicting electrodiagnostic outcome in patients with upper limb symptoms: are the history and physical examination helpful? *Arch Phys Med Rehabil.* 2000; 81:436–441.

21. Marin R, Dillingham TR, Chang A, Belandres P. Extensor digitorum brevis reflex in normals and patients with radiculopathies. *Muscle Nerve.* 1995;18:52–59.

22. Matsumoto M, Fujimura Y, Toyama Y. Usefulness and reliability of neurological signs for level diagnosis in cervical myelopathy caused by soft disc herniation. *J Spinal Disord.* 1996; 9(4):317–21.

23. Matsumoto M, Ishikawa M, Ishii K, Nishizawa T, Maruiwa H, Nakamura M, Chiba K, Toyama Y. Usefulness of neurological examination for diagnosis of the affected level in patients with cervical compressive myelopathy: prospective comparative study with radiological evaluation. *J Neurosurg Spine.* 2005;2(5):535–539.

24. Miller T, Johnston SC. Should the Babinski sign be part of the routine neurological examination? *Neurology.* 2005;65:1165–1168.

25. Olaleye D, Perkins BA, Bril V. Evaluation of three screening tests and a risk assessment model for diagnosing peripheral neuropathy in the diabetes clinic. *Diabetes Res Clin Pract.* 2001;54(2):115–128.

26. Peeters GG, Aufdemkampe G, Oostendorp RA. Sensibility testing in patients with a lumbosacral radicular syndrome. *J Manipulative Physiol Ther.* 1998;21(2):81–88.

27. Perkins BA, Olaleye D, Zinman B, Bril V. Simple screening tests for peripheral neuropathy in the diabetes clinic. *Diabetes Care.* 2001;24(2): 250–256.

28. Porchet F, Fankhauser H, de Tribolet N. Extreme lateral lumbar disc herniation: clinical presentation in 178 patients. *Acta Neurochir (Wien).* 1994;127(3-4):203–209.

29. Rico RE, Jonkman EJ. Measurement of the Achilles tendon reflex for the diagnosis of lumbosacral root compression syndromes. *J Neurol Neurosurg Psychiatry.* 1982;45(9):791–795.

30. Spangfort E. The lumbar disc herniations—a computer aided analysis of 2,504 operations. *Acta Orthop Scand.* 1972;(Suppl 142):1–93.

31. Spurling RG, Scoville WB. Lateral rupture of the cervical intervertebral disc. *Surg Gynecol Obstet.* 1944;78:350–358.

32. Sung R, Wang J. Correlation between a positive Hoffmann's reflex and cervical pathology in asymptomatic individuals. *Spine.* 2001;26:67–70.

33. Tokuhashi Y, Satoh K, Funami S. A quantitative evaluation of sensory dysfunction in lumbosacral radiculopathy. *Spine.* 1991;16(11):1321–1328.

34. Uchihara T, Furukawa T, Tsukagoshi H. Compression of brachial plexus as a diagnostic test of cervical cord lesion. *Spine.* 1994;19(19):2170–2173.

35. Vroomen P, de Krom M, Wilmink J, Kester A, Knottnerus J. Diagnostic value of history and physical examination in patients suspected of lumbosacral nerve root compression. *J Neurol Neurosurg Psychiatry.* 2002;72:630–634.

36. Wainner R, Fritz J, Irrgang J, Boninger M, Delitto A, Allison S. Reliability and diagnostic accuracy of the clinical examination and patient self-report measures for cervical radiculopathy. *Spine.* 2003;28:52–62.

37. Wong TM, Leung HB, Wong WC. Correlation between magnetic resonance imaging and radiographic measurement of cervical spine in cervical myelopathic patients. *J Orthop Surg.* 2004;12:239–242.

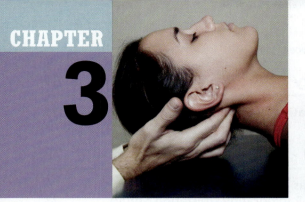

Physical Examination Tests for the Cervical Spine

TESTS FOR CERVICAL RADICULOPATHY

Spurling's Compression Test

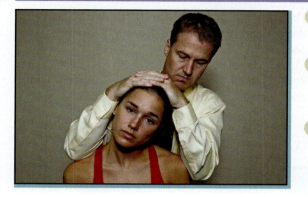

1 The patient assumes a neutral cervical posture while in sitting. Assess resting symptoms.

2 The patient is instructed to side flex his or her head to the side of his or her referred symptoms. If radicular pain is present, the test is positive.

3 (If no symptoms up to this point) The examiner then applies a combined compression and side flexion force in the direction of side flexion. If radicular pain is present, the test is positive.

UTILITY SCORE   2

Study	Reliability	Sensitivity	Specificity	LR+	LR−	DOR	QUADAS Score (0–14)
Bertilson et al.[2]	.14 to .28 kappa	NT	NT	NA	NA	NT	NA
Spurling & Scoville[17]	NT	100	NT	NA	NA	NA	4
Uchihara et al.[21]	NT	11	100	NA	NA	NA	8
Tong et al.[20]	NT	30	93	4.3	.75	5.69	9
Shah & Rajshekhar[14]	NT	93	95	18.6	0.07	256.4	9
Wainner et al.[26]	.60 kappa	50	86	3.57	0.58	6.14	10
Wainner et al.[26] (Included Side Flexion Toward the Rotation and Extension)	.62 kappa	50	74	1.92	0.67	2.85	10
Viikari-Juntura et al.[24] (Right Side)	NT	36	92	4.5	0.69	6.47	11
Viikari-Juntura et al.[24] (Left Side)	NT	39	92	4.87	0.66	7.35	11
Sandmark & Nisell[13] (Not for Radiculopathy)	NT	77	92	9.62	0.25	38.5	9

Comments: The Spurling's maneuver appears to be specific but not sensitive and would not function well as a screen. Some have described the test by including ipsilateral rotation with side flexion while others have included extension. The description provided is the original description from Spurling and Scoville.[17]

TESTS FOR CERVICAL RADICULOPATHY

Valsalva Maneuver

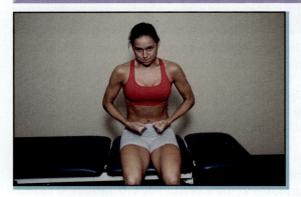

1. The patient assumes a sitting position.

2. The patient is instructed to hold his or her breath then "bear down" as in performing a toileting procedure.

3. Reproduction of concordant pain during bearing down is considered a positive response.

UTILITY SCORE 2

Study	Reliability	Sensitivity	Specificity	LR+	LR−	DOR	QUADAS Score (0–14)
Wainner et al.[26]	.69 kappa	22	94	3.67	0.82	4.41	10

Comments: The test appears to be moderately reliable and specific for patients with cervical radiculopathy. The test should not be used as a screen.

Brachial Plexus Compression Test

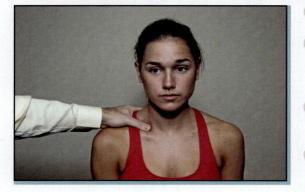

1. The patient assumes a sitting position.

2. The examiner applies a compressive force with his or her hand, just above the clavicle on the symptomatic side.

3. Special effort to apply compression lateral to the scalenes is made to apply traction to the nerve bundle.

4. A positive test is reproduction of radicular symptoms.

UTILITY SCORE 2

Study	Reliability	Sensitivity	Specificity	LR+	LR−	DOR	QUADAS Score (0–14)
Uchihara et al.[21]	NT	69	83	4.1	0.37	10.8	8

Comments: The test mimics those of thoracic outlet syndrome. It is doubtful that the test could discriminate between cervical radiculopathy and thoracic outlet syndrome, and may demonstrate false positives if localized pain only is queried.

TESTS FOR CERVICAL RADICULOPATHY

Cervical Hyperflexion

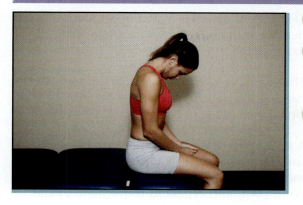

1 The patient assumes a sitting position.

2 The patient is instructed to flex his or her neck to the first point of pain. If no pain, the patient is instructed to flex toward end range.

3 Reproduction of radicular symptoms during hyperflexion is considered a positive response.

UTILITY SCORE 2

Study	Reliability	Sensitivity	Specificity	LR+	LR−	DOR	QUADAS Score (0–14)
Uchihara et al.[21]	NT	8	100	NA	NA	NA	8
Wainner et al.[26] (limited <55°)	.60 kappa	89	41	1.51	0.27	5.6	10

Comments: The dramatic differences in values are unexplained. Wainner et al.[26] provided better methodology for their study and the results are likely more transferable to a population with cervical radiculopathy.

TESTS FOR CERVICAL RADICULOPATHY

Cervical Distraction Test

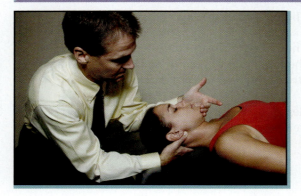

1) The patient assumes a supine position. The patient's symptoms require assessment prior to the examination.

2) The examiner uses a chin cradle grip around the head of the patient, specifically targeting the occipital shelf of the neck.

3) A traction force is applied and the patient's symptoms are reassessed. Pain is respected and the same pattern of movement to pain, movement beyond pain, and repeated movement should be implemented.

4) A positive test is reduction of symptoms during traction.

UTILITY SCORE   2

Study	Reliability	Sensitivity	Specificity	LR+	LR−	DOR	QUADAS Score (0–14)
Bertilson et al.[2]	.63 to .43 kappa	NT	NT	NA	NA	NA	NA
Wainner et al.[26]	.88 kappa	44	90	4.4	0.62	7.1	10
Viikari-Juntura et al.[24]	NT	40	100	NA	NA	NA	11

Comments: Though only moderate, this test provides one of the best diagnostic scores of the tests for cervical radiculopathy. The test is highly specific for cervical radiculopathy.

Upper Limb Tension Test (ULTT)

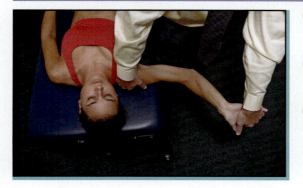

1) The patient assumes a supine position. The examiner assesses resting symptoms.

2) The examiner blocks the shoulder girdle to stabilize the scapulae. Symptoms are again assessed.

3) If no reproduction of symptoms has occurred, the glenohumeral joint is abducted to 110 degrees with slight coronal plane extension. Symptoms are again assessed.

TESTS FOR CERVICAL RADICULOPATHY

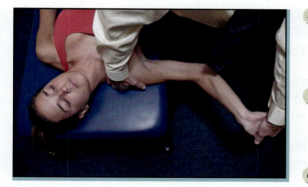

4 If no reproduction of symptoms has occurred, the forearm is supinated completely and the wrist and fingers are extended. Ulnar deviation is implemented. Symptoms are again assessed.

5 If no reproduction of symptoms has occurred, elbow extension is applied. Symptoms are again assessed. One may measure the degree of elbow extension if range of motion is an objective.

6 Lateral flexion of the neck is used to sensitize the procedure. A positive test is reproduction of symptoms during distal movement.

UTILITY SCORE 2

Study	Reliability	Sensitivity	Specificity	LR+	LR−	DOR	QUADAS Score (0–14)
Wainner et al.[26] (Median Nerve Bias)	.76 kappa	97	22	1.24	.14	9.1	10
Wainner et al.[26] (Radial Nerve Bias)	.83 kappa	72	33	1.07	.84	1.26	10
Bertilson et al.[2] (Median Nerve Bias)	.03 kappa	NT	NT	NA	NA	NA	NA
Bertilson et al.[2] (Radial Nerve Bias)	.11 kappa	NT	NT	NA	NA	NA	NA
Bertilson et al.[2] (Ulnar Nerve Bias)	NT	NT	NT	NA	NA	NA	NA
Sandmark & Nisell[13] (Not for Radiculopathy)	NT	77	94	12.8	.24	52.4	9

Comments: This sensitive test is most likely associated with a number of dysfunctions. Studies have supported that a positive ULTT is not specific to a selected disorder secondary to anatomical considerations. To increase the specificity of the test, one should look for concordant symptoms, sensitization, and asymmetry from side to side. The test should be considered an excellent screen for radiculopathy as a negative finding is compelling toward the lack of existence of radiculopathy.

TESTS FOR CERVICAL RADICULOPATHY

Cervical Hyperextension (Jackson's Test)

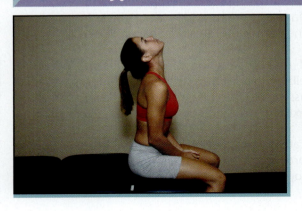

1 The patient assumes a sitting position.

2 The patient is instructed to extend his or her neck to the first point of pain. If no pain, the patient is instructed to extend toward end range.

3 Reproduction of symptoms is considered a positive response.

UTILITY SCORE 3

Study	Reliability	Sensitivity	Specificity	LR+	LR−	DOR	QUADAS Score (0–14)
Uchihara et al.[21]	NT	25	90	2.5	0.83	3	8
Sandmark & Nisell[13] (Not for Radiculopathy)	NT	27	90	2.7	0.81	3.32	9

Comments: Although the test is specific, the examiner would be best served to differentiate localized pain compared to radicular symptoms.

TESTS FOR CERVICAL RADICULOPATHY

Shoulder Abduction Test

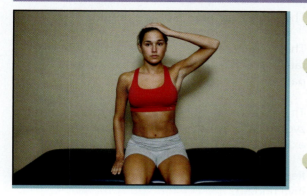

1 The patient assumes a sitting position. The examiner assesses resting symptoms.

2 The patient actively places his or her arm on top of his or her head. The examiner then determines the presence or absence of the symptoms. It is unlikely that causative level of the cervical radiculopathy can be discriminated with this test.

3 A positive test is identified by reduction of the patient's concordant pain.

UTILITY SCORE 3

Study	Reliability	Sensitivity	Specificity	LR+	LR−	DOR	QUADAS Score (0–14)
Davidson et al.[4]	NT	68	NT	NA	NA	NA	8
Wainner et al.[26]	.20 kappa	17	92	2.12	0.90	2.35	10
Viikari-Juntura et al.[24] (Right Side)	NT	38	80	1.9	0.77	2.45	11
Viikari-Juntura et al.[24] (Left Side)	NT	43	80	2.2	0.71	3	11

Comments: The test is not considered a good screen but is moderately specific. Overall, the diagnostic value is not compelling for diagnosis.

TESTS FOR CERVICAL RADICULOPATHY

▶ Quadrant Test

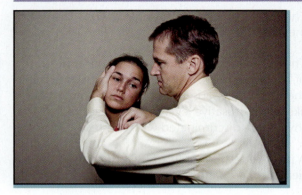

1 The patient assumes a sitting position.

2 The examiner instructs the patient to side flex, rotate and extend his or her neck toward the side of pain.

3 The examiner gently provides overpressure to the zygomatic process toward side flexion, rotation and extension.

4 Reproduction of arm symptoms is considered a positive finding.

UTILITY SCORE ?

Study	Reliability	Sensitivity	Specificity	LR+	LR−	DOR	QUADAS Score (0–14)
Uchihara et al.[21]	NT	NT	NT	NA	NA	NA	NT
Comments: This test is commonly used to "rule out" cervical dysfunction but at present is untested.							

▶ Cervical Compression Test

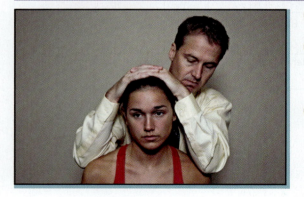

1 The patient assumes a sitting position.

2 The examiner stands behind the patient. With the elbows on each shoulder, the examiner applies a downward force through the head.

3 Reproduction of symptoms is considered a positive response.

UTILITY SCORE ?

Study	Reliability	Sensitivity	Specificity	LR+	LR−	DOR	QUADAS Score (0–14)
Bertilson et al.[2]	.44 kappa	NT	NT	NA	NA	NA	NA
Comments: The Kappa value suggests the test has only fair agreement. The diagnostic value remains untested.							

TESTS FOR UPPER CERVICAL INSTABILITY

Modified Sharp Purser Test

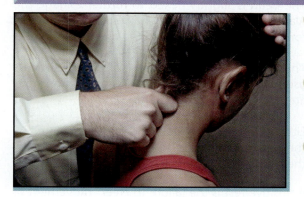

1 The patient assumes a sitting position. The patient's head should be slightly flexed. The examiner assesses resting symptoms.

2 The examiner stands to the side of the patient and stabilizes the C2 spinous process using a pincer grasp.

3 Gently at first, the examiner applies a posterior translation force from the palm of the hand on the patient's forehead toward a posterior direction.

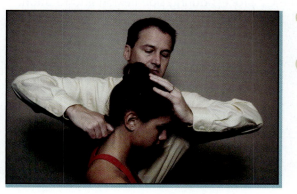

4 Symptoms are assessed for both degree of linear displacement (palpated) or symptom provocation.

5 Collectively, a positive test is identified either by reproduction of myelopathic symptoms during forward flexion or decrease in symptoms during an anterior to posterior movement or excess displacement during the AP movement.

UTILITY SCORE   2

Study	Reliability	Sensitivity	Specificity	LR+	LR−	DOR	QUADAS Score (0–14)
Cattrysse et al.[3] (includes only those that were significantly related)	NT	NT	NA	NA	NA	NA	.67 kappa
Uitvlugt & Indenbaum[22]	NT	69	96	17.3	0.32	53.4	8

Comments: Uitvlugt and Indenbaum[22] found high specificity with the Sharp Purser and described the test as "symptom reduction upon posterior force through the head." The test differs from the original Sharp Purser, which was poorly defined and only consisted of upper cervical flexion. Precautions should be taken prior to use on patients who may have a dens fracture.

TESTS FOR UPPER CERVICAL INSTABILITY

Alar Ligament Stability Test

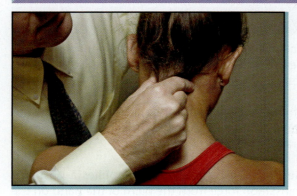

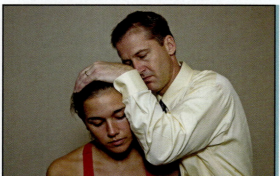

1 The patient assumes a sitting or supine position. The head is slightly flexed to further engage the Alar ligament. The examiner assesses resting symptoms.

2 The examiner stabilizes the C2 spinous process using a pincer grasp. A firm grip ensures appropriate assessment of movement.

3 Either side flexion or rotation is passively initiated by the examiner. During these passive movements, the examiner attempts to feel movement of C2.

4 A positive test is the failure to "feel" movement of the C2 process during side flexion and rotation.

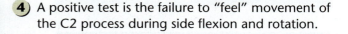

UTILITY SCORE ?

Study	Reliability	Sensitivity	Specificity	LR+	LR−	DOR	QUADAS Score (0–14)
Not tested	NT	NT	NT	NA	NA	NA	NA

Comments: Precautions should be taken prior to use on patients who may have a dens fracture. There are several considerations associated with the Alar ligament test. First, any movement of C2 during side flexion or rotation should be considered normal. Second, the patient may experience some discomfort during the procedure, specifically posttrauma, and this finding should be considered a "red flag" for high-velocity techniques. Finally, some individuals have recommended using the coupling pattern of C0-1 or C1-2 to identify pathology; however, since the coupling pattern is inconsistent, this is not advised. Others suggest that selected range of motion losses are indicative of capsular restrictions or hypermobility but this line of thought has not been tested.

TESTS FOR UPPER CERVICAL INSTABILITY

Upper Cervical Flexion Test

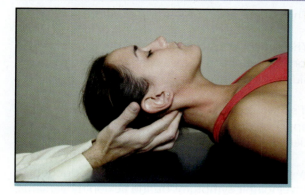

1. The patient assumes a supine position. The examiner assesses resting symptoms.

2. Using a friction massage grip (digits 2 and 3 are held tightly together) the examiner contacts the posterior aspect of the bilateral C1 transverse processes. The palms of the examiner are placed under the occiput of the patient.

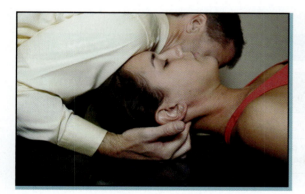

3. The examiner then applies an anterior force to the C1 transverse processes, lifting the head as the force is applied. This position is held for 15 to 20 seconds.

4. If no symptoms occur, the examiner can apply a downward force on the patient's forehead using the anterior aspect of the shoulder. This position is held for 15 to 20 seconds.

5. A positive test is identified by excessive translation or reproduction of instability-related symptoms.

UTILITY SCORE ?

Study	Reliability	Sensitivity	Specificity	LR+	LR−	DOR	QUADAS Score (0–14)
Cattrysse et al.[3] (includes only those that were significantly related among raters)	.64 to 1.00 kappa	NT	NT	NA	NA	NA	NA

Comments: This test exhibits moderate to strong reliability but has not been tested for validity. The test is similar in construct to the Sharp Purser test. Precautions should be taken prior to use on patients who may have a dens fracture.

TESTS FOR UPPER CERVICAL INSTABILITY

Original Sharp Purser Test

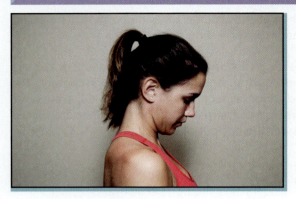

1 The patient assumes a sitting position.

2 The patient is instructed to nod the head into flexion. Reproduction of myelopathic symptoms is considered a positive test.

3 If no symptoms are encountered, the examiner can apply very gentle flexion to the forehead of the patient.

4 A positive test is identified by reproduction of myelopathic symptoms during flexion movements.

UTILITY SCORE ?

Study	Reliability	Sensitivity	Specificity	LR+	LR−	DOR	QUADAS Score (0–14)
Sharp et al.[15]	NT	NT	NT	NA	NA	NA	NA

Comments: Sharp et al.[15] provided a very poor description of the procedure in the seminal paper. The manner in which this test is commonly taught is not the description provided by the original authors.

TESTS FOR UPPER CERVICAL INSTABILITY

Anterior Stability Test of the Atlanto-Occipital Joint

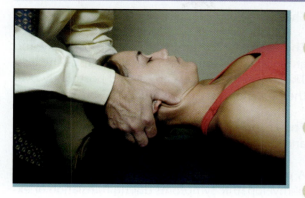

1 The patient assumes a supine position.

2 The cranium of the patient is supported with the examiner's finger under the occiput. The thumbs of the examiner are placed medially on the anterior aspect of the patient's C1-2 transverse processes.

3 The examiner lifts the occiput while simultaneously applying pressure to the anterior aspect of C1-2 transverse processes.

4 A positive test is identified either by reproduction of myelopathic symptoms during anterior translation or excess displacement during the PA movement.

UTILITY SCORE ?

Study	Reliability	Sensitivity	Specificity	LR+	LR−	DOR	QUADAS Score (0–14)
Dobbs[6]	NT	NT	NT	NA	NA	NA	NA

Comments: Precautions should be taken prior to use on patients who may have a dens fracture. This is another of the many cervical spine instability tests that remain uninvestigated.

TESTS FOR UPPER CERVICAL INSTABILITY

Direct Anterior Translation Stress Test

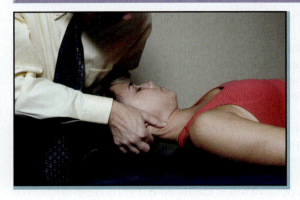

1 The patient assumes a supine position.

2 The examiner's thumbs are placed medially and anteriorly over the anterolateral aspect of the axis. The examiner's fingers are placed posteriorly over the posterior arch of the atlas.

3 The examiner applies a stress between the fingers and the thumbs.

4 A positive test is identified either by reproduction of myelopathic symptoms during translation or excess displacement during the movement.

UTILITY SCORE ?

Study	Reliability	Sensitivity	Specificity	LR+	LR−	DOR	QUADAS Score (0–14)
Dobbs[6]	NT	NT	NT	NA	NA	NA	NA

Comments: Another poorly investigated cervical spine instability test. Precautions should be taken prior to use on patients who may have a dens fracture. This technique is difficult to perform and may not provide information beyond the modified Sharp Purser test.

TESTS FOR UPPER CERVICAL INSTABILITY

Lateral Shear Test of the Atlanto-Axial Articulation

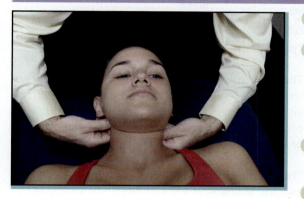

1 The patient assumes a supine position.

2 The examiner uses a "key fob" grip and stabilizes/contacts the C1 transverse process on one side. Using a key fob grip, the examiner applies the same form of grip on the opposite side of the neck at the transverse aspect of C2.

3 The examiner applies a stress between the two grips incorporating a transverse shear force.

4 A positive test is identified either by reproduction of myelopathic symptoms during translation or excess displacement during the movement.

UTILITY SCORE ?

Study	Reliability	Sensitivity	Specificity	LR+	LR−	DOR	QUADAS Score (0–14)
Dobbs[6]	NT	NT	NT	NA	NA	NA	NA

Comments: Precautions should be taken prior to use on patients who may have a dens or a Jefferson's fracture. This is another poorly studied cervical spine instability test.

TESTS FOR MID-CERVICAL INSTABILITY

AP and PA Stress Testing of the Mid-Cervical Spine

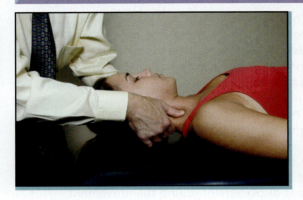

1 The patient assumes a supine position.

2 The examiner's thumbs are placed medially and anteriorly over the anterolateral aspect of the mid-cervical segments. The examiner's fingers are placed posteriorly over the posterior arch of segment above or below the tested mid-cervical segment.

3 The examiner applies a stress between the fingers and the thumbs.

4 A positive test is identified either by reproduction of myelopathic symptoms during translation or excess displacement during the movement.

UTILITY SCORE **?**

Study	Reliability	Sensitivity	Specificity	LR+	LR−	DOR	QUADAS Score (0–14)
Dobbs[6]	NT	NT	NT	NA	NA	NA	NA
Comments: This is an untested stress test of the mid-cervical spine.							

TESTS FOR MID-CERVICAL INSTABILITY

Lateral Stress Testing of the Mid-Cervical Spine

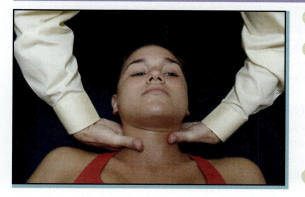

1 The patient assumes a supine position.

2 The examiner's lateral border of his or her metacarpalphalangeal joint is placed against the transverse process of a selected mid-cervical level. On the opposite side of the cervical spine, the opposite hand of the examiner provides a similar MCP grip on a mid-cervical level above or below the previous level.

3 The examiner applies a medial force to the patient's neck with each hand.

4 A positive test is identified either by reproduction of myelopathic symptoms during translation or excess displacement during the movement.

UTILITY SCORE ?

Study	Reliability	Sensitivity	Specificity	LR+	LR−	DOR	QUADAS Score (0–14)
Dobbs[6]	NT	NT	NT	NA	NA	NA	NA
Comments: This is an untested stress test of the mid-cervical spine.							

TEST FOR POTENTIAL VERTEBRAL ARTERY DYSFUNCTION

Vertebral Basilar Insufficiency (VBI) Test

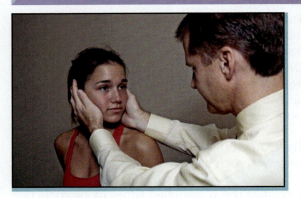

1. The patient is interviewed to extract signs and symptoms of VBI. If remarkable, the patient is referred out for appropriate medical consult.

2. Prior to a comprehensive clinical examination, the examiner performs end-range cervical rotation tests on the patient in a sitting or supine position. The position is held for 10 seconds with observation for signs and symptoms of VBI.

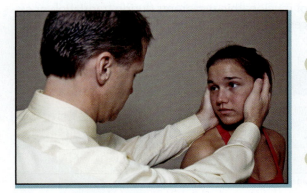

3. The head is returned to a neutral position and held for a minimum of 10 seconds.

4. Rotation is repeated to the opposite side and the position is held for 10 seconds. The examiner observes for signs and symptoms of VBI. If remarkable, the patient is referred for appropriate medical consult.

5. A positive test is identified by initiation of symptoms such as dizziness, diploplia, dysphasia, dysarthria, drop attacks, nausea, and nystagmus.

UTILITY SCORE ?

Study	Reliability	Sensitivity	Specificity	LR+	LR−	DOR	QUADAS Score (0–14)
Not tested	NT	NT	NT	NA	NA	NA	NA

Comments: Much debate exists on the safety and applicability of the VBI tests. We recommend that it is inappropriate to perform the VBI if significant signs are present during the patient history. The test may reproduce symptoms and can be dangerous if applied injudiciously. In addition to the patient complaints listed above, numbness around the mouth, anxiety, and other neurological sensations should be investigated. The protocol selected is associated with literature that promotes end-range rotation. Others have described tests that include extension, rotation and extension, and traction. All are likely beneficial. Although VBI testing has been associated with measured reductions in blood flow, patients rarely demonstrate clinical symptoms, leading to potential finding of false positives.

TESTS FOR CERVICOGENIC HEADACHE

Flexion-Rotation Test

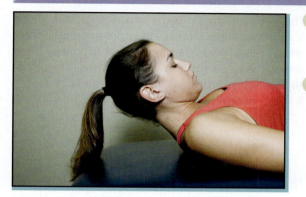

1 The patient assumes a supine position. The examiner stands at the head of the patient. Resting symptoms are assessed.

2 The patient actively fixes his or her neck into maximum flexion.

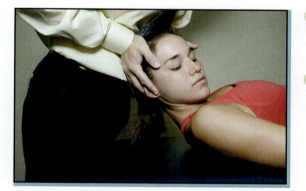

3 Second, the examiner applies a full rotational force to both sides. Symptoms are queried to determine if concordant.

4 The test is both a pain provocation test and a test for range of motion loss. If a loss of 10 degrees or greater is noted, the test is considered positive.

UTILITY SCORE   1

Study	Reliability	Sensitivity	Specificity	LR+	LR−	DOR	QUADAS Score (0–14)
Hall & Robinson[7]	NT	86	100	NA	NA	NA	12

Comments: The design of Hall and Robinson's[7] study was fairly good, using standardized criteria to outline cervicogenic headache findings. The test likely isolates C1–C2, and most likely does not assess the presence of cervicogenic headache at other levels.

TESTS FOR CERVICOGENIC HEADACHE

Neck Flexor Muscle Endurance Test

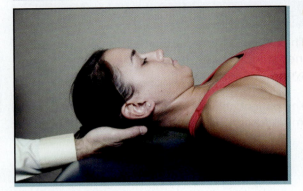

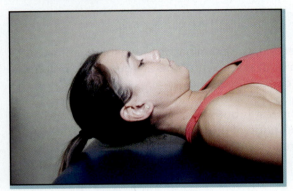

(1) The patient lies in a supine position.

(2) The examiner positions the patient so that the head is actively retracted and held approximately 2.5 cm off the plinth (the examiner places his or her hand under the head for knowledge of position). Visually a skin fold is present in the anterior lateral neck. A line is drawn on this skin fold.

(3) The patient is instructed to hold this position. If the patient's head touches the examiner's hand or he or she loses the skin folds, he or she is instructed to hold the head or tuck the chin.

(4) A positive test is undefined but the test is terminated if the patient cannot hold the lines of the skin fold or cannot hold his or her head up any longer for over a second.

UTILITY SCORE   ?

Study	Reliability	Sensitivity	Specificity	LR+	LR−	DOR	QUADAS Score (0–14)
Harris et al.[8] (Without Neck Pain)	.82–91 ICC	NT	NT	NA	NA	NA	NA
Harris et al.[8] (With Neck Pain)	.67 ICC	NT	NT	NA	NA	NA	NA
Olsen et al.[12] (With Neck Pain)	.83, .85, .88 ICC	NT	NT	NA	NA	NA	NA

Comments: This test would benefit from a validity investigation for patients with cervicogenic headaches. It is likely that this test reflects lower cervical flexor strength, not upper cervical.

TESTS FOR LEVEL OF DYSFUNCTION OR STABILITY

Posterior Anterior Mobilization

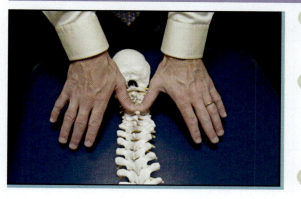

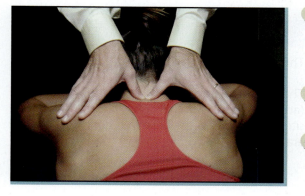

1 The patient may lie in prone or sidelying. The neck is positioned in neutral and resting symptoms are assessed.

2 The examiner palpates the C2 spinous process using the tips of the thumb. Using a thumb-to-thumb application, the examiner applies a gentle downward force up to the first point of the patient's complaint of pain and the pain response is assessed.

3 The examiner then pushes beyond the first point of pain, toward end range, and reassesses pain and quality of movement. Additionally, one should assess splinting or muscle spasm. The clinician should assess if pain is concordant.

4 The examiner repeats the movements toward end range while assessing pain. One should use caution if the patient reports significant pain that is unrelenting.

5 The process is repeated on each spinous process to T4 to identify the concordant segment.

6 A positive test is identified by reproduction of the patient's concordant pain.

TESTS FOR LEVEL OF DYSFUNCTION OR STABILITY

Study	Reliability	Sensitivity	Specificity	LR+	LR−	DOR	QUADAS Score (0–14)
Jull, Bogduk, & Marsland[11]	NT	100	100	NA	NA	NA	9
Van Suijlekom et al.[23] (Upper Cervical Tenderness)	.14 kappa	NT	NT	NA	NA	NA	8
Van Suijlekom et al.[23] (Mid-Cervical Tenderness)	.37 kappa	NT	NT	NA	NA	NA	8
Van Suijlekom et al.[23] (Lower Cervical Tenderness)	.31 kappa	NT	NT	NA	NA	NA	8

Comments: The test results may vary based on application force, determination of what is considered a positive finding, and the examiner's conception of stiffness. It is likely that this test is highly sensitive at implicating the level of a disorder, but is not specific for a pathological process.

Palpation of Physiological Movement

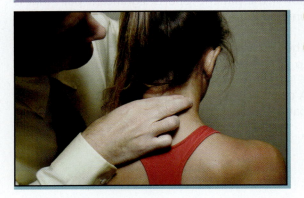

1. The patient is placed in a sitting position.

2. The examiner palpates the lateral aspect of C2-3 (articular pillars) with his or her fingers. The opposite hand stabilizes the head in order to apply a lateral/extension movement.

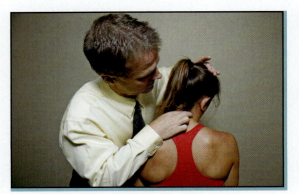

3. The examiner applies a series of lateral/extension movements to feel the amount of motion at that segment. The same procedure can be used for lower segments.

4. Increased movement at one level versus another is considered positive.

TESTS FOR LEVEL OF DYSFUNCTION OR STABILITY

UTILITY SCORE 2

Study	Reliability	Sensitivity	Specificity	LR+	LR−	DOR	QUADAS Score (0–14)
Smedmark et al.[16] (C1-2 Rotation)	.28 kappa	NT	NT	NA	NA	NA	NA
Smedmark et al.[16] (C2-3 Rotation)	.43 kappa	NT	NT	NA	NA	NA	NA
Smedmark et al.[16] (C7 Flex-Extension)	.36 kappa	NT	NT	NA	NA	NA	NA
Humphreys et al.[10] (C2-3 Block)	.76 kappa	98	91	10.9	0.02	495.8	11
Humphreys et al.[10] (C5-6 Block)	.46 kappa	78	55	1.7	0.4	4.3	11
Sandmark & Nisell[13] (Not for Radiculopathy)	NT	82	79	3.9	0.23	17.1	9
Comments: The testing procedure appears to be sensitive in identifying fused joint levels.							

TESTS TO DETERMINE IF A RADIOGRAPH IS REQUIRED

Canadian C-Spine Rules

1 Patients who are cognitively intact and have no neurological symptoms; or

2 Patients who are under the age of 65; or

3 Patients who are not fearful of moving the head upon command; or

4 Patients who were not involved in a distraction-based injury; or

5 Patients who demonstrate no midline pain do not need a radiograph.

6 Any positive finding in any of the above five categories should result in a radiographic test.

UTILITY SCORE **1**

Study	Reliability	Sensitivity	Specificity	LR+	LR−	DOR	QUADAS Score (0–14)
Stiell et al.[18] (Not Including Indeterminate Cases)	NT	99	45	1.81	0.01	136.1	12
Stiell et al.[18] (Not Including Indeterminate Cases)	NT	99	45	1.81	0.01	136.1	12
Stiell et al.[18] (Including Indeterminant Cases)	NT	99	91	10.7	0.01	1615.7	12
Stiell et al.[19]	.6 kappa	100	43	NT	NT	NT	12
Bandiera et al.[1]	.6 kappa	100	43	NT	NT	NT	9

Comments: Because the test is designed as a screen it is imperative that the findings exhibit high sensitivity. In order to rule out the need for an x-ray, all five categories should be negative. The decision rules are designed to be used in the acute stage of the injury.

TESTS TO DETERMINE IF A RADIOGRAPH IS REQUIRED

NEXUS (National Emergency X-Radiography Utilization Study)

1 Patients who do not have tenderness at posterior midline of the cervical spine.

2 Patients who have no focal neurological deficit.

3 Patients who have a normal level of alertness.

4 Patients who have no evidence of intoxication.

5 Patients who do not have a clinically apparent, painful injury that may distract them from a cervical injury.

6 Any positive finding in any of the above five categories should result in a radiographic test.

UTILITY SCORE 2

Study	Reliability	Sensitivity	Specificity	LR+	LR−	DOR	QUADAS Score (0–14)
Stiell et al.[18]	.52 to .72 kappa	91	37	1.43	0.25	5.7	12
Dickinson et al.[5]	.23 to .78 kappa	93	38	1.49	0.19	7.7	9
Hoffman et al.[9]	NT	99	13	1.14	0.08	14.7	11

Comments: Note the lower sensitivity values, suggesting this "screen" is less effective than the Canadian C-Spine rules. Nonetheless, the test still demonstrates value.[25] The rules are designed to be used in the acute stage of the injury.

Key Points

1. The majority of clinical special tests for cervical radiculopathy have been investigated within the literature.

2. Many of the clinical special tests for cervical instability have not been investigated for diagnostic accuracy. Those that have been studied may be influenced by bias.

3. Tests such as the ULTT and Brachial Plexus Compression have high sensitivity for detection of cervical radiculopathy.

4. The Spurling's compression test demonstrates variable findings, depending on the studies cited.

5. Although untested for diagnostic accuracy, the vertebral basilar insufficiency test is likely not sensitive but a specific test, albeit of high risk if findings are noted.

6. Prior to administration of cervical spine instability tests, specifically after trauma, one should perform the Canadian C-Spine rules.

7. The Canadian C-Spine rules used to detect who would benefit from a radiograph are highly sensitive and function very well as a screen in the acutely injured patient.

8. The flexion-rotation test for cervicogenic headaches detection is likely diagnostic because the criteria included for patients with cervicogenic headaches was very specific.

References

1. Bandiera G, Stiell IG, Wells GA, Clement C, De Maio V, Vandemheen KL, Greenberg GH, Lesiuk H, Brison R, Cass D, Dreyer J, Eisenhauer MA, Macphail I, McKnight RD, Morrison L, Reardon M, Schull M, Worthington J; Canadian C-Spine and CT Head Study Group. The Canadian C-spine rule performs better than unstructured physician judgment. *Ann Emerg Med.* 2003;42(3):395–402.

2. Bertilson B, Grunnesjo M, Strender LE. Reliability of clinical tests in the assessment of patient with neck/shoulder problems—impact of history. *Spine.* 2003;19:2222–2231.

3. Cattrysse E, Swinkels RA, Oostendorp RA, Duquet W. Upper cervical instability: are clinical tests reliable? *Man Ther.* 1997;2(2):91–97.

4. Davidson R, Dunn E, Metzmaker J. The shoulder abduction test in the diagnosis of radicular pain in cervical extradural compression monoradiculopathies. *Spine.* 1981;6:441–445.

5. Dickinson G, Stiell IG, Schull M, Brison R, Clement CM, Vandemheen KL, Cass D, McKnight D, Greenberg G, Worthington JR, Reardon M, Morrison L, Eisenhauer MA, Dreyer J, Wells GA. Retrospective application of the NEXUS low-risk criteria for cervical spine radiography in Canadian emergency departments. *Ann Emerg Med.* 2004;43(4):507–514.

6. Dobbs A. Manual therapy assessment of cervical instability. *Orthopaedic Physical Therapy Clinics of North America.* 2001;10:431–454.

7. Hall T, Robinson K. The flexion-rotation test and active cervical mobility—a comparative measurement study in cervicogenic headache. *Man Ther.* 2004;9(4):197–202.

8. Harris KD, Heer DM, Roy TC, Santos DM, Whitman JM, Wainner RS. Reliability of a measurement of neck flexor muscle endurance. *Phys Ther.* 2005;85(12):1349–1355.

9. Hoffman JR, Mower WR, Wolfson AB, Todd KH, Zucker MI. Validity of a set of clinical criteria to rule out injury to the cervical spine in patients with blunt trauma. National Emergency X-Radiography Utilization Study Group. *N Engl J Med.* 2000;343(2):94–99.

10. Humphreys BK, Delahaye M, Peterson CK. An investigation into the validity of cervical spine

motion palpation using patients with congenital block vertebrae as a "gold standard". *BMC Musculoskelet Disord.* 2004;5:19.

11. Jull G, Bogduk N, Marsland A. The accuracy of manual diagnosis for cervical zygapophysial joint pain syndromes. *Med J Aust.* 1988;148(5): 233–236.

12. Olsen L, Millar L, Dunker J, Hicks J, Glanz D. Reliability of a clinical test for deep cervical flexor endurance. *J Manipulative Physiol Therapeutics.* 2006;29:134–138.

13. Sandmark H, Nisell R. Validity of five common manual neck pain provoking tests. *Scand J Rehabil Med.* 1995;27(3):131–136.

14. Shah KC, Rajshekhar V. Reliability of diagnosis of soft cervical disc prolapse using Spurling's test. *Br J Neurosurg.* 2004;18(5):480–483.

15. Sharp J, Purser DW, Lawrence JS. Rheumatoid arthritis of the cervical spine in the adult. *Ann Rheum Dis.* 1958;17(3):303–13.

16. Smedmark V, Wallin M, Arvidsson I. Inter-examiner reliability in assessing passive intervertebral motion of the cervical spine. *Man Ther.* 2000;5(2):97–101.

17. Spurling RG, Scoville WB. Lateral rupture of the cervical intervertebral disc. *Surg Gynecol Obstet.* 1944;78:350–358.

18. Stiell IG, Clement CM, McKnight RD, Brison R, Schull MJ, Rowe BH, Worthington JR, Eisenhauer MA, Cass D, Greenberg G, MacPhail I, Dreyer J, Lee JS, Bandiera G, Reardon M, Holroyd B, Lesiuk H, Wells GA. The Canadian C-spine rule versus the NEXUS low-risk criteria in patients with trauma. *N Engl J Med.* 2003;349(26):2510–2518.

19. Stiell IG, Wells GA, Vandemheen KL, Clement CM, Lesiuk H, De Maio VJ, Laupacis A, Schull M, McKnight RD, Verbeek R, Brison R, Cass D, Dreyer J, Eisenhauer MA, Greenberg GH, MacPhail I, Morrison L, Reardon M, Worthington J. The Canadian C-spine rule for radiography in alert and stable trauma patients. *JAMA.* 2001;286(15):1841–1848.

20. Tong HC, Haig AJ, Yamakawa K. The Spurling test and cervical radiculopathy. *Spine.* 2002; 27(2):156–159.

21. Uchihara T, Furukawa T, Tsukagoshi H. Compression of brachial plexus as a diagnostic test of cervical cord lesion. *Spine.* 1994;19(19): 2170–2173.

22. Uitvlugt G, Indenbaum S. Clinical assessment of atlantoaxial instability using the Sharp-Purser test. *Arthritis Rheum.* 1988;31(7): 918–922.

23. Van Suijlekom HA, De Vet HC, Van Den Berg SG, Weber WE. Interobserver reliability in physical examination of the cervical spine in patients with headache. *Headache.* 2000;40 (7):581–586.

24. Viikari-Juntura E, Porras M, Laasonen EM. Validity of clinical tests in the diagnosis of root compression in cervical disc disease. *Spine.* 1989;14(3):253–257.

25. Viikari-Juntura E, Takala E, Riihimaki H, Martikainen R, Jappinen P. Predictive validity of symptoms and signs in the neck and shoulders. *J Clin Epidemiol.* 2000;53(8):800–808.

26. Wainner RS, Fritz JM, Irrgang JJ, Boninger ML, Delitto A, Allison S. Reliability and diagnostic accuracy of the clinical examination and patient self-report measures for cervical radiculopathy. *Spine.* 2003;28(1):52–62.

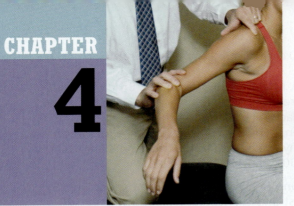

CHAPTER 4

Physical Examination Tests for the Shoulder Complex

Tests for Acromioclavicular (AC) Joint Pathology   124

Tests for Axillary Nerve Palsy   127

TESTS FOR A TORN ROTATOR CUFF/IMPINGEMENT

Rent Test (Rotator Cuff [RC] Tear)

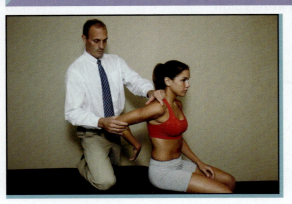

1 The patient is seated with arm relaxed while the examiner stands to the rear.

2 The examiner palpates anterior to the anterior edge of the acromion with one hand while grasping the patient's flexed elbow with the other.

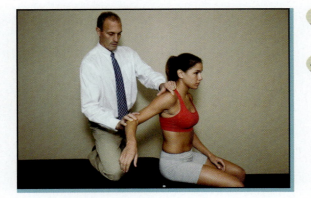

3 The examiner extends the patient's arm and then slowly internally and externally rotates the shoulder.

4 An eminence (prominent greater tuberosity) and a rent (depression of about 1 finger width) will be felt in the presence of a rotator cuff tear.

UTILITY SCORE 2

Study	Reliability	Sensitivity	Specificity	LR+	LR−	DOR	QUADAS Score (0–14)
Wolf & Agrawal[54]	NT	96	97	32	0.04	800	9
Lyons & Tomlinson[33]	NT	91	75	3.64	0.12	30.33	6

Comments: The Rent Test[5] should not be used to judge the size of a rotator cuff tear but rather the absence or presence of a rotator cuff tear. The quality of the studies keeps this Utility Score from being a 1.

TESTS FOR A TORN ROTATOR CUFF/IMPINGEMENT

Supine Impingement Test (RC Tear)

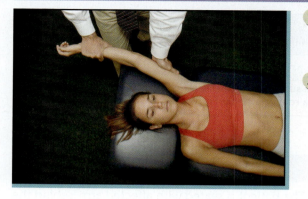

1 The patient assumes a supine position. The examiner stands to the side of the patient's involved shoulder.

2 The examiner grasps the patient's wrist and distal humerus and elevates the patient's arm to end range (170 degrees or greater).

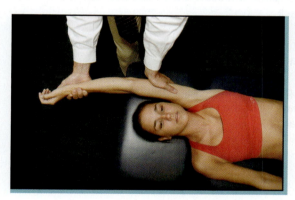

3 The examiner next moves the patient's arm into external rotation then adducts the arm to the patient's ear.

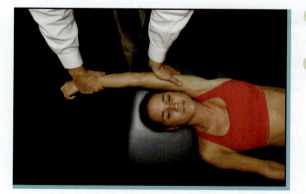

4 The examiner now internally rotates the patient's arm.

5 The Supine Impingement test is positive if the patient reports a significant increase in shoulder pain.

(continued)

TESTS FOR A TORN ROTATOR CUFF/IMPINGEMENT

UTILITY SCORE **2**

Study	Reliability	Sensitivity	Specificity	LR+	LR−	DOR	QUADAS Score (0–14)
Litaker et al.[30]	NT	97	9	1.07	0.33	3.24	11

Comments: This study was designed well but retrospectively. The supine impingement test does not appear diagnostic but may have value as a screen since a negative finding may rule out a rotator cuff tear. Further research needs to be performed.

Lift-Off Test (Subscapularis Tear)

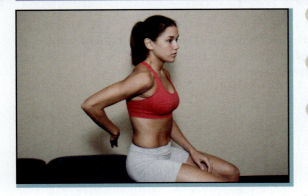

1. The patient is seated with affected arm behind the back.

2. The patient is asked to lift his or her arm off of the back.

3. A positive test for subscapularis tear is indicated by inability of the patient to lift his or her arm off of the back.

UTILITY SCORE **2**

Study	Reliability	Sensitivity	Specificity	LR+	LR−	DOR	QUADAS Score (0–14)
Gerber & Krushell[11]	NT	92	NT	NA	NA	NA	9
Hertel et al.[16]	NT	62	100	NA	NA	NA	8
Ostor et al.[44]	κ = .28–.32	NT	NT	NT	NT	NT	NA

Comments: The study by Gerber and Krushell[11] had a sample size of 16 subjects, all men, but referenced another study of 162 subjects with very little detail. One study shows high specificity, meaning this test has value when positive, of ruling in a subscapularis tear; more research needs to be performed, especially in light of the quality of this study. Of some concern is fair interobserver agreement.

TESTS FOR A TORN ROTATOR CUFF/IMPINGEMENT

Internal Rotation Lag Sign (Subscapularis Tear)

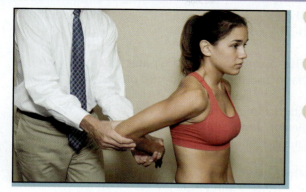

1 The patient is seated with affected arm behind the back.

2 The examiner grasps the patient's elbow with one hand and the wrist with the other.

3 The examiner lifts the patient's arm off of the back.

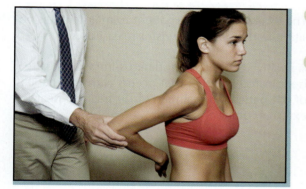

4 The examiner asks the patient to maintain this position as the patient's wrist is released.

5 A positive test for subscapularis tear is indicated by a lag that occurs with the inability of the patient to maintain his or her arm off of the back.

UTILITY SCORE 2

Study	Reliability	Sensitivity	Specificity	LR+	LR−	DOR	QUADAS Score (0–14)
Hertel et al.[16]	NT	97	96	24.25	0.03	808.33	8

Comments: Despite the solid statistical numbers, the Utility Score is only a 2 due to potential for bias in the conduct of this study or incomplete reporting of the study findings. More research needs to be performed, especially in light of the quality of this study.

TESTS FOR A TORN ROTATOR CUFF/IMPINGEMENT

External Rotation Lag Sign (Supraspinatus/Infraspinatus Tear)

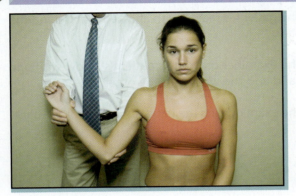

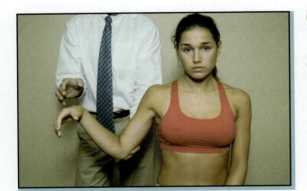

① The patient is seated with the examiner standing to the rear.

② The examiner grasps the patient's elbow with one hand and the wrist with the other.

③ The examiner places the elbow in 90 degrees of flexion and the shoulder in 20 degrees of elevation in the scapular plane.

④ The examiner passively externally rotates the shoulder to near end range.

⑤ The examiner asks the patient to maintain this position as the patient's wrist is released.

⑥ A positive test for supraspinatus/infraspinatus tear is indicated by a lag that occurs with the inability of the patient to maintain his or her arm near full external rotation.

UTILITY SCORE | **2**

Study	Reliability	Sensitivity	Specificity	LR+	LR−	DOR	QUADAS Score (0–14)
Hertel et al.[16]	NT	70	100	NA	NA	NA	8
Walch et al[52]	NT	100	100	NA	NA	NA	6

Comments: Despite the solid statistical numbers, the Utility Score is only a 2 due to potential for bias in the conduct of these studies or incomplete reporting of the study findings. More research needs to be performed, especially in light of the quality of these studies.

TESTS FOR A TORN ROTATOR CUFF/IMPINGEMENT

Drop Sign (Infraspinatus Tear, Irreparable Fatty Degeneration of Infraspinatus)

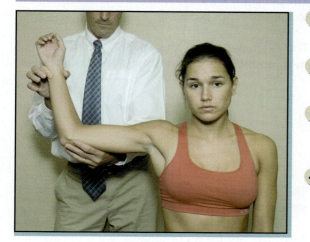

1 The patient is seated with the examiner standing to the rear.

2 The examiner grasps the patient's elbow with one hand and the wrist with the other.

3 The examiner places the elbow in 90 degrees of flexion and the shoulder in 90 degrees of elevation in the scapular plane.

4 The examiner passively externally rotates the shoulder to near end range.

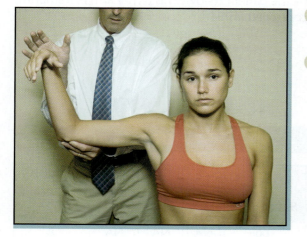

5 The examiner asks the patient to maintain this position as the patient's wrist is released.

6 A positive test for infraspinatus tear is indicated by a lag that occurs with the inability of the patient to maintain his or her arm near full external rotation.

UTILITY SCORE   2

Study	Reliability	Sensitivity	Specificity	LR+	LR−	DOR	QUADAS Score (0–14)
Hertel et al.[16]	NT	20	100	NA	NA	NA	8
Walch et al.[52]	NT	100	100	NA	NA	NA	6

Comments: Despite the solid statistical numbers, the Utility Score is only a 2 due to potential for bias in both studies secondary to research design flaws. Walch et al.[52] performed the Drop Sign with the arm at the patient's side, which is not the original description. More research needs to be performed, especially in light of the quality of these studies.

TESTS FOR A TORN ROTATOR CUFF/IMPINGEMENT

Drop Arm Test (Supraspinatus Tear, Subacromial Impingement)

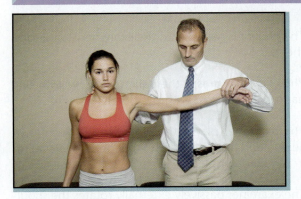

1 The patient is standing with the examiner standing to the front (not pictured).

2 The examiner grasps the patient's wrist and passively abducts the patient's shoulder to 90 degrees.

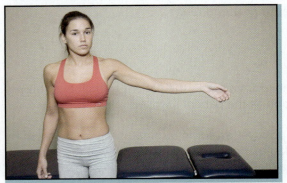

3 The examiner releases the patient's arm with instructions to slowly lower the arm.

4 A positive test for supraspinatus tear is the inability by the patient to lower his or her arm in a smooth, controlled fashion.

UTILITY SCORE 3

Study	Reliability	Sensitivity	Specificity	LR+	LR−	DOR	QUADAS Score (0–14)
Calis et al.[3] (Supraspin. Tear Impingement)	NT NT	15 8	100 97	NA 2.66	NA .94	NA 2.83	8 8
Murrell & Walton[40] (RC Tear)	NT	10	98	5.00	.92	5.43	5
Park et al.[46] (Impingement or Rotator Cuff Disease)	NT	27	88	2.25	.83	2.71	10
Ostor et al.[44] (Supraspinatus Tear)	κ = .28–.66	NT	NT	NA	NA	NA	NA

Comments: Calis et al.[3] used subacromial injection as the criterion standard whereas surgery is the better choice. Park et al.[46] used this as an active test where the patient moved the arm through "elevation" and looked for a "drop" as the patient lowered the arm. If this test has value, it is in a positive finding to rule in either a rotator cuff tear or impingement. The likelihood ratios indicate this is only a modest diagnostic test at best despite fair to significant interobserver agreement.

TESTS FOR A TORN ROTATOR CUFF/IMPINGEMENT

Empty Can Test/Supraspinatus Test (Rotator Cuff Tear, All Stages of Impingement Syndrome from Bursitis Through a Rotator Cuff Tear)

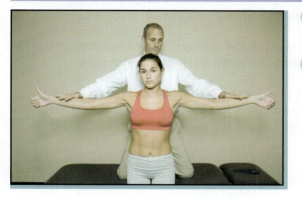

1 The patient elevates the arms to 90 degrees with thumbs up (full can position).

2 The examiner provides downward pressure on the arms and notes the patient's strength.

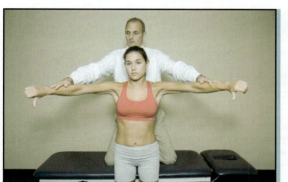

3 The patient elevates the arms to 90 degrees and horizontally adducts 30 degrees (scapular plane) with thumbs pointed down as if "emptying a can."

4 The examiner provides downward pressure on the arms and notes the patient's strength.

5 A positive test for rotator cuff tear is examiner assessment of more weakness in the empty can position versus the full can position, patient complaint of pain, or both.

UTILITY SCORE 2

Study	Reliability	Sensitivity	Specificity	LR+	LR−	DOR	QUADAS Score (0–14)
Itoi et al.[19] (Supraspinatus Tear)	NT	89	50	1.78	0.22	8.09	9
Park et al.[46] (Impingement or Rotator Cuff Disease)	NT	44	90	4.2	0.63	6.67	10
Ostor et al.[44] (Supraspinatus Tear)	κ = .44–.49	NT	NT	NA	NA	NA	NA

Comments: This test was originally described by Jobe and Moynes[22] as a supraspinatus strength test only, without a provocation component. Itoi et al.[19] used weakness, pain, or both as a positive sign and looked at the ability of the test to detect damage in any of the rotator cuff muscles. Park et al.[46] performed the test as originally described, which may explain high specificity in one study and high sensitivity in the other. Unfortunately, these divergent results leave the examiner unsure as to whether this test should be used to screen for or diagnose impingement and rotator cuff tear.

TESTS FOR A TORN ROTATOR CUFF/IMPINGEMENT

Full Can/Supraspinatus Test (Supraspinatus Tear)

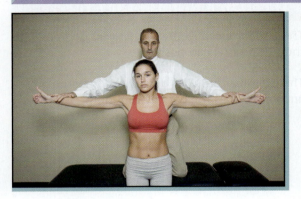

1. The patient elevates the arms to 90 degrees with thumbs up (full can position).

2. The examiner provides downward pressure on the arms and notes the patient's strength.

3. A positive test for rotator cuff tear is examiner assessment of more weakness in the involved shoulder, patient complaint of pain, or both.

UTILITY SCORE 3

Study	Reliability	Sensitivity	Specificity	LR+	LR−	DOR	QUADAS Score (0–14)
Itoi et al.[19]	NT	86	57	2.00	0.25	8.00	9

Comments: Kelly et al.[23] first described this test as a less painful alternative test to the Empty Can Test. Like the Empty Can Test, this test was originally designed as a supraspinatus strength test only, but now is a poor test for both rotator cuff tear and impingement. More research needs to be performed, especially in light of the quality of this study.

TESTS FOR A TORN ROTATOR CUFF/IMPINGEMENT

Posterior Impingement Sign (Rotator Cuff Tear and/or Posterior Labral Tear)

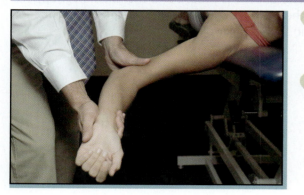

1 With the patient in supine, the shoulder is placed in 90–110 degrees of abduction, 10–15 degrees of extension, and maximum external rotation.

2 A positive test is indicated by complaints of pain in the deep posterior shoulder.

UTILITY SCORE **3**

Study	Reliability	Sensitivity	Specificity	LR+	LR−	DOR	QUADAS Score (0–14)
Meister et al.[37]	NT	76	85	5.06	0.28	18.07	6

Comments: Despite good statistical numbers, the gender of the patients in this study was not specified and other design flaws leave a great potential for bias. More research needs to be performed, especially in light of the quality of this study.

TESTS FOR A TORN ROTATOR CUFF/IMPINGEMENT

Hornblower's Sign (Irreparable Fatty Degeneration of Teres Minor)

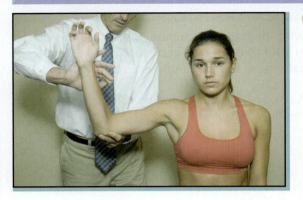

1 The patient is seated and the examiner supports the patient's shoulder in 90 degrees of abduction in the scapular plane.

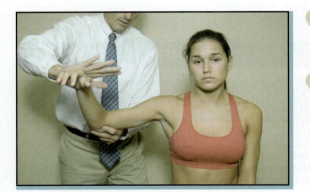

2 The elbow is flexed to 90 degrees and the patient is asked to forcefully externally rotate the shoulder against the examiner's resistance.

3 A positive test is indicated by the inability of the patient to maintain external rotation against examiner resistance.

UTILITY SCORE | **3**

Study	Reliability	Sensitivity	Specificity	LR+	LR−	DOR	QUADAS Score (0–14)
Walch et al.[52]	NT	100	93	NA	NA	NA	6

Comments: Despite the solid statistical numbers, the Utility Score is only a 3 due to potential for bias in the conduct of this study or incomplete reporting of the study findings. More research needs to be performed, especially in light of the quality of this study.

TESTS FOR A TORN ROTATOR CUFF/IMPINGEMENT

Belly Press Test (Subscapularis Tear)

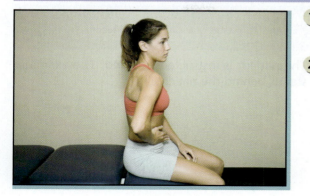

1 The patient can sit or stand with elbow flexed to 90 degrees.

2 The patient internally rotates the shoulder, causing the palm of the hand to be pressed into the stomach.

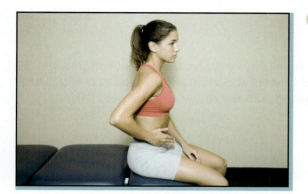

3 A positive test is indicated by the elbow dropping behind the body into extension.

UTILITY SCORE ?

Study	Reliability	Sensitivity	Specificity	LR+	LR−	DOR	QUADAS Score (1–14)
Gerber et al.[10]	NT	NT	NT	NA	NA	NA	NA

Comments: The Belly Press Test[10] was originally described as an alternative to the Lift-off Test in those patients without adequate internal shoulder rotation. Research needs to be performed to investigate the diagnostic accuracy of this test.

TESTS FOR IMPINGEMENT

Internal Rotation Resisted Strength Test (IRRST) (Internal/Intraarticular vs. External/Subacromial Impingement)

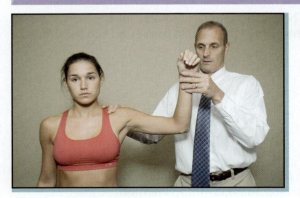

1 The patient is instructed to stand. The examiner stands behind the patient.

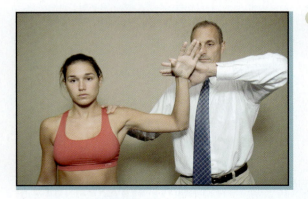

2 The examiner places the patient's shoulder in 90 degrees of abduction and 80 degrees of external rotation with the elbow at 90 degrees flexion.

TESTS FOR IMPINGEMENT

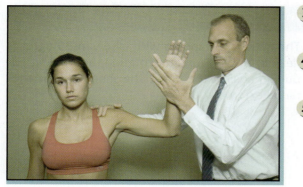

3 The examiner applies manual resistance to the wrist, first to test isometric external rotation.

4 The examiner applies manual resistance to the wrist, next to test isometric internal rotation.

5 The examiner compares the results of these isometric tests. If internal rotation strength is weaker than external rotation, the IRRST test is considered positive and the patient purportedly has internal impingement.

UTILITY SCORE | 2

Study	Reliability	Sensitivity	Specificity	LR+	LR−	DOR	QUADAS Score (0–14)
Zaslav[56]	NT	88	96	22	0.12	183.33	8

Comments: Despite the great statistical numbers, the Utility Score is only a 2 due to potential for bias in the conduct of this study and/or incomplete reporting of the study findings. More research needs to be performed, especially in light of the quality of this study.

TESTS FOR IMPINGEMENT

Infraspinatus Test (All Stages of Subacromial Impingement)

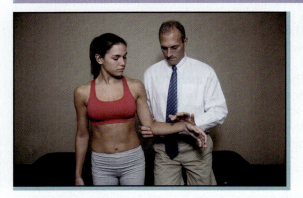

1 The patient is standing with elbow in 90 degrees flexion, neutral forearm rotation, and elbow adducted against the body. The shoulder is in end-range external rotation.

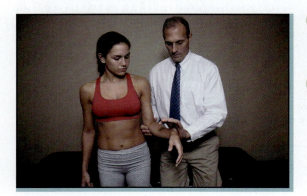

2 The examiner stands to the side of the patient and provides an internal rotation force while the patient resists.

3 A positive test is indicated by patient giving way due to either pain or weakness or if there is a positive External Rotation Lag Sign.

UTILITY SCORE   2

Study	Reliability	Sensitivity	Specificity	LR+	LR−	DOR	QUADAS Score (0–14)
Park HB et al.[46]	NT	42	90	4.20	0.65	6.46	10
Ostor et al.[44]	κ = .18–.45	NT	NT	NA	NA	NA	NA

Comments: Park et al.[46] incorporated the External Rotation Lag Sign as part of the assessment of the infraspinatus in effect, combining two tests. Unfortunately, the test has only a small effect on posttest probability when trying to find any stage of impingement (bursitis through full-thickness rotator cuff tear).

TESTS FOR IMPINGEMENT

Neer Test (Subacromial Impingement, Subacromial Bursitis [SAB], Rotator Cuff Tear, Superior Labral Tear)

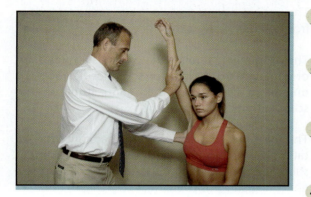

1 The patient is seated while the examiner stands to the side of the involved shoulder.

2 The examiner raises the patient's arm into flexion with one hand while the other hand stabilizes the scapula.

3 The examiner applies forced flexion toward end range in an attempt to reproduce the shoulder pain.

4 If concordant shoulder pain is present, the test is positive.

UTILITY SCORE 3

Study	Reliability	Sensitivity	Specificity	LR+	LR−	DOR	QUADAS Score (0–14)
MacDonald et al.[34] (SAB	NT	75	48	1.40	0.52	2.69	7
Rotator Cuff Tear)	NT	83	51	1.69	0.33	5.12	7
Park et al.[46]	NT	68	69	2.20	0.46	4.78	10
Calis et al.[3]	NT	89	31	1.28	0.35	3.66	8
Parentis et al.[45] (Superior Labral Tear)	NT	48	51	.98	1.02	.96	5
Bak & Fauno[1] (Impingement)	NT	0	100	NA	NA	NA	6
Nakagawa et al.[42] (Superior Labral Tear)	NT	33	60	.83	1.11	.75	10

Comments: The test was originally described by Neer in 1983 and a positive test was confirmed by injecting 10ml of xylocaine into the subacromial space and repeating steps 1–4 above in a pain-free fashion. This test is, at best, mediocre with little effect on posttest probability of diagnosing impingement syndrome and the diagnosis of impingement itself may not be useful since it covers a broad spectrum of pathology. The ability of this test to detect a superior labral tear is worse than chance.

TESTS FOR IMPINGEMENT

Hawkins-Kennedy Test (Subacromial Impingement, Subacromial Bursitis, Rotator Cuff Tear, Superior Labral Tear)

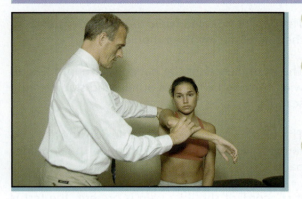

1. The patient is seated while the examiner stands in front of the involved shoulder.

2. The examiner first raises the patient's arm into approximately 90 degrees of shoulder flexion with one hand while the other hand stabilizes the scapula (typically superiorly).

3. The examiner applies forced humeral internal rotation in an attempt to reproduce the concordant shoulder pain. If concordant shoulder pain is present, the test is positive.

UTILITY SCORE 3

Study	Reliability	Sensitivity	Specificity	LR+	LR−	DOR	QUADAS Score (0–14)
MacDonald et al.[34] (Bursitis,	NT	92	44	1.64	0.18	9.11	7
Rotator Cuff Tear)	NT	88	43	1.54	0.27	5.70	7
Park HB et al.[46] (Impingement)	NT	72	66	2.11	0.42	5.02	10
Calis et al.[3] (Impingement,	NT	92	25	1.22	0.32	3.81	8
Rotator Cuff Tear)	NT	100	36	NA	NA	NA	8
Parentis et al.[45] (Superior Labral Tear)	NT	65	30	.94	1.15	.82	5
Bak & Fauno[1] (Impingement)	NT	80	76	3.33	0.26	12.81	6
Ostor et al.[44] (Impingement)	κ = .18–.43	NT	NT	NA	NA	NA	NA
Nakagawa et al.[42] (Superior Labral Tear)	NT	50	67	1.52	.75	2.03	10

Comments: The Hawkins-Kennedy Test[15] is probably a more sensitive test suitable for screening for either impingement or rotator cuff tear than it is a specific test suitable for ruling in a finding. Furthermore, in the best performed/reported study, the test has mediocre value and may not be a good screening or diagnostic test.

Painful Arc Test (All Stages of Subacromial Impingement, Acromioclavicular [AC] Joint Disorder)

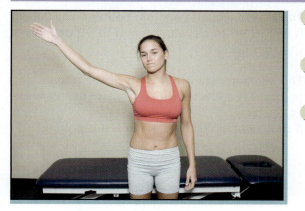

1 The patient is standing. The examiner faces the patient to observe shoulder motion.

2 The patient is instructed to actively abduct the involved shoulder.

3 A positive test is indicated by patient report of concordant pain in the 60- to 120-degree range. Pain outside of this range is considered a negative test. Pain that increases in severity as the arm reaches 180 degrees is indicative of a "disorder of the acromioclavicular joint."

UTILITY SCORE 3

Study	Reliability	Sensitivity	Specificity	LR+	LR−	DOR	QUADAS Score (0–14)
Park HB[46] (Impingement)	NT	74	81	3.89	0.32	12.17	10
Calis et al.[3] (Impingement, Rotator Cuff Tear)	NT NT	33 45	81 79	1.73 2.14	0.82 0.70	2.11 3.06	8 8
Litaker et al.[30] (Rotator Cuff Tear)	NT	98	10	1.09	0.20	5.45	11

Comments: The Painful Arc Test[24] modifies posttest probability very little. Furthermore, the broad cluster of diagnoses captured under "impingement" may not aid the examiner with intervention.

TESTS FOR IMPINGEMENT

Cross-Body Adduction Test (Subacromial Impingement, Acromioclavicular [AC] Joint Damage)

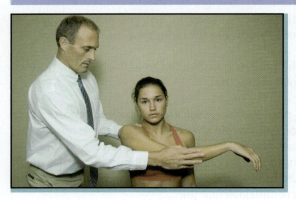

(1) The patient assumes a sitting position. The patient is instructed to elevate the arm to 90 degrees of shoulder flexion.

(2) The examiner stands in front of the patient and horizontally adducts the patient's arm to end range.

(3) If shoulder pain is present, the test is positive.

UTILITY SCORE 3

Study	Reliability	Sensitivity	Specificity	LR+	LR−	DOR	QUADAS Score (0–14)
Park HB et al.[46] (Impingement)	NT	23	82	1.27	0.93	1.37	10
Calis et al.[3] (Impingement, Rotator Cuff Tear)	NT NT	82 90	28 29	1.13 1.27	0.64 0.35	1.77 3.63	8 8
Chronopoulos et al.[4] (AC Joint Pathology)	NT	77	79	3.66	0.29	12.62	10
Ostor et al.[44] (AC Joint Pathology)	κ = .08–.29	NT	NT	NT	NT	NT	NA

Comments: The Cross-Body Test[36] appears to be a stronger indicator of AC joint pathology than impingement but the interobserver agreement of this test may negatively affect clinical application.

TESTS FOR A TORN LABRUM/INSTABILITY

Biceps Load Test II (SLAP Lesion)

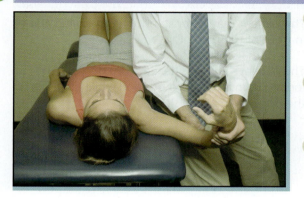

1 The patient assumes a supine position. The examiner sits on the side of the patient's involved extremity.

2 The examiner places the patient's shoulder in 120 degrees of abduction, the elbow in 90 degrees of flexion, and the forearm in supination.

3 The examiner moves the patient's shoulder to end-range external rotation (apprehension position).

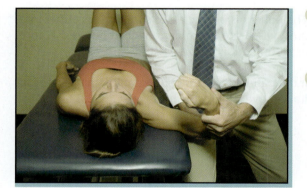

4 At end-range external rotation, the examiner asks the patient to flex his or her elbow while the examiner resists this movement.

5 A positive test is indicated as a reproduction of concordant pain during resisted elbow flexion.

UTILITY SCORE   1

Study	Reliability	Sensitivity	Specificity	LR+	LR−	DOR	QUADAS Score (0–14)
Kim et al.[27] (SLAP)	κ = .82	90	97	26.38	.11	239.82	10

Comments: This sequel to the Biceps Load Test[28] was performed in a broader spectrum of patients with blinding of the testers. Although the test requires further validation in more studies, these test results seem to indicate that the Biceps Load Test II is reliable and useful in diagnosing SLAP lesions of the shoulder. However, more research needs to be performed.

TESTS FOR A TORN LABRUM/INSTABILITY

Yergason's Test (Subacromial Impingement, Superior Labral Anterior to Posterior [SLAP] Lesion, Any Labral Lesion, Long Head of Biceps Pathology)

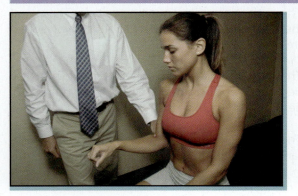

1 The patient may sit or stand. The examiner stands in front of the patient.

2 The patient's elbow is flexed to 90 degrees and the forearm is in a pronated position while maintaining the upper arm at the side.

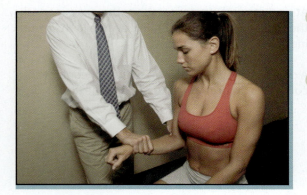

3 The patient is instructed to supinate his or her forearm, while the examiner concurrently resists forearm supination at the wrist.

4 If the patient localizes concordant pain to the bicipital groove, the test is positive.

TESTS FOR A TORN LABRUM/INSTABILITY

UTILITY SCORE **2**

Study	Reliability	Sensitivity	Specificity	LR+	LR−	DOR	QUADAS Score (0–14)
Calis et al.[3] (Impingement, Rotator Cuff Tear)	NT NT	37 50	86 86	2.64 3.57	0.73 0.58	3.62 6.16	8 8
Holtby & Razmjou[18] (SLAP)	NT	43	79	2.05	.72	2.85	12
Guanche & Jones[13] (SLAP, Any Labral Lesion)	NT NT	12 9	96 93	3.00 1.29	.92 .98	3.26 1.32	12 12
Parentis et al.[45] (SLAP)	NT	13	93	1.78	.94	1.89	5
Ostor et al.[44] (Long Head of Biceps Pathology)	κ = .28	NT	NT	NA	NA	NA	NA

Comments: The better studies show Yergason's Test[55] to have high specificity and therefore, a positive test may help rule in a labral tear but the likelihood ratios indicate that overall, the test is minimally helpful in diagnosis of a SLAP lesion. The interobserver agreement of this test is fair when detecting pathology of the long head of the biceps.

TESTS FOR A TORN LABRUM/INSTABILITY

Crank Test (Labral Tear, SLAP Lesion)

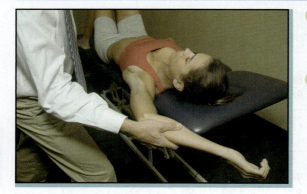

(1) The patient assumes either a sitting or supine position. The examiner either stands or sits at the side of the involved extremity.

(2) The examiner places the patient's shoulder in 160 degrees of elevation in the scapular plane and elbow in 90 degrees of flexion.

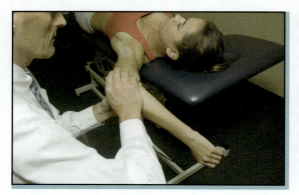

(3) The examiner first applies a compression force to the humerus and then rotates the humerus repeatedly into internal rotation and external rotation in an attempt to pinch the torn labrum.

(4) A positive test is indicated by the production of pain either with or without a click in the shoulder or by reproduction of the patient's concordant complaint (usually pain or catching).

UTILITY SCORE 2

Study	Reliability	Sensitivity	Specificity	LR+	LR−	DOR	QUADAS Score (0–14)
Parentis et al.[45] (SLAP)	NT	9	83	.50	1.10	.45	5
Stetson & Templin[51] (Labral Tear)	NT	46	56	1.04	.96	1.08	10
Myers et al.[41] (SLAP)	NT	35	70	.87	2	.44	8
Liu et al.[31] (Labral Tear)	NT	91	93	7.0	.10	70	11
Nakagawa et al.[42] (Superior Labral Tear)	NT	58	72	2.1	.58	3.62	10

Comments: There is uncertainty in use for the Crank Test[31] in diagnosing SLAP lesions, according to available research, and its use to detect any labral tear is mixed, according to two stronger studies. More well-designed research is needed.

TESTS FOR A TORN LABRUM/INSTABILITY

Kim Test (Posteroinferior Labral Lesion)

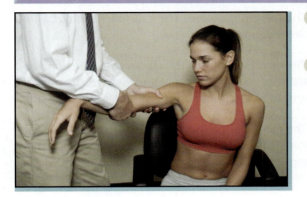

1. The patient is seated in a chair with his or her back supported.

2. The examiner stands to the side of the involved shoulder and faces the patient. The examiner grasps the elbow with one hand and the mid-humeral region with the other and elevates the patient's arm to 90 degrees abduction.

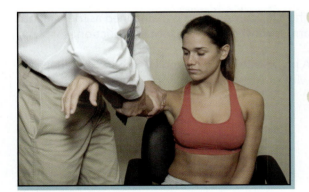

3. Simultaneously the examiner provides an axial load to the humerus and a 45-degree diagonal elevation to the distal humerus concurrent with a posteroinferior glide to the proximal humerus.

4. A positive test is indicated by a sudden onset of posterior shoulder pain.

UTILITY SCORE **2**

Study	Reliability	Sensitivity	Specificity	LR+	LR−	DOR	QUADAS Score (0–14)
Kim et al.[29]	NT	80	94	13.33	0.21	63.48	9

Comments: More research with more strict methodology needs to be done to corroborate these statistics, but as of now, the Kim Test is a significant indicator of a posteroinferior labral lesion. However, the Jerk Test[29] is easier to perform and performs better statistically.

TESTS FOR A TORN LABRUM/INSTABILITY

Jerk Test (Posteroinferior Labral Lesion)

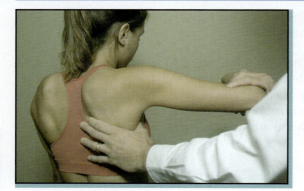

1. The patient is seated. The examiner stands behind the patient.

2. The examiner grasps the elbow with one hand and the scapula with the other and elevates the patient's arm to 90 degrees abduction and internal rotation.

3. The examiner provides an axial compression-based load to the humerus through the elbow maintaining the horizontally abducted arm.

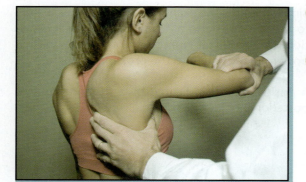

4. The axial compression is maintained as the patient's arm is moved into horizontal adduction.

5. A positive test is indicated by a sharp shoulder pain with or without a clunk or click.

UTILITY SCORE **2**

Study	Reliability	Sensitivity	Specificity	LR+	LR−	DOR	QUADAS Score (0–14)
Kim et al.[26]	NT	73	98	36.5	0.27	135.19	9
Nakagawa et al.[42] (Superior Labral Tear)	NT	25	80	1.25	.94	1.33	10

Comments: More research with more strict methodology needs to be done to corroborate these statistics, but as of now, the Jerk Test[26,29] is a significant indicator of a posteroinferior labral lesion and a nondescript test for superior labral tear (not the original purpose of the test).

TESTS FOR A TORN LABRUM/INSTABILITY

Anterior Release/Surprise Test (Anterior Instability)

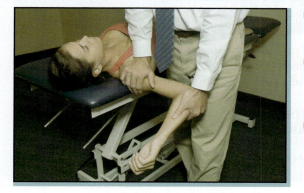

1 The patient assumes a supine position. The examiner stands beside the patient.

2 The examiner grasps the forearm with one hand and provides a posterior force on the humerus with the other.

3 The posterior force on the proximal humerus is maintained while the examiner moves the patient's shoulder into the apprehension position of 90 degrees abduction and end-range external rotation.

4 The posterior force on the humerus is then released.

5 A positive test is indicated if the patient reports sudden pain, an increase in pain, or by reproduction of the patient's concordant symptoms.

UTILITY SCORE **2**

Study	Reliability	Sensitivity	Specificity	LR+	LR−	DOR	QUADAS Score (0–14)
Gross & Distefano[12]	NT	92	89	8.36	0.08	104.5	9
Lo et al.[32]	NT	64	99	64	0.36	177.78	7
Comments: Despite the apparently good statistics, the quality of these two studies is poor so the examiner should be guarded about the results.							

TESTS FOR A TORN LABRUM/INSTABILITY

Speed's Test (All Stages of Subacromial Impingement, Superior Labral Anterior to Posterior [SLAP] Lesion, Any Labral Lesion, Biceps Pathology)

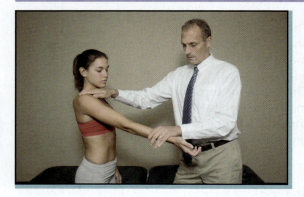

1. The patient assumes a standing position. The patient is instructed to extend his or her elbow and fully supinates the forearm.

2. The examiner, standing in front of the patient, resists shoulder flexion from zero to 60 degrees.

3. If the patient localizes concordant pain to the bicipital groove, the test is positive.

UTILITY SCORE 3

Study	Reliability	Sensitivity	Specificity	LR+	LR−	DOR	QUADAS Score (0–14)
Park et al.[46] (Impingement)	NT	38	83	2.23	0.74	3.01	10
Calis et al.[3] (Impingement, Rotator Cuff Tear)	NT	69	56	1.56	0.55	2.84	8
	NT	85	57	1.98	0.26	7.62	8
Holtby & Razmjou[18] (SLAP)	NT	32	75	1.28	0.91	1.41	12
Bennett[2] (SLAP + Biceps Pathology)	NT	90	14	1.04	0.72	1.44	9
Guanche & Jones[13] (SLAP, Any Labral Lesion)	NT	9	74	.35	1.23	.28	12
	NT	18	87	1.38	.94	1.45	12
Morgan et al.[39] (Ant. Labrum, Posterior Labrum, SLAP)	NT	100	70	NA	NA	NA	11
	NT	29	11	.32	6.32	.05	11
	NT	78	37	1.23	0.60	2.05	11
Parentis et al.[45] (SLAP)	NT	48	68	1.49	0.77	1.94	5
Ostor et al.[44] (Long Head of Biceps Pathology)	κ = .17–.32	NT	NT	NT	NT	NT	NA
Nakagawa et al.[42] (Superior Labral Tear)	NT	4	100	NA	NA	NA	10

Comments: Speed's Test[6] was originally used to test for long head bicipital tenosynovitis but its use has expanded to many pathologies. Unfortunately, in the well-performed studies, it seems a poor test for any of those pathologies with the exception of an anterior labral tear, where one study showed it may be used as a screening tool due to high sensitivity. Ironically, Speed's Test[6] has never been studied as a test for tenosynovitis.

TESTS FOR A TORN LABRUM/INSTABILITY

Apprehension Test (Anterior Instability)

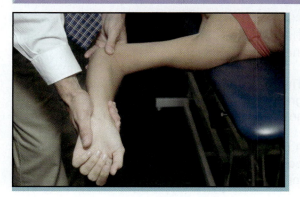

1 The patient is either standing or supine. The examiner stands either behind or at the involved side of the patient.

2 The examiner grasps the wrist with one hand and maximally externally rotates the humerus with the shoulder in 90 degrees of abduction.

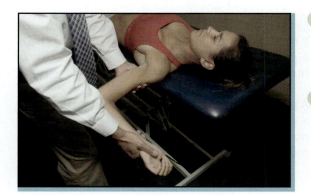

3 Forward pressure is then applied to the posterior aspect of the humeral head by either the examiner (if patient is standing) or the examination table (if the patient is in supine).

4 A positive test for anterior instability is indicated by a show of apprehension by the patient or a report of pain.

UTILITY SCORE 3

Study	Reliability	Sensitivity	Specificity	LR+	LR−	DOR	QUADAS Score (0–14)
Guanche & Jones[13] (SLAP	NT	30	63	.81	1.11	.73	12
Any Labral Lesion)	NT	40	87	3.08	.69	4.46	12
Lo et al.[32]	NT	53	99	53	0.47	112.77	7

Comments: The Apprehension Test[47] was originally described in 1981 by Rowe and Zarins[47] to detect anterior instability but interestingly, only Lo et al.[32] have studied this test in context. Unfortunately, the Lo et al.[32] study had many design/reporting faults. Therefore, the use of this test to rule in anterior instability is unknown. Furthermore, this test is of minimal use to diagnose any labral lesion and no use in diagnosing a SLAP lesion.

TESTS FOR A TORN LABRUM/INSTABILITY

Apprehension-Relocation Test/Jobe Relocation Test (Anterior Instability, Labral Tear, SLAP Lesion)

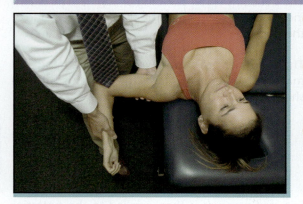

1. The patient assumes a supine position. The examiner stands beside the patient.

2. The examiner pre-positions the shoulder at 90 degrees of abduction then grasps the patient's forearm and maximally externally rotates the humerus.

3. A posterior to anterior force is then applied to the posterior aspect of the humeral head by the examiner.

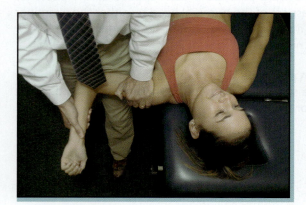

4. If the patient displays apprehension or reports pain, a posterior force is then applied to the proximal humerus.

5. A positive test for anterior instability is indicated by a decrease in the pain or apprehension, whereas no change in pain symptoms indicates impingement.

TESTS FOR A TORN LABRUM/INSTABILITY

UTILITY SCORE 3

Study	Reliability	Sensitivity	Specificity	LR+	LR−	DOR	QUADAS Score (0–14)
Guanche & Jones[13] (SLAP	NT	36	63	.97	1.02	.95	12
Any Labral Lesion)	NT	44	87	3.38	.64	5.28	12
Morgan et al.[39]							
(Ant. Labral Tear	NT	4	27	.05	3.52	.01	11
Posterior Labral Tear	NT	85	68	2.67	.21	12.71	11
Combined [SLAP])	NT	59	54	1.28	.76	1.68	11
Parentis et al.[45] (SLAP)	NT	44	51	.90	1.10	.82	5
Nakagawa et al.[42] (Superior Labral Tear)	NT	75	40	1.25	.63	1.98	10
Lo et al.[32] (Anterior Instability)	NT	46	54	1.0	1.0	1.0	7
Speer et al.[50]							
(Anterior Instability)	NT	54	44	.96	1.05	.91	9
(Pain Apprehension)	NT	68	100	NA	NA	NA	9

Comments: Originally described by Jobe et al. in 1989,[21] the Relocation Test was supposed to differentiate between impingement and anterior instability. The Speer et al.[50] study would seem to indicate that the Relocation Test has value as a positive test in ruling in anterior instability when the patient emotes "apprehension." However, the Speer et al.[50] study had significant limitations with regard to blinding and description of the spectrum of patients so the numbers are to be taken with caution. Research does not support the use of this test to differentiate impingement from instability or to diagnose any type of labral tear.

TESTS FOR A TORN LABRUM/INSTABILITY

Modified Relocation Test/Modified Jobe Relocation Test (Labral Pathology)

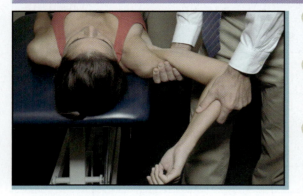

1. The patient assumes a supine position. The examiner stands beside the patient.

2. The examiner prepositions the shoulder at 120 degrees of abduction then grasps the patient's forearm and maximally externally rotates the humerus.

3. A posterior to anterior force is then applied to the posterior aspect of the humeral head by the examiner.

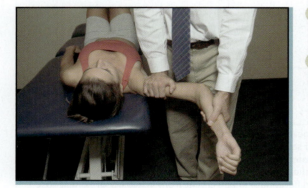

4. If the patient reports pain, a posterior force is then applied to the proximal humerus.

5. A positive test for labral pathology is indicated by a report of pain with the anterior-directed force and relief of pain with the posterior-directed force.

UTILITY SCORE 3

Study	Reliability	Sensitivity	Specificity	LR+	LR−	DOR	QUADAS Score (0–14)
Hamner et al.[14]	NT	92	100	92	0.08	1150	7

Comments: Great statistics but only 14 subjects, all overhead-throwing athletes ages 21–31, and many other design faults that lead to potential bias. At best, the Modified Relocation Test[14] would be an intriguing test for further research.

TESTS FOR A TORN LABRUM/INSTABILITY

Forced Shoulder Abduction and Elbow Flexion Test (Superior Labral Tear)

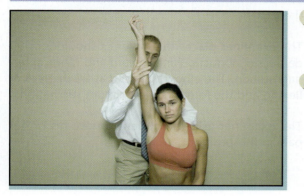

1 The patient assumes a sitting position. The examiner typically stands at the side of the involved extremity.

2 The examiner places the patient's shoulder in maximum abduction with full elbow extension and notes pain in the posterior-superior aspect of the shoulder.

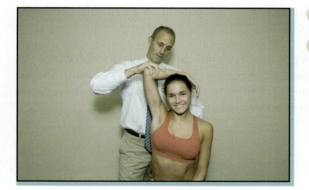

3 The examiner then flexes the patient's elbow.

4 A positive test is indicated by the production of pain in the posterior-superior aspect of the shoulder during shoulder abduction with elbow extension that is diminished or relieved by elbow flexion.

UTILITY SCORE **3**

Study	Reliability	Sensitivity	Specificity	LR+	LR−	DOR	QUADAS Score (0–14)
Nakawaga et al.[42]	NT	67	67	2.0	.49	4.0	10

Comments: The one study to examine the Forced Shoulder Abduction and Elbow Flexion Test[42] had some design and reporting flaws. Most notably, all subjects were young throwing athletes and only 2 of 54 subjects were female, leading to spectrum bias. More well-designed research is needed.

TESTS FOR A TORN LABRUM/INSTABILITY

Pain Provocation Test (SLAP Lesion)

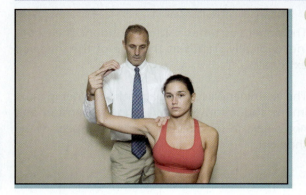

1 The patient is seated. The examiner stands behind the patient.

2 The examiner places the patient's shoulder in 90 degrees of abduction and toward end-range external rotation. The elbow is placed at 90 degrees of flexion and the forearm in maximum supination.

3 The examiner asks the patient to rate his or her pain in this position.

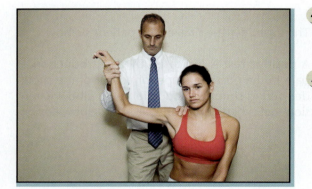

4 The examiner then fully pronates the patient's forearm and asks the patient to again rate his or her pain.

5 A positive test is indicated by production of the patient's concordant pain in the forearm-pronated position or when the patient's pain is worse in pronation than in supination.

UTILITY SCORE 3

Study	Reliability	Sensitivity	Specificity	LR+	LR−	DOR	QUADAS Score (0–14)
Mimori et al.[38] SLAP	NT	100	90	NA	NA	NA	7
Parentis et al.[45] SLAP	NT	17	90	1.72	.92	1.87	5

Comments: Despite the great numbers reported by Mimori et al.,[38] their study had many design faults, including a criterion standard (arthroscopy) that was given to only 11 of 32 patients. Even if the numbers were not suspicious, the test would only be useful in diagnosing SLAP tears in young, male baseball players—quite a limited population.

TESTS FOR A TORN LABRUM/INSTABILITY

Sulcus Sign (Inferior Laxity, Superior Labral Tear)

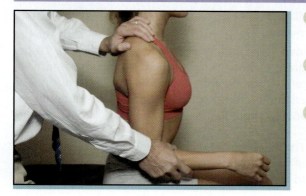

1 The patient is seated. The examiner stands behind the patient.

2 The examiner grasps the elbow and pulls down, causing an inferior traction force.

3 The examiner notes, in centimeters, the distance between the inferior surface of the acromion and the superior portion of the humeral head.

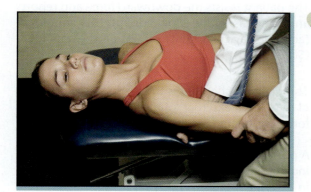

4 The examiner repeats the test in supine with the shoulder in 20 degrees of abduction and in forward flexion while maintaining a neutral rotation.

UTILITY SCORE **3**

Study	Reliability	Sensitivity	Specificity	LR+	LR−	DOR	QUADAS Score (0–14)
Silliman & Hawkins[48]	NT	NT	NT	NA	NA	NA	NA
Nakagawa et al.[42] (Superior Labral Tear)	NT	17	93	2.43	.89	2.73	10

Comments: The sulcus sign is often used clinically but, amazingly, only researched in one study.[42] The use of this sign to detect inferior instability is not supported but the sulcus sign may be a specific test that rules in a superior labral tear when positive.

TESTS FOR A TORN LABRUM/INSTABILITY

Active Compression Test/O'Brien's Test (Labral Tear, SLAP Lesion, Labral Abnormality, Acromioclavicular [AC] Joint Pathology)

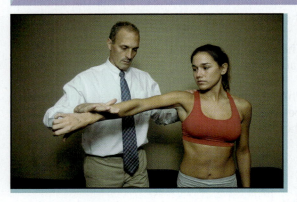

1. The patient is instructed to stand with his or her involved shoulder at 90 degrees of flexion, 10 degrees of horizontal adduction, and maximum internal rotation with the elbow in full extension. The examiner stands directly behind the patient's involved shoulder.

2. The examiner applies a downward force at the wrist of the involved extremity. The patient is instructed to resist the force.

3. The patient resists the downward force and reports any pain as either "on top of the shoulder" (acromioclavicular joint) or "inside the shoulder" (SLAP lesion).

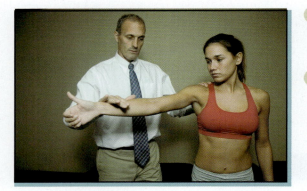

4. The patient's shoulder is then moved to a position of maximum external rotation, and the downward force is repeated.

5. A positive test is indicated by pain or painful clicking in shoulder internal rotation and less or no pain in external rotation.

TESTS FOR A TORN LABRUM/INSTABILITY

UTILITY SCORE **3**

Study	Reliability	Sensitivity	Specificity	LR+	LR−	DOR	QUADAS Score (0–14)
O'Brien[43] (Labral Abnormality, AC Joint Pathology)	NT NT	100 100	99 97	NA NA	NA NA	NA NA	3 3
Guanche & Jones[13] (SLAP, Any Labral Lesion)	NT NT	54 63	47 73	1.01 2.33	.98 .51	1.03 4.57	12 12
Morgan et al.[39] (Anterior Labral, Posterior Labral Tear, Combined [SLAP])	NT	88 32 85	42 13 41	1.52 .37 1.44	.28 5.14 .36	5.43 .07 4.00	11 11 11
Parentis et al.[45] (SLAP)	NT	65	49	1.27	.72	1.76	5
McFarland et al.[35] (SLAP)	NT	47	55	1.04	.96	1.08	11
Stetson & Templin[51] (Labral Tear)	NT	54	31	.78	1.48	.53	10
Myers et al.[41] (SLAP)	NT	78	11	.88	2	.44	8
Walton et al.[53] (AC Joint)	NT	16	90	1.6	0.93	1.72	13
Nakagawa et al.[42] (Superior Labral Tear)	NT	54	60	1.35	.77	1.75	10

Comments: The original optimistic statistical numbers presented by O'Brien et al.[43] were most likely the result of poor study design. Better conducted studies have shown little to no value in the use of the Active Compression Test in diagnosis of either a labral tear or an AC joint problem or, as originally intended, to differentiate a labral tear from an AC joint problem.

TESTS FOR A TORN LABRUM/INSTABILITY

Resisted Supination External Rotation Test (RSERT)

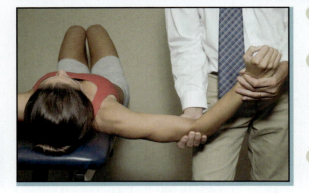

(1) The patient assumes a supine position. The examiner stands beside the patient's involved extremity.

(2) The examiner grasps the patient's hand and supports the elbow. The examiner then places the patient's shoulder in 90 degrees of abduction and neutral rotation, the elbow in 65–70 degrees of flexion, and the forearm in neutral pronation/supination.

(3) The examiner instructs the patient to attempt to supinate his or her arm.

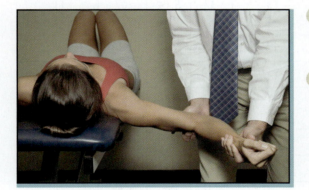

(4) The examiner resists supination while gradually moving the patient's shoulder to end range of external rotation.

(5) A positive test is indicated by the production of pain in the anterior or deep shoulder, clicking or catching in the shoulder, or by reproduction of the patient's concordant symptoms.

UTILITY SCORE **3**

Study	Reliability	Sensitivity	Specificity	LR+	LR−	DOR	QUADAS Score (0–14)
Myers et al.[41] (SLAP)	NT	83	82	4.61	.20	23.05	8

Comments: The RSERT has only a small to moderate effect on the posttest probability of having a SLAP lesion. Additionally, there is only one study (and it involved numerous design and reporting limitations) that looked at this test. More research needs to be performed, especially in light of the quality of this study.

TESTS FOR A TORN LABRUM/INSTABILITY

Compression-Rotation Test (SLAP Lesion)

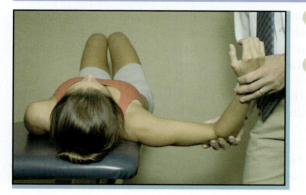

1 The patient assumes a supine position. The examiner stands to the side of the involved extremity.

2 The examiner passively places the patient's shoulder in 90 degrees of abduction and the elbow in 90 degrees of flexion.

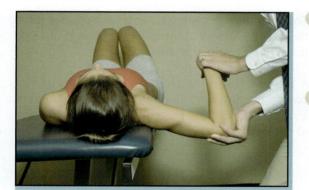

3 The examiner first applies a compression force to the humerus and rotates the humerus back and forth from internal rotation to external rotation in an attempt to pinch the torn labrum.

4 A positive test is indicated by the production of a catching or snapping in the shoulder.

UTILITY SCORE **3**

Study	Reliability	Sensitivity	Specificity	LR+	LR−	DOR	QUADAS Score (0–14)
McFarland et al.[35] (SLAP)	NT	24	76	1.0	1.0	1.0	11

Comments: The Compression-Rotation Test was originally reported by Snyder et al.[49] The one study to examine the Compression-Rotation Test was performed well. There appears to be little use for this test in the clinic to detect SLAP lesions.

TESTS FOR A TORN LABRUM/INSTABILITY

Anterior Slide Test

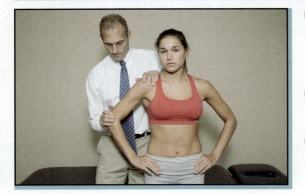

1. The patient is in either standing or sitting with his or her hands on the hips so that the thumb is positioned posteriorly. The examiner stands behind the patient.

2. The examiner places one hand superior on the shoulder to stabilize the scapula and clavicle.

3. The examiner places his or her opposite hand on the patient's elbow with the palm of the hand cupping the olecranon.

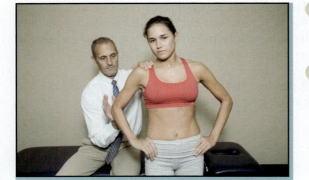

4. The examiner provides an anterior-superior force through the elbow to the glenohumeral joint while the patient resists this movement.

5. A positive test is indicated by the production of pain in the anterior shoulder, by the production of a pop or click in the shoulder, or by reproduction of the patient's concordant symptoms.

UTILITY SCORE **3**

Study	Reliability	Sensitivity	Specificity	LR+	LR−	DOR	QUADAS Score (0–14)
McFarland et al.[35] (SLAP)	NT	8	84	.50	1.10	.45	11
Kibler[25] (SLAP)	NT	78	92	9.75	.24	40.63	6
Parentis et al.[45] (SLAP)	NT	13	84	.79	1.04	.76	5
Nakagawa et al.[42] (Superior Labral Tear)	NT	5	93	.71	1.0	.71	10

Comments: The original author's solid statistical numbers may be the result of poor study design and reporting. The one well-performed study to examine the Anterior Slide Test seems to indicate that there is little use for this test in the clinic to detect SLAP lesions.

TESTS FOR A TORN LABRUM/INSTABILITY

Biceps Load Test (SLAP Lesion with Anterior Shoulder Dislocation)

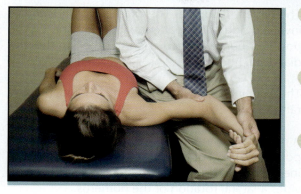

1. The patient assumes a supine position. The examiner sits on the side of the patient's involved extremity.

2. The examiner places the patient's shoulder in 90 degrees of abduction, the elbow in 90 degrees of flexion, and the forearm in supination.

3. The examiner moves the patient's shoulder to end-range external rotation (apprehension position).

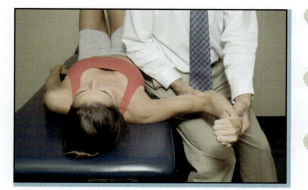

4. At end-range external rotation, the examiner asks the patient to flex his or her elbow while the examiner resists this movement.

5. The examiner queries the patient if and how his or her apprehension has changed after flexion of the elbow.

6. A positive test is indicated by either no change in apprehension or pain that is worsened with resisted elbow flexion.

UTILITY SCORE   3

Study	Reliability	Sensitivity	Specificity	LR+	LR−	DOR	QUADAS Score (0–14)
Kim et al.[28] (SLAP)	κ = .85	91	97	29.32	.09	325.77	9

Comments: The great numbers reported by Kim et al.[28] would seem to warrant a better "Utility Score," but their study had many design faults, including the fact that only patients with repeated anterior dislocations were studied. The fact that all patients had repetitive dislocations may have been a more important predictor of a SLAP lesion than the Biceps Load Test.[28] The authors may have recognized these shortcomings since they developed the Biceps Load II Test.[27]

TESTS FOR A TORN LABRUM/INSTABILITY

Clunk Test (Labral Tear, Superior Labral Tear)

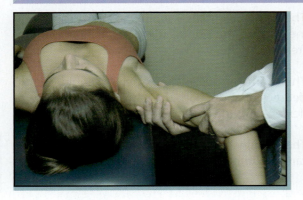

1. The patient is supine. The examiner stands to the involved side of the patient with one hand on the posterior humeral head and the other on the medial distal humerus.

2. The examiner abducts the patient's shoulder to end range.

3. A posterior to anterior force is then applied to the posterior aspect of the humeral head by the examiner's one hand while the hand at the elbow provides a lateral rotation of the humerus.

4. A positive test is indicated by a "clunk" or a grinding.

UTILITY SCORE | **3**

Study	Reliability	Sensitivity	Specificity	LR+	LR−	DOR	QUADAS Score (0–14)
Nakagawa et al.[42] (Superior Labral Tear)	NT	44	68	1.38	.82	1.68	10

Comments: Based on this one study with a limited patient population (52 male, 2 female throwing athletes), this often-used clinical test for labral tear has little merit.

TESTS FOR A TORN LABRUM/INSTABILITY

Biceps Tension Test (Unstable Superior Labrum Lesions/SLAP Lesions)

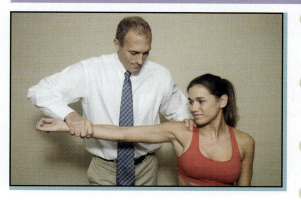

1 The patient assumes a sitting or standing position. The examiner stands in front of the patient (not pictured).

2 The patient places his or her arm in 90 degrees of shoulder abduction, with a fully extended elbow and forearm supinated.

3 The examiner applies a downward-directed force to the distal forearm.

4 A positive test is indicated by patient report of pain.

UTILITY SCORE 3

Study	Reliability	Sensitivity	Specificity	LR+	LR−	DOR	QUADAS Score (0–14)
Field & Savoie[7]	NT	NT	NT	NA	NA	NA	NA
Kim et al[28]	NT	73	78	3.32	.35	9.4	9

Comments: The original description of the test is very limited. The one study to examine this test consisted of patients only with shoulder dislocation. More research needs to be performed to validate this test.

TESTS FOR A TORN LABRUM/INSTABILITY

Hyperabduction Test

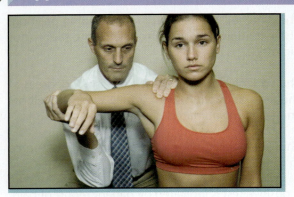

① The patient is seated. The examiner stands behind the patient.

② The examiner stabilizes the scapula with a downward force on the supraclavicular region and passively places the patient's elbow in 90 degrees of flexion and the patient's forearm in pronation.

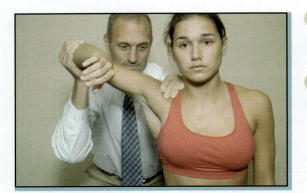

③ The examiner moves the patient's arm to maximum abduction, stabilizing the scapula to reduce rotation.

④ A positive test is indicated by passive abduction greater than 105 degrees.

UTILITY SCORE ?

Study	Reliability	Sensitivity	Specificity	LR+	LR−	DOR	QUADAS Score (0–14)
Gagey & Gagey[8]	NT	NT	NT	NA	NA	NA	NA

Comments: This is a very interesting test studied in cadavers, normal volunteers, and patients undergoing surgery for instability but neither diagnostic accuracy nor reliability was established. The clinician using this test may also find that patients with inferior instability report pain, apprehension, and even symptoms of brachial plexus impingement.

TESTS FOR A TORN LABRUM/INSTABILITY

Anterior Drawer Test (Anterior Laxity)

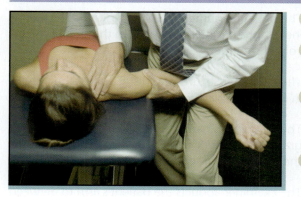

1. The patient assumes a supine position.

2. The examiner secures the distal arm of the patient in his or her axillary region (not pictured).

3. The examiner's hands are placed so that one hand stabilizes the scapula and the other grasps the proximal humerus.

4. The examiner abducts the patient's arm to between 80 and 100 degrees, and then applies a posterior-to-anterior force (traction force) to the humerus. The examiner carefully notes the amount of translation of the glenohumeral joint compared to the uninvolved shoulder.

UTILITY SCORE ?

Study	Reliability	Sensitivity	Specificity	LR+	LR−	DOR	QUADAS Score (0–14)
Gerber & Ganz[9]	NT	NT	NT	NA	NA	NA	NA

Comments: The Anterior Drawer is often used clinically but amazingly has never been researched, perhaps because of the difficulty of establishing a criterion standard for "instability."

TESTS FOR A TORN LABRUM/INSTABILITY

Posterior Drawer Test (Posterior Laxity)

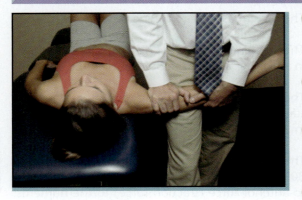

1. The patient assumes a supine position. The examiner stands beside the patient to the side of the involved shoulder.

2. The examiner secures the distal arm of the patient in his or her axillary region.

3. The examiner's hands are placed so that one hand grasps the anterior humerus, while the other grasps the posterior humerus.

4. The examiner abducts the patient's arm to between 80 and 100 degrees, and then applies an anterior-to-posterior force to the humerus. The examiner carefully notes the amount of translation of the glenohumeral joint compared to the uninvolved shoulder.

UTILITY SCORE ?

Study	Reliability	Sensitivity	Specificity	LR+	LR−	DOR	QUADAS Score (0–14)
Gerber & Ganz[9]	NT	NT	NT	NA	NA	NA	NA

Comments: The Posterior Drawer is often used clinically but amazingly has never been researched, perhaps because of the difficulty of establishing a criterion standard for "instability."

TESTS FOR A TORN LABRUM/INSTABILITY

Load and Shift Test (Anterior, Posterior, Inferior Laxity)

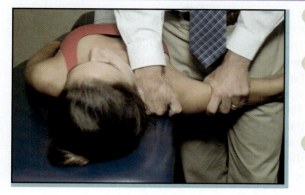

1 The patient assumes a supine position. The examiner stands to the side of the patient's involved shoulder.

2 The examiner grasps the proximal humerus with one hand, providing a compression force and "loading" the humerus into the glenoid fossa. The examiner's other hand stabilizes the scapula.

3 The examiner applies an anterior-to-posterior force, noting the amount of translation as either I (to the posterior rim of the glenoid) or II (beyond the rim of the glenoid).

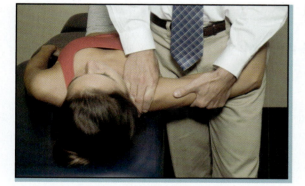

4 The examiner applies a posterior-to-anterior force, noting the amount of translation as either I (to the anterior rim of the glenoid) or II (beyond the rim of the glenoid).

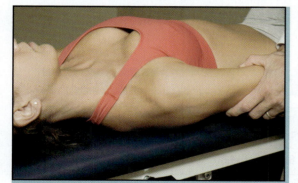

5 A *sulcus sign* (see page 111) is then performed to assess the full excursion of the humeral head in the glenoid fossa.

UTILITY SCORE ?

Study	Reliability	Sensitivity	Specificity	LR+	LR−	DOR	QUADAS Score (0–14)
Silliman & Hawkins[48]	NT	NT	NT	NA	NA	NA	NA

Comments: This test is currently unstudied, even though it has been in use for 15 years.

TESTS FOR ACROMIOCLAVICULAR (AC) JOINT PATHOLOGY

AC Resisted Extension Test (AC Joint Abnormality)

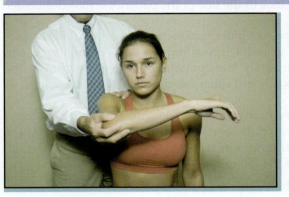

1 The patient is seated with his or her shoulder in 90 degrees of flexion and internal rotation, and his or her elbow in 90 degrees of flexion.

2 The examiner, standing beside the patient, asks the patient to horizontally abduct his or her arm while the examiner provides an isometric resistance to this movement.

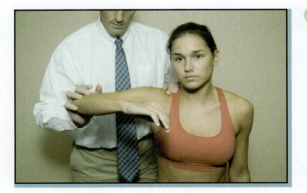

3 A positive test is indicated by pain at the AC joint.

UTILITY SCORE **2**

Study	Reliability	Sensitivity	Specificity	LR+	LR−	DOR	QUADAS Score (0–14)
Chronopoulos et al.[4]	NT	72	85	4.80	0.32	15	10

Comments: This study had some design features, like lack of blinding and not reporting patient inclusion/exclusion criteria, that the examiner should view with caution despite the likelihood ratios indicating that the AC Resisted Extension Test[20] has a moderate effect on the posttest probability of the patient having an AC joint pathology.

TESTS FOR ACROMIOCLAVICULAR (AC) JOINT PATHOLOGY

AC Joint Palpation (AC Joint Pain)

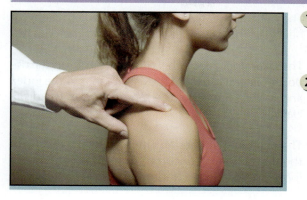

1 The patient is seated with the involved arm at his or her side. The examiner stands behind the patient and palpates the AC joint.

2 Production of the concordant sign is a positive test.

UTILITY SCORE   2

Study	Reliability	Sensitivity	Specificity	LR+	LR−	DOR	QUADAS Score (0–14)
Walton et al.[53]	NT	96	10	1.07	.40	2.68	13

Comments: Based on this one well-performed study, AC joint palpation should not be used as a diagnostic tool but may be a valuable screen as a negative test to rule out the AC joint. More research needs to be performed.

TESTS FOR ACROMIOCLAVICULAR (AC) JOINT PATHOLOGY

Paxinos Sign (AC Joint Pain)

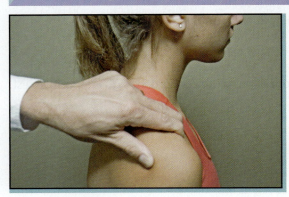

1 The patient is seated with the involved arm at his or her side. The examiner stands behind the patient.

2 The examiner places his or her thumb under the posterolateral aspect of the acromion and the index and middle fingers of the same hand on the distal clavicle.

3 The examiner applies an anterosuperior force with the thumb while concurrently applying an inferior force with the index and middle fingers.

4 A positive test is indicated by pain reproduction or an increase in pain at the AC joint.

UTILITY SCORE 3

Study	Reliability	Sensitivity	Specificity	LR+	LR−	DOR	QUADAS Score (0–14)
Walton et al.[53]	NT	79	50	1.58	0.42	3.76	13

Comments: Based on this one well-performed study, the Paxinos Test/Sign[53] modifies the posttest probability of detecting AC joint pain minimally and should not be used as a diagnostic tool.

TEST FOR AXILLARY NERVE PALSY

Deltoid Extension Lag Sign

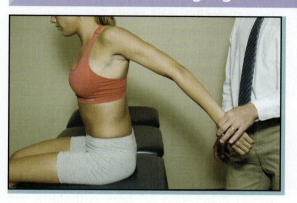

1 The patient is seated. The examiner stands behind the patient.

2 The examiner grasps the patient's wrist and pulls the arm into near full extension.

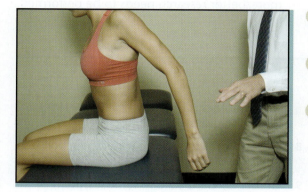

3 The examiner instructs the patient to maintain this arm position, then releases the wrists.

4 The inability to maintain the shoulder extension is considered a positive test.

5 The examiner records any lag to the nearest 5 degrees.

UTILITY SCORE ?

Study	Reliability	Sensitivity	Specificity	LR+	LR−	DOR	QUADAS Score (0–14)
Hertel et al.[17]	NT	NT	NT	NA	NA	NA	NA

Comments: This study was performed with only five male patients after acute traumatic anterior dislocation of the shoulder to monitor recovery of the axillary nerve.

Key Points

1. For rotator cuff tears:
   - The Rent Test, Lift-off Test, Internal Rotation Lag Sign, and External Rotation Lag Sign show promise as diagnostic tools in the clinical examination but more and better-designed research is warranted.
   - The Supine Impingement Test has promise as a screening examination technique where a negative test would rule out a rotator cuff tear.
   - The Drop Sign may have value as a positive test to rule in an infraspinatus tear.

2. Impingement is a broad diagnosis that captures a range of pathologies from subacromial bursitis, to partial rotator cuff tear, to a full thickness rotator cuff tear, making its value as a diagnostic label questionable.

3. There are no clinical examination tests of diagnostic value in patients with impingement.

4. For detecting laxity/instability, only one test, the Anterior Release/Surprise Test, shows some promise but more/better research is required.

5. For SLAP lesions, the Biceps Load Test II is a good diagnostic tool.

6. For posteroinferior labral tears, both the Kim Test and Jerk Test show promise, but more/better research is needed.

7. Pain with palpation is a good screen as a negative test to rule out AC joint pathology.

8. The Resisted Extension Test may be of some use in diagnosing AC joint pathology, but more/better research needs to be performed.

References

1. Bak K, Faunl P. Clinical findings in competitive swimmers with shoulder pain. *Am J Sports Med.* 1997;25:254–260.

2. Bennett WF. Specificity of the Speed's test: arthroscopic technique for evaluating the biceps tendon at the level of the bicipital groove. *Arthroscopy.* 1998;14:789–796.

3. Calis M, Akgun K, Birtane M, Karacan I, Calis H, Tuzun F. Diagnostic values of clinical diagnostic tests in subacromial impingement syndrome. *Ann Rheum Dis.* 2000;59:44–47.

4. Chronopoulos E, Kim TK, Park HB, Ashenbrenner D, McFarland EG. Diagnostic value of physical tests for isolated chronic acromioclavicular lesions. *Am J Sports Med.* 2004;32:655–661.

5. Codman EA. Rupture of the supraspinatus tendon. 1911. *Clin Orthop Relat Res.* 1990:3–26.

6. Crenshaw AH, Kilgore WE. Surgical treatment of bicipital tenosynovitis. *J Bone Joint Surg Am.* 1966;48:1496–1502.

7. Field LD, Savoie FH, 3rd. Arthroscopic suture repair of superior labral detachment lesions of the shoulder. *Am J Sports Med.* 1993;21:783–790; discussion 790.

8. Gagey OJ, Gagey N. The hyperabduction test. *J Bone Joint Surg Br.* 2001;83:69–74.

9. Gerber C, Ganz R. Clinical assessment of instability of the shoulder. With special reference to anterior and posterior drawer tests. *J Bone Joint Surg Br.* 1984;66:551–556.

10. Gerber C, Hersche O, Farron A. Isolated rupture of the subscapularis tendon. *J Bone Joint Surg Am.* 1996;78:1015–1023.

11. Gerber C, Krushell RJ. Isolated rupture of the tendon of the subscapularis muscle. Clinical features in 16 cases. *J Bone Joint Surg Br.* 1991;73:389–394.

12. Gross ML, Distefano MC. Anterior release test. A new test for occult shoulder instability. *Clin Orthop Relat Res.* 1997:105–108.

13. Guanche CA, Jones DC. Clinical testing for tears of the glenoid labrum. *Arthroscopy.* 2003;19:517–523.

14. Hamner DL, Pink MM, Jobe FW. A modification of the relocation test: arthroscopic findings associated with a positive test. *J Shoulder Elbow Surg.* 2000;9:263–267.

15. Hawkins RJ, Kennedy JC. Impingement syndrome in athletes. *Am J Sports Med.* 1980;8:151–158.

16. Hertel R, Ballmer FT, Lombert SM, Gerber C. Lag signs in the diagnosis of rotator cuff rupture. *J Shoulder Elbow Surg.* 1996;5:307–313.

17. Hertel R, Lambert SM, Ballmer FT. The deltoid extension lag sign for diagnosis and grading of axillary nerve palsy. *J Shoulder Elbow Surg.* 1998;7:97–99.

18. Holtby R, Razmjou H. Accuracy of the Speed's and Yergason's tests in detecting biceps pathology and SLAP lesions: comparison with arthroscopic findings. *Arthroscopy.* 2004;20:231–236.

19. Itoi E, Kido T, Sano A, Urayama M, Sato K. Which is more useful, the "full can test" or the "empty can test," in detecting the torn supraspinatus tendon? *Am J Sports Med.* 1999;27:65–68.

20. Jacob AK, Sallay PI. Therapeutic efficacy of corticosteroid injections in the acromioclavicular joint. *Biomed Sci Instrum.* 1997;34:380–385.

21. Jobe FW, Kvitne RS, Giangarra CE. Shoulder pain in the overhand or throwing athlete: the relationship of anterior instability and rotator cuff impingement. *Orthop Rev.* 1989;18:963–975.

22. Jobe FW, Moynes DR. Delineation of diagnostic criteria and a rehabilitation program for rotator cuff injuries. *Am J Sports Med.* 1982;10:336–339.

23. Kelly BT, Kadrmas WR, Speer KP. The manual muscle examination for rotator cuff strength: an electromyographic investigation. *Am J Sports Med.* 1996;24:581–588.

24. Kessel L, Watson M. The painful arc syndrome. Clinical classification as a guide to management. *J Bone Joint Surg Br.* 1977;59:166–172.

25. Kibler WB. Specificity and sensitivity of the anterior slide test in throwing athletes with superior glenoid labral tears. *Arthroscopy.* 1995;11:296–300.

26. Kim KH, Cho JG, Lee KO, et al. Usefulness of physical maneuvers for prevention of vasovagal syncope. *Circ J.* 2005;69:1084–1088.

27. Kim SH, Ha KI, Ahn JH, Kim SH, Choi HJ. Biceps load test II: a clinical test for SLAP lesions of the shoulder. *Arthroscopy.* 2001;17:160–164.

28. Kim SH, Ha KI, Han KY. Biceps load test: a clinical test for superior labrum anterior and posterior lesions in shoulders with recurrent anterior dislocations. *Am J Sports Med.* 1999;27:300–303.

29. Kim SH, Park JS, Jeong WK, Shin SK. The Kim test: a novel test for posteroinferior labral lesion of the shoulder—a comparison to the jerk test. *Am J Sports Med.* 2005;33:1188–1192.

30. Litaker D, Pioro M, El Bilbeisi H, Brems J. Returning to the bedside: using the history and physical examination to identify rotator cuff tears. *J Am Geriatr Soc.* 2000;48:1633–1637.

31. Liu SH, Henry MH, Nuccion SL. A prospective evaluation of a new physical examination in predicting glenoid labral tears. *Am J Sports Med.* 1996;24:721–725.

32. Lo IK, Nonweiler B, Woolfrey M, Litchfield R, Kirkley A. An evaluation of the apprehension, relocation, and surprise tests for anterior shoulder instability. *Am J Sports Med.* 2004;32:301–307.

33. Lyons AR, Tomlinson JE. Clinical diagnosis of tears of the rotator cuff. *J Bone Joint Surg Br.* 1992;74:414–415.

34. MacDonald PB, Clark P, Sutherland K. An analysis of the diagnostic accuracy of the Hawkins and Neer subacromial impingement signs. *J Shoulder Elbow Surg.* 2000;9:299–301.

35. McFarland EG, Kim TK, Savino RM. Clinical assessment of three common tests for superior labral anterior-posterior lesions. *Am J Sports Med.* 2002;30:810–815.

36. McLaughlin H. On the frozen shoulder. *Bull Hosp Joint Dis.* 1951;12:383–393.

37. Meister K, Buckley B, Batts J. The posterior impingement sign: diagnosis of rotator cuff and posterior labral tears secondary to internal impingement in overhand athletes. *Am J Orthop.* 2004;33:412–415.

38. Mimori K, Muneta T, Nakagawa T, Shinomiya K. A new pain provocation test for superior labral tears of the shoulder. *Am J Sports Med.* 1999;27:137–142.

39. Morgan CD, Burkhart SS, Palmeri M, Gillespie M. Type II SLAP lesions: three subtypes and their relationships to superior instability and rotator cuff tears. *Arthroscopy.* 1998;14:553–565.

40. Murrell GA, Walton JR. Diagnosis of rotator cuff tears. *Lancet.* 2001;357:769–770.

41. Myers TH, Zemanovic JR, Andrews JR. The resisted supination external rotation test: a new test for the diagnosis of superior labral anterior posterior lesions. *Am J Sports Med.* 2005;33:1315–1320.

42. Nakagawa S, Yoneda M, Hayashida K, Obata M, Fukushima S, Miyazaki Y. Forced shoulder abduction and elbow flexion test: a new simple clinical test to detect superior labral injury in the throwing shoulder. *Arthroscopy.* 2005;21:1290–1295.

43. O'Brien SJ, Pagnani MJ, Fealy S, McGlynn SR, Wilson JB. The active compression test: a new and effective test for diagnosing labral tears and acromioclavicular joint abnormality. *Am J Sports Med.* 1998;26:610–613.

44. Ostor AJ, Richards CA, Prevost AT, Hazleman BL, Speed CA. Interrater reproducibility of clinical tests for rotator cuff lesions. *Ann Rheum Dis.* 2004;63:1288–1292.

45. Parentis MA, Mohr KJ, ElAttrache NS. Disorders of the superior labrum: review and treatment guidelines. *Clin Orthop Relat Res.* 2002:77–87.

46. Park HB, Yokota A, Gill HS, El Rassi G, McFarland EG. Diagnostic accuracy of clinical tests for the different degrees of subacromial impingement syndrome. *J Bone Joint Surg Am.* 2005;87:1446–1455.

47. Rowe CR, Zarins B. Recurrent transient subluxation of the shoulder. *J Bone Joint Surg Am.* 1981;63:863–872.

48. Silliman JF, Hawkins RJ. Current concepts and recent advances in the athlete's shoulder. *Clin Sports Med.* 1991;10:693–705.

49. Snyder SJ, Karzel RP, Del Pizzo W, Ferkel RD, Friedman MJ. SLAP lesions of the shoulder. *Arthroscopy.* 1990;6:274–279.

50. Speer KP, Hannafin JA, Altchek DW, Warren RF. An evaluation of the shoulder relocation test. *Am J Sports Med.* 1994;22:177–183.

51. Stetson WB, Templin K. The crank test, the O'Brien test, and routine magnetic resonance imaging scans in the diagnosis of labral tears. *Am J Sports Med.* 2002;30:806–809.

52. Walch G, Boulahia A, Calderone S, Robinson AH. The "dropping" and "hornblower's" signs in evaluation of rotator-cuff tears. *J Bone Joint Surg Br.* 1998;80:624–628.

53. Walton J, Mahajan S, Paxinos A, et al. Diagnostic values of tests for acromioclavicular joint pain. *J Bone Joint Surg Am.* 2004;86-A:807–812.

54. Wolf EM, Agrawal V. Transdeltoid palpation (the rent test) in the diagnosis of rotator cuff tears. *J Shoulder Elbow Surg.* 2001;10:470–473.

55. Yergason R. Supination sign. *J Bone Joint Surg.* 1931;13:160–165.

56. Zaslav KR. Internal rotation resistance strength test: a new diagnostic test to differentiate intra-articular pathology from outlet (Neer) impingement syndrome in the shoulder. *J Shoulder Elbow Surg.* 2001;10:23–27.

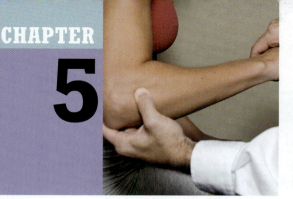

Physical Examination Tests for the Elbow, Wrist, and Hand

SPECIAL TESTS FOR THE ELBOW
TESTS FOR ULNAR NERVE ENTRAPMENT

Elbow Flexion Test (Cubital Tunnel Syndrome)

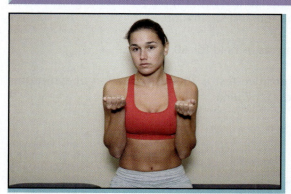

1 Patient is sitting with both arms and shoulders in the anatomic position. Both elbows are fully but not forcibly flexed with full wrist extension.

2 Patients are asked to describe any symptoms following holding this position for 3 minutes.

3 A positive test is the reproduction of pain, tingling, or numbness along the ulnar nerve distribution.

UTILITY SCORE   2

Study	Reliability	Sensitivity	Specificity	LR+	LR−	DOR	QUADAS Score (0–14)
Buehler & Thayer[9]	NT	93	NT	NA	NA	NA	NT
Novak et al.[51]	NT	75	99	75	0.25	297	7

Comments: Buehler & Thayer[9] studied 15 subjects with suspected cubital tunnel syndrome confirmed by NCS without a control group. Novak et al.[51] performed the elbow flexion test without wrist extension and with wrist supination held for 60 seconds.

TESTS FOR ULNAR NERVE ENTRAPMENT

Pressure Provocation Test (Cubital Tunnel Syndrome)

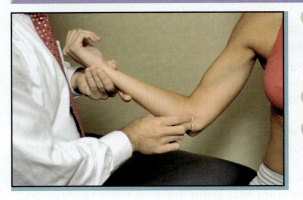

1. The examiner places his or her first and second fingers over the patient's ulnar nerve proximal to the cubital tunnel with the elbow in 20 degrees flexion and forearm supination.

2. The test is held for 60 seconds.

3. A positive test is the reproduction of symptoms along the ulnar nerve.

UTILITY SCORE 2

Study	Reliability	Sensitivity	Specificity	LR+	LR−	DOR	QUADAS Score (0–14)
Novak et al.[51]	NT	.89	98	45	0.11	396	7
Comments: This test should be used with caution secondary to potential bias of the single study.							

TESTS FOR ULNAR NERVE ENTRAPMENT

Percussion Test/Tinel's Sign (Cubital Tunnel Syndrome)

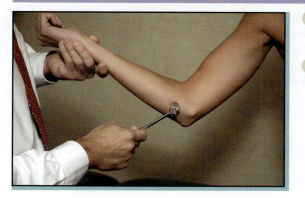

1 The examiner applies four to six taps to the patient's ulnar nerve just proximal to the cubital tunnel.

2 A positive test is the reproduction of symptoms along the ulnar nerve.

UTILITY SCORE 2

Study	Reliability	Sensitivity	Specificity	LR+	LR−	DOR	QUADAS Score (0–14)
Novak et al.[51]	NT	70	98	35	0.31	114	7
Rayan et al.[61]	NT	NT	24	NA	NA	NA	NT
Comments: Rayan et al.[61] observed the presence of a positive elbow percussion test in 48 of 204 asymptomatic elbows.							

TESTS FOR ULNAR NERVE ENTRAPMENT

Elbow Flexion Test (Ulnar Nerve Neuropathy)

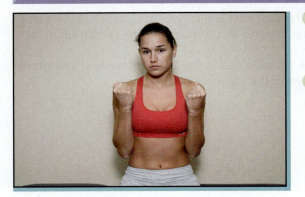

(1) Patient is instructed to fully flex the elbows with the wrists and shoulders in neutral. This position is held for 60 seconds.

(2) Full elbow flexion is maintained for 60 seconds with the shoulders in neutral and wrist in full extension.

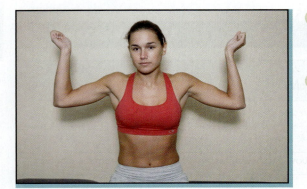

(3) The patient is asked to abduct the shoulders to 90 degrees with the elbows in full flexion and wrist in full extension for 90 seconds.

(4) A positive test is reproduction of ulnar nerve symptoms (paresthesia) along the ulnar nerve distribution.

UTILITY SCORE **?**

Study	Reliability	Sensitivity	Specificity	LR+	LR−	DOR	QUADAS Score (0–14)
Rayan et al.[61]	NT	NT	13	NA	NA	NA	NT

Comments: Rayan et al.[61] studied this test in a population of 204 elbows of patients without upper extremity diagnosis. The study used a combination of four movements: (1) full elbow flexion passively with wrist in neutral was positive in 10%; (2) same test with the wrist in full extension was positive in 7%; (3) same test with the shoulder in 90 degrees of abduction was positive in 11%; (4) same test with the shoulder in 90 degrees of abduction and wrist in full extension was positive in 13%.

TEST FOR ELBOW FRACTURE

Elbow Extension Test

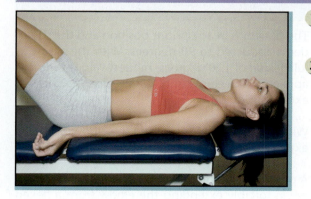

1 Patient lies supine and is asked to fully extend the elbow.

2 A positive test is indicated by the patient's inability to fully extend the elbow.

UTILITY SCORE 2

Study	Reliability	Sensitivity	Specificity	LR+	LR−	DOR	QUADAS Score (0–14)
Docherty et al.[15]	NT	97	69	3.1	0.04	72	10

Comments: This test was designed as a clinical screening test for radiographic evaluation of elbow fractures. A single false positive was present in the Docherty et al.[15] study with the patient being able to fully extend the elbow with radiographic evidence of a nondisplaced radial head fracture.

TESTS FOR ELBOW INSTABILITY

Moving Valgus Stress Test (Chronic Medial Collateral Ligament Tear of the Elbow)

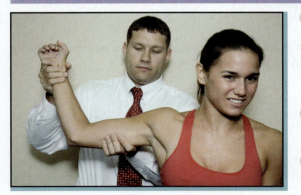

1 The patient is in an upright position and the shoulder is abducted to 90 degrees. With the elbow in full flexion of 120 degrees, modest valgus torque is applied to the elbow until the shoulder reaches full external rotation.

2 With a constant valgus torque the elbow is quickly extended to 30 degrees.

3 A positive test is reproduction of medial elbow pain when forcibly extending the elbow from a flexed position between 120 to 70 degrees.

UTILITY SCORE **2**

Study	Reliability	Sensitivity	Specificity	LR+	LR−	DOR	QUADAS Score (0–14)
O'Driscoll et al.[53]	NT	100	75	4	0	NA	10
Comments: Spectrum bias exists within this study: low study population with 19 of 21 patients being male.							

Posterior Lateral Rotary Instability (Posterior Lateral Instability of the Radius)

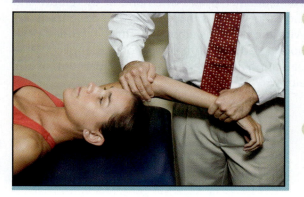

1 The patient lies supine.

2 The examiner flexes the shoulder until the arm is above the patient's head with the elbow in full extension. One hand of the examiner prevents external rotation of the humerus.

3 The examiner's other hand grasps the patient's forearm into full supination.

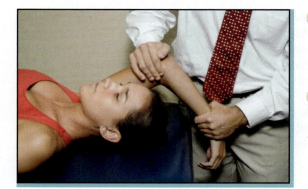

4 The examiner brings the patient's elbow into flexion while applying a supinatory force at the forearm and a valgus stress and axial compression at the elbow.

5 A positive test is posterior lateral displacement or apprehension of the radius followed by reduction of the radius as the elbow approaches 90 degrees.

UTILITY SCORE **?**

Study	Reliability	Sensitivity	Specificity	LR+	LR–	DOR	QUADAS Score (0–14)
O'Driscoll et al.[52]	NT	NT	NT	NA	NA	NA	NT

Comments: O'Driscoll et al.[52] performed this test on a case series of five patients who demonstrated apprehension with testing and posterolateral dislocation of the radial head under anesthesia. All five patients underwent operative restoration to improve functional integrity of the ulnar part of the lateral collateral ligament. Four of the five patients returned to normal function.

TESTS FOR ELBOW INSTABILITY

Varus Stress Test (Integrity of the Lateral Collateral Complex)

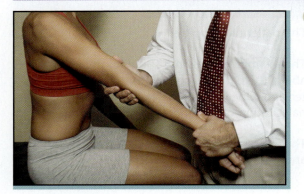

1 The examiner places one hand at the elbow and the other hand is placed over the patient's wrist. With the patient's elbow in a fully extended position, an adduction or varus force is applied while palpating the lateral collateral ligament of the elbow.

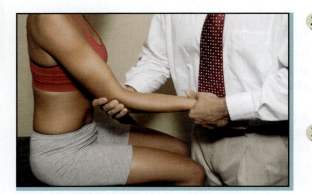

2 The examiner places one hand at the elbow and the other hand is placed over the patient's wrist. With the patient's elbow in 20–30 degrees of flexion, an adduction or varus force is applied while palpating the lateral collateral ligament of the elbow.

3 A positive test is reproduction of distraction pain laterally and compression pain medially at the joint line and laxity with stress.

UTILITY SCORE ?

Study	Reliability	Sensitivity	Specificity	LR+	LR−	DOR	QUADAS Score (0–14)
NA	NT	NT	NT	NA	NA	NA	NT

Comments: No diagnostic accuracy studies have been performed to determine the sensitivity or specificity of the Varus Stress Test of the elbow. Authors have suggested that placing the elbow in a slight degree of flexion will assist in differentiating ligamentous versus bony joint involvement.

Valgus Stress Test

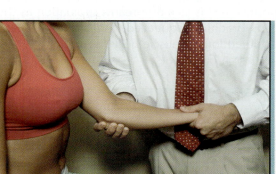

1 The examiner places one hand at the elbow and the other hand is placed over the patient's wrist. With the patient's elbow in a fully extended position, an abduction or valgus force is applied while palpating the medial collateral ligament of the elbow.

2 The examiner places one hand at the elbow and the other hand is placed over the patient's wrist. With the patient's elbow in 20–30 degrees of flexion, an abduction or valgus force is applied while palpating the medial collateral ligament of the elbow.

3 A positive test is reproduction of distraction pain medially and compression pain laterally at the elbow joint line with stress.

UTILITY SCORE ?

Study	Reliability	Sensitivity	Specificity	LR+	LR−	DOR	QUADAS Score (0–14)
NA	NT	NT	NT	NA	NA	NA	NT

Comments: No diagnostic accuracy studies have been performed to determine the sensitivity or specificity of the valgus Stress Test of the elbow. It is suggested that placing the elbow in a slight degree of flexion will assist in differentiating ligamentous versus bony joint involvement.

TEST FOR BICEPS TEAR

Biceps Squeeze Test (Distal Bicep Tendon Rupture)

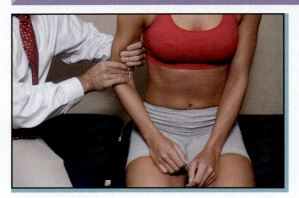

1 Patient is seated and the forearm resting comfortably in the patient's lap with the elbow flexed to approximately 60–80 degrees and forearm in slight pronation.

2 The examiner stands on the affected side and squeezes the biceps firmly with both hands with one hand at the distal myotendinous junction and the other around the belly of the biceps brachii.

3 A positive test is lack of forearm supination as the biceps brachii is squeezed, indicating a biceps brachii tendon or muscle belly rupture.

UTILITY SCORE | **3**

Study	Reliability	Sensitivity	Specificity	LR+	LR−	DOR	QUADAS Score (0–14)
Ruland et al.[63]	NT	96	100	NA	0.04	NA	9

Comment: This study only included 25 male patients referred for suspected biceps tendon rupture. It is unclear regarding the interpretation of the index and reference test without knowledge of results.

TESTS FOR LATERAL EPICONDYLITIS

Cozen's Test

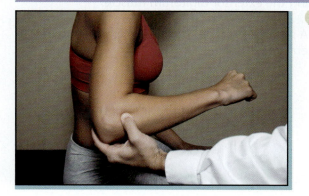

(1) The examiner palpates the lateral epicondyle with his or her thumb. The patient makes a fist with the forearm in pronation and radial deviation of the wrist.

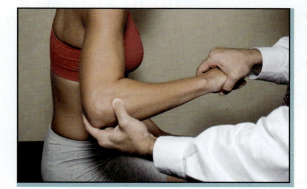

(2) The patient extends the wrist against a force applied by the examiner.

(3) A positive test is reproduction of pain along the lateral epicondyle.

UTILITY SCORE ?

Study	Reliability	Sensitivity	Specificity	LR+	LR−	DOR	QUADAS Score (0–14)
Cozen[13]	NT	NT	NT	NA	NA	NA	NT
Comments: No diagnostic accuracy studies have been performed to determine the sensitivity and specificity of this test.							

TESTS FOR LATERAL EPICONDYLITIS

Lateral Epicondylitis/Maudsley's Test

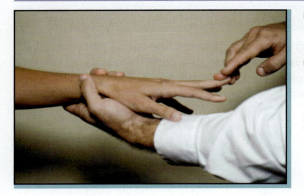

1. The examiner resists third digit extension, stressing the extensor digitorum muscle.

2. A positive test is reproduction of pain along the lateral epicondyle.

UTILITY SCORE ?

Study	Reliability	Sensitivity	Specificity	LR+	LR−	DOR	QUADAS Score (0–14)
NA	NT	NT	NT	NA	NA	NA	NT
Comments: No diagnostic accuracy testing has been performed to determine the sensitivity or specificity of this test.							

Key Points

1. There are few well-designed diagnostic accuracy studies assessing the elbow for pathology.

2. The common diagnostic clinical tests used in clinical practice for the elbow, such as the varus and valgus stress and medial and lateral epicondylitis, have not been studied for diagnostic accuracy.

3. Those tests that have been studied for diagnostic accuracy, such as cubital tunnel syndrome and moving valgus stress testing, demonstrate several procedural biases.

SPECIAL TESTS FOR THE WRIST AND HAND
TEST FOR THUMB INSTABILITY

Gamekeeper's or Skier's Thumb/Ulnar Collateral Ligament (UCL) Test

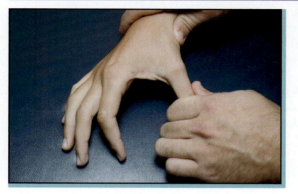

1 The patient sits while the examiner stabilizes the patient's hand with one hand and takes the patient's thumb into extension with the other hand.

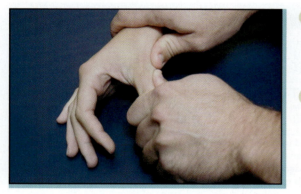

2 While holding the thumb into extension, the examiner applies a valgus stress to the metacarpal-phalangeal joint of thumb to stress the ulnar collateral ligament.

3 A positive test is present if the valgus movement is greater than 30 to 35 degrees, indicating a complete tear of the ulnar collateral ligament and accessory collateral ligaments.

UTILITY SCORE   ?

Study	Reliability	Sensitivity	Specificity	LR+	LR−	DOR	QUADAS Score (0–14)
Heyman et al.[33]	NT	94	NT	NA	NA	NA	NT

Comments: Heyman et al.[33] reported a 100% sensitivity and 46% specificity for detection of a palpable mass proximal to the MCP joint to indicate a complete tear of the UCL of the thumb.

TEST FOR THUMB TENOSYNIVITIS

Finkelstein's Test

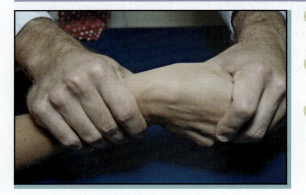

1 The patient makes a fist with the thumb inside the fingers.

2 The examiner stabilizes the forearm and deviates the wrist toward the ulnar side.

3 A positive test is indicated by pain over the abductor pollicis longus and extensor pollicis brevis tendons at the wrist, and is indicative of paratendonitis.

UTILITY SCORE   2

Study	Reliability	Sensitivity	Specificity	LR+	LR−	DOR	QUADAS Score (0–14)
Finkelstein[22]	NT	NT	NT	NA	NA	NA	NT
Alexander et al.[2]	NT	81	50	1.62	0.38	4.26	9

Comments: No diagnostic accuracy studies have been performed in order to determine the sensitivity and specificity of the original Finkelstein Test for de Quevain's syndrome. Alexander et al.[2] performed an extensor pollicis brevis test to determine a septum between the EPB and APL, which led to the diagnosis and surgical intervention for de Quervain's disease. Testing consisted of two parts: the examiner resisted thumb metacarpalphalangeal joint extension, then the examiner resisted thumb palmar abduction. A positive test was if pain was reproduced during resistance of thumb extension greater than abduction. A positive test may indicate a separate compartment for the EPB.

TEST FOR CENTRAL SLIP RUPTURE

Integrity of the Central Slip Test

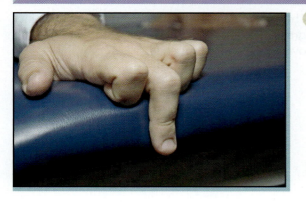

1 The patient flexes the finger to 90 degrees at the proximal interphalangeal joint over the edge of the table.

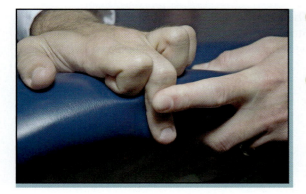

2 The patient is then asked to extend the proximal interphalangeal joint while the examiner palpates the middle phalanx.

3 A positive test is the examiner's feeling of little pressure from the middle phalanx while the distal interphalangeal joint is extending.

UTILITY SCORE ?

Study	Reliability	Sensitivity	Specificity	LR+	LR−	DOR	QUADAS Score (0–14)
Elson[20]	NT	NT	NT	NA	NA	NA	NT
Comments: No diagnostic accuracy studies have been performed to determine sensitivity and specificity of this clinical test.							

TESTS FOR WRIST INSTABILITY

Watson Scaphoid Test (Scaphoid Instability)

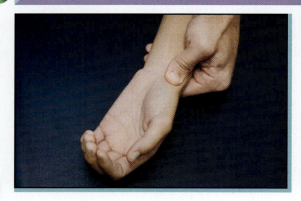

1 The patient's arm is slightly pronated. The examiner grasps the wrist from the radial side with thumb over the scaphoid tubercle.

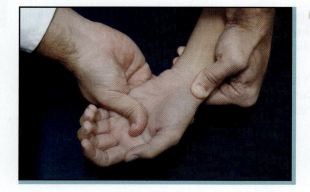

2 The examiner's other hand grasps the metacarpals. Starting in ulnar deviation and slight extension, the wrist is moved into radial deviation and slight flexion.

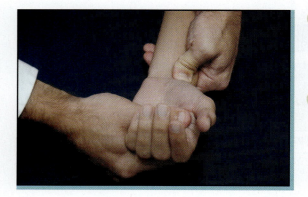

3 The examiner's thumb presses the scaphoid out of normal alignment when laxity exists and when the thumb is released there is a "thunk" as the scaphoid moves back in place.

4 A positive test is identified by subluxation or clunk over the examiner's thumb and patient reports pain.

TESTS FOR WRIST INSTABILITY

UTILITY SCORE 2

Study	Reliability	Sensitivity	Specificity	LR+	LR−	DOR	QUADAS Score (0–14)
LaStayo & Howell[45]	NT	69	66	2.0	0.47	4.3	12

Comments: Easterling & Wolfe[18] demonstrated a 34% prevalence of the painless but positive for laxity Watson tests in a population of 100 uninjured wrists. Lane[44] described a modification of the Watson Test and named this test the Scaphoid Shift Test. The positioning is the same as the Watson Test, however, with the wrist in neutral to slight (0–10) degree of radial deviation and neutral wrist flexion/extension, the examiner quickly pushes the tubercle of the scaphoid in a dorsal direction, noting a clunk, crepitus, or pain in comparison to the opposite wrist.

Ulnomeniscotriquetral Dorsal Glide (TFCC Tear or Triquetral Instability)

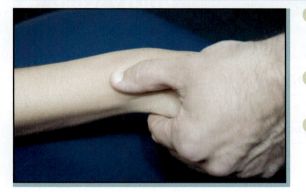

1. The examiner places his or her thumb dorsally over the ulna while placing the PIP of the index finger over the piso-triquetral complex.

2. Produce a dorsal glide of the piso-triquetral complex.

3. A positive test is reproduction of pain or laxity in the ulnomeniscotriquetral region.

UTILITY SCORE 2

Study	Reliability	Sensitivity	Specificity	LR+	LR−	DOR	QUADAS Score (0–14)
LaStayo & Howell[45]	NT	66	64	1.8	0.5	3.4	12

Comments: This test is commonly referred to as the Piano Key Test.

TESTS FOR WRIST INSTABILITY

Ballottement (Reagan's) Test (Lunotriquetral Ligament Integrity)

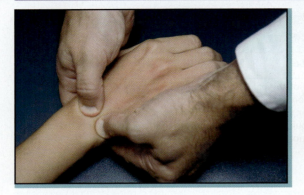

1 The examiner grasps the triquetrum between the thumb and second finger of one hand and the lunate with the thumb and second finger of the other hand.

2 The examiner moves the lunate palmar and dorsal with respect to the triquetrum.

3 A positive test is laxity, crepitus, or reproduction of the patient's pain during anterior posterior movement.

UTILITY SCORE 3

Study	Reliability	Sensitivity	Specificity	LR+	LR−	DOR	QUADAS Score (0–14)
Reagan et al.[62]	NT	NT	NT	NA	NA	NA	NT
LaStayo & Howell[45]	NT	64	44	1.14	0.82	1.40	12
Comments: It is unclear if the index test and reference test was interpreted without knowledge of either result.							

TESTS FOR WRIST INSTABILITY

Wrist-Flexion and Finger-Extension Test (Scapholunate Pathology)

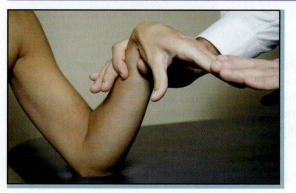

1 The patient is placed in the sitting position with the elbow placed on the table.

2 The examiner holds the patient's wrist in flexion and asks the patient to extend the fingers against resistance.

3 A positive test is identified by pain over the scaphoid.

UTILITY SCORE **?**

Study	Reliability	Sensitivity	Specificity	LR+	LR−	DOR	QUADAS Score (0–14)
Truong et al.[71]	NT	NT	NT	NA	NA	NA	NT

Comments: No diagnostic accuracy studies have been performed to determine the sensitivity and specificity of this particular clinical test. Truong et al.[71] described this test for use in determining scapholunate pathology using a composite of five clinical exam techniques and tests.

Dorsal Capitate Displacement Apprehension Test (To Determine Stability of the Capitate Bone)

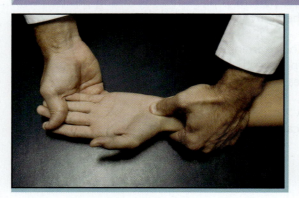

1. The patient sits facing the examiner.

2. The examiner holds the patient's hand with one hand. The thumb of the examiner is placed over the patient's palmer aspect of the capitate while the other hand holds the patient's hand in neutral and applies a counterpressure when the examiner pushes the capitate posterior with the thumb.

3. A positive test is identified by reproduction of the patient's concordant pain or apprehension. A positive test may also be if half of the proximal pole of the capitate is displaced outside of the lunate fossa.

UTILITY SCORE ?

Study	Reliability	Sensitivity	Specificity	LR+	LR−	DOR	QUADAS Score (0–14)
Johnson & Carrera[34]	NT	NT	NT	NA	NA	NA	NT

Comments: No diagnostic accuracy studies have been performed to determine sensitivity and specificity of this particular test in isolation. Truong et al.[71] performed a similar test named the Capitolunate Instability Pattern Wrist Maneuver in order to determine scapholunate instability in a series of tests. However, sensitivity and specificity cannot be calculated from this study. Johnson and Carrera[34] examined 12 patients under fluoroscopic control demonstrating dorsal subluxation of the capitate out of the cup of the lunate. Eleven patients underwent surgical intervention in order to shorten the radio-capitate ligament.

TESTS FOR TRIANGULAR FIBROCARTILAGE COMPLEX

Press Test

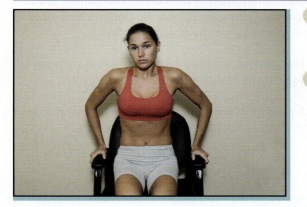

(1) The patient places both hands on the arms of a stable chair and pushes off to suspend the body using only the hands.

(2) A positive test is the reproduction of wrist pain while pressing up the patient's body weight.

UTILITY SCORE ?

Study	Reliability	Sensitivity	Specificity	LR+	LR−	DOR	QUADAS Score (0–14)
Lester et al.[46]	NT	100	NT	NA	NA	NA	NT

Comments: Lester et al.[46] reported 100% sensitivity compared with arthroscopic surgery and a 79% sensitivity compared to MRI arthrogram. Specificity could not be determined based on the methodology of this test design.

TESTS FOR TRIANGULAR FIBROCARTILAGE COMPLEX

Supination Lift Test

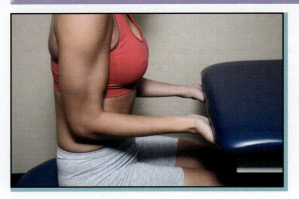

1. The patient is seated with elbows flexed to 90 degrees and forearms supinated. The patient is asked to place the palms flat on the underside of a heavy table or against the examiner's hands.

2. The patient is asked to lift the table or push up against the resisting examiner's hands.

3. A positive test is pain localized to the ulnar side of the wrist or difficulty applying force.

UTILITY SCORE ?

Study	Reliability	Sensitivity	Specificity	LR+	LR−	DOR	QUADAS Score (0–14)
Buterbaugh et al.[11]	NT	NT	NT	NA	NA	NA	NT
Comments: No diagnostic accuracy studies have been performed to determine the sensitivity and specificity of this clinical test.							

TESTS FOR CARPAL TUNNEL SYNDROME

Composite Physical Exam and History

1. Examination by neurologist or standardized questionnaire to gather history of presenting symptoms prior to NCS.

2. A positive test is the ability of a physical exam, history, or questionnaire to predict the diagnosis of CTS in relation to the reference standard of NCS.

UTILITY SCORE 1

Study	Reliability	Sensitivity	Specificity	LR+	LR−	DOR	QUADAS Score (0–14)
*Katz et al.[36]	NT	84	72	3.0	0.2	14	13
*Gunnarsson et al.[29]	NT	94	80	4.7	0.1	63	13
*Bland[5]	NT	79	56	1.8	0.4	4.8	11
*Wainner et al.[73]	NT	18	99	18	0.8	22	12

Comments: No specific detail was given by Katz et al.[36] or Gunnarsson et al.[29] to the content of the physical exam other than an exam by a board-certified neurologist. The Bland[5] study provided a questionnaire, including the Levine Questionnaire and Symptoms Severity Scale, to describe a collection of CTS history symptoms and collect information from patients. Wainner et al.[73] developed a clinical prediction rule including a positive Flick sign, Symptom Severity Scale of greater than 1.9, decreased sensibility testing, age greater than 45, and wrist ratio index greater than 0.67 for the above diagnostic accuracy.

*Indicates those studies using EMG/NCS as inclusion criteria.

Katz Hand Diagram

1 The patient is asked to fill out a diagram using a key of numbness, pain, tingling, and decreased sensation.

2 The Katz Hand Diagram is subdivided into those patients to have "classic," "probable," "possible," and "unlikely" based on completion of the diagram.

UTILITY SCORE 2

Study	Reliability	Sensitivity	Specificity	LR+	LR−	DOR	QUADAS Score (0–14)
*Szabo et al.[69]	NT	76	98	38	0.2	155	9
*Katz et al.[36]	NT	61	71	2.1	0.5	3.8	13
*Katz & Stirrat[37]	NT	80	90	3.6	0.1	65	11
Atroshi et al.[4]	NT	80	90	8.0	0.2	36	8
*Gunnarsson et al.[29]	NT	66	69	2.1	0.5	4.3	13
O'Gradaigh & Merry[54]	NT	72	53	1.5	0.5	2.9	8

Comments: With the exception of reporting intermediate results, the Katz Hand Diagram is an excellent method of collecting patient information with consistent diagnostic accuracy to support its use.

*Indicates those studies using EMG/NCS as inclusion criteria.

TESTS FOR CARPAL TUNNEL SYNDROME

Wrist Ratio Index

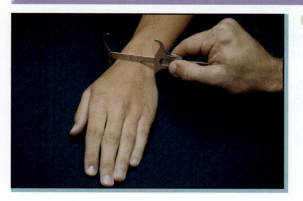

1 Sliding calipers are used to measure the medio-lateral (ML) wrist width in centimeters.

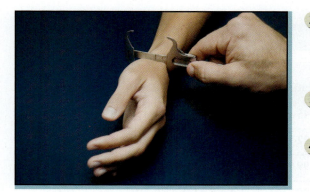

2 Next, sliding calipers are used to measure the anteroposterior height (AP) in centimeters. Caliper jaws are aligned with the distal wrist crease for both measurements.

3 Wrist ratio index is computed by dividing the AP wrist width by the ML wrist width.

4 A positive test is a wrist ratio of greater than 0.67.

UTILITY SCORE 2

Study	Reliability	Sensitivity	Specificity	LR+	LR−	DOR	QUADAS Score (0–14)
*Kuhlman & Hennessey[41]	NT	69	73	2.6	0.4	6.0	10
Radecki[60]	NT	47	83	2.8	0.6	4.3	10
*Wainner et al.[73]	ICC .77 (AP) .86 (ML)	93	26	1.3	0.3	4.7	12

Comments: Wainner et al.[73] used the wrist ratio index as part of the clinical prediction rule to diagnose CTS. As a test in isolation the wrist ratio index does not appear to have strong diagnostic accuracy.

*Indicates those studies using EMG/NCS as inclusion criteria.

TESTS FOR CARPAL TUNNEL SYNDROME

Thenar Atrophy

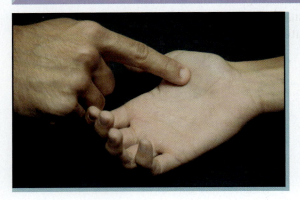

1 The examiner observes the patient's thenar eminence in comparison to the contralateral thenar eminence for signs of atrophy.

2 A positive test is the presence of observable atrophy in the thenar eminence.

UTILITY SCORE **2**

Study	Reliability	Sensitivity	Specificity	LR+	LR−	DOR	QUADAS Score (0–14)
*de Krom et al.[14]	NT	70	45	1.3	0.7	1.9	10
*Gerr & Letz[25]	NT	28	82	1.6	0.9	1.8	12
*Golding et al.[27]	NT	04	99	4.0	1.0	4.1	7
*Katz et al.[36]	NT	14	90	1.4	1.0	1.5	13

Comments: There is little evidence to support the use of thenar atrophy in the diagnosis of CTS. Thenar atrophy is a sign of CTS, however, these patients are generally in the later stages of CTS and have not been part of diagnostic accuracy studies.

*Indicates those studies using EMG/NCS as inclusion criteria.

TESTS FOR CARPAL TUNNEL SYNDROME

Wrist Flexion (Phalen's)

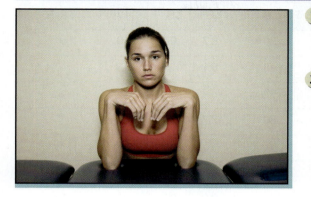

1 The patient is asked to hold the forearms vertically and allow both hands to drop into complete flexion at the wrist for approximately 60 seconds.

2 A positive test is the reproduction of symptoms along the distribution of the median nerve.

UTILITY SCORE 2

Study	Reliability	Sensitivity	Specificity	LR+	LR−	DOR	QUADAS Score (0–14)
Phalen[58]	NT	74	NT	NA	NA	NA	NT
Mossman & Blau[50]	NT	33	NT	NA	NA	NA	6
Seror[64]	NT	62	90?	6.2	0.42	15	6
*Buch-Jaeger & Foucher[8]	NT	58	54	1.3	0.8	1.6	9
*Gerr & Letz[25]	NT	75	33	1.1	0.7	1.5	12
*Heller et al.[32]	NT	67	59	1.6	0.6	2.9	5
*Katz et al.[36]	NT	75	47	1.4	0.5	2.7	13
*Kuhlman & Hennessey[41]	NT	51	76	2.1	0.6	3.3	10
*Golding et al.[27]	NT	10	86	0.7	1.0	.68	7
Burke et al.[10]	NT	49	54	1.1	0.9	1.2	6
Ahn[1]	NT	68	91	7.4	.4	21	8
*Amirfeyz et al.[3]	NT	83	98	41.5	.17	239.2	7
*Hansen et al.[31]	NT	34	74	1.3	0.9	1.5	11
*Tetro et al.[70]	NT	61	83	3.6	0.5	7.6	9

(continued)

TESTS FOR CARPAL TUNNEL SYNDROME

Study	Reliability	Sensitivity	Specificity	LR+	LR−	DOR	QUADAS Score (0–14)
*Gonzalez del Pino et al.[28]	NT	87	90	8.7	0.1	60	10
*de Krom et al.[14]	NT	49	48	0.9	1.1	0.9	10
*Mondelli et al.[49]	NT	59	93	8.4	0.4	19	8
LaJoie et al.[43]	NT	92	88	7.7	0.1	84	5
*Szabo et al.[69]	NT	75	95	15	0.3	57	9
*Gellman et al.[23]	NT	71	80	3.6	0.4	9.8	9
*Fertl et al.[21]	NT	79	92	9.9	0.2	43	13
*Durkan[17]	NT	70	84	4.4	0.4	5.7	7
Borg & Lindblom[7]	NT	83	67	2.5	0.3	9.9	7
Gunnarsson et al.[29]	NT	86	48	1.7	0.3	5.7	13
Williams et al.[77]	NT	88	100	NA	0.12	NA	11
O'Gradaigh & Merry[54]	NT	72	53	1.5	0.5	2.9	8
*Yii & Elliot[78]	NT	87	93	12	0.1	89	8
*Wainner et al.[73]	0.79	77	40	1.29	0.58	2.23	12

Comments: Phalen originally described this test for carpal tunnel syndrome in 1966. Some studies have varied this test to be performed by the patient with wrist in complete flexion and elbow extended, bilateral wrist flexion with the dorsal aspect of the hand pressing against one another, or passive wrist flexion by the examiner. However, there have been no studies to verify these alterations in wrist or elbow movement or studies that compare these alterations for the diagnostic accuracy of CTS.

*Indicates those studies using EMG/NCS as inclusion criteria.

TESTS FOR CARPAL TUNNEL SYNDROME

Flick Maneuver

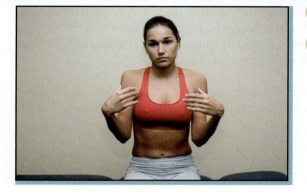

1. The patient vigorously shakes his or her hand(s).

2. A positive test is the resolution of paresthesia symptoms associated with carpal tunnel syndrome during or following administration of "flicking the wrist."

UTILITY SCORE 2

Study	Reliability	Sensitivity	Specificity	LR+	LR−	DOR	QUADAS Score (0–14)
*Hansen et al.[31]	NT	37	74	1.4	0.9	1.7	11
*Pryse-Phillips[59]	NT	93	96	23	0.1	319	6
*de Krom et al.[14]	NT	50	61	1.3	0.8	1.6	10
Gunnarsson et al.[29]	NT	90	30	1.3	0.3	3.9	13

Comments: These studies vary greatly in what constitutes a positive Flick Maneuver in the manner in which the data is collected. Some studies define a flick as a rapid, alternating movement up and down of the wrist whereas others describe a positive flick with as little movement as elbow extension.

*Indicates those studies using EMG/NCS as inclusion criteria.

TESTS FOR CARPAL TUNNEL SYNDROME

Percussion (Tinel's)

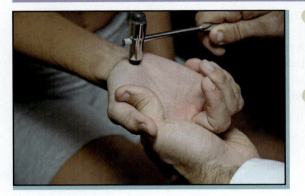

1 The patient's wrist is placed in a neutral position. The examiner use his or her finger or a reflex hammer (pictured) to tap on the median nerve where it enters the carpal tunnel.

2 A positive test reproduces symptoms of paresthesia along the median nerve distribution.

UTILITY SCORE **2**

Study	Reliability	Sensitivity	Specificity	LR+	LR−	DOR	QUADAS Score (0–14)
*Gerr & Letz[25]	NT	25	67	0.7	1.1	0.67	12
Golding et al.[27]	NT	26	80	1.3	0.9	1.4	7
*Heller et al.[32]	NT	60	77	2.7	0.5	5.0	5
*Katz et al.[36]	NT	60	67	1.8	0.6	2.9	13
*Kuhlman & Hennessey[41]	NT	23	87	1.8	0.9	1.9	10
*Buch-Jaeger & Foucher[8]	NT	42	64	1.1	0.9	1.3	9
*Ahn[1]	NT	68	90	6.8	0.4	18.7	8
Amirfeyz et al.[3]	NT	48	94	8.0	0.6	14.5	7
*Hansen et al.[31]	NT	27	91	3.0	0.8	3.7	11
*Tetro et al.[70]	NT	74	91	8.2	0.3	29	9
**Gonzalez del Pino et al.[28]	NT	33	97	11	0.7	16	10
*de Krom et al.[14]	NT	35	53	0.7	1.2	0.6	10
*Mondelli et al.[49]	NT	41	90	4.1	0.7	6.3	8
LaJoie et al.[43]	NT	97	91	11	0.03	327	5

TESTS FOR CARPAL TUNNEL SYNDROME

Study	Reliability	Sensitivity	Specificity	LR+	LR−	DOR	QUADAS Score (0–14)
**Szabo et al.[69]	NT	64	99	64	0.4	176	9
*Gellman et al.[23]	NT	44	94	7.3	0.6	12	9
*MacDermid et al.[47]	0.81	59;41	92;94	7.4/6.8	0.5/0.6	17/11	9
*Seror[65]	NT	63	45	1.1	0.8	1.4	4
*Gunnarsson et al.[29]	NT	62	57	1.4	0.7	2.2	13
*Walters & Rice[74]	NT	64;57	40;31	1.1/0.8	0.9/1.4	1.2/0.6	9
*Durkan[17]	NT	56	80	2.8	0.6	5.1	7
*O'Gradaigh & Merry[54]	NT	55	72	2.0	0.6	3.1	8
Borg & Lindblom[7]	NT	64	62	1.7	0.6	2.9	7
*Gelmers[24]	NT	43	74	1.7	0.8	2.1	10
*Stewart & Eisen[67]	NT	40	71	1.4	0.8	1.6	8
*Mossman & Blau[50]	NT	79	NT	NA	NA	NA	6
Williams et al.[77]	NT	67	100	NA	0.3	NA	11
*Yii & Elliot[78]	NT	42	100	NA	0.6	NA	8
*Wainner et al.[73]	0.47	41	58	0.98	1.01	0.96	12

Comments: Variations exist between studies on the location and number of taps necessary to elicit a positive response. Some studies performed by tapping the median nerve in 20 degrees of extension, others tap along the path of the median nerve up to where the median nerve enters the carpal tunnel. In a few studies the examiners used a reflex hammer to tap rather than the examiner's finger. Gonzalez del Pino et al.[28] and Szabo et al.[69] used surgical outcomes as the reference standard. MacDermid et al.[47] calculated the sensitivity and specificity separately for two testers used in the reliability study. Walters and Rice[74] divided the sensitivity and specificity into groups of those patients with positive NCS for distal sensory latency and distal motor latency, respectfully.

*Indicates those studies using EMG/NCS as inclusion criteria.

Wrist Flexion and Median Nerve Compression

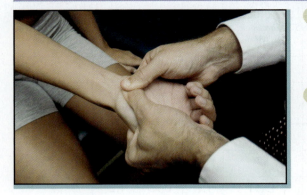

1 The patient sits with elbow fully extended, forearm in supination and wrist flexed to 60 degrees. Even, constant pressure is applied by the examiner over the median nerve at the carpal tunnel.

2 A positive test is the reproduction of symptoms along the median nerve distribution within 30 seconds.

UTILITY SCORE **2**

Study	Reliability	Sensitivity	Specificity	LR+	LR−	DOR	QUADAS Score (0–14)
*Tetro et al.[70]	NT	86	95	17	0.1	117	9
Edwards[19]	NT	62	92	7.8	0.4	19	4

Comments: Tetro et al.[70] originally performed this study to validate a new provocation test, which involved wrist flexion and nerve compression. Edwards[19] studied a population of diabetic patients only without blinding. In addition, he used a reference standard of a questionnaire as inclusion criteria that would not accurately classify the target disorder.

*Indicates those studies using EMG/NCS as inclusion criteria.

TESTS FOR CARPAL TUNNEL SYNDROME

Median Nerve Compression Test/Pressure Provocation Test

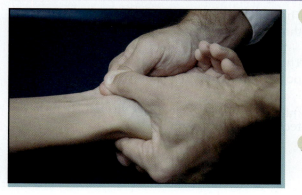

1 The examiner sits opposite the patient and holds the patient's hands with the examiner's thumbs directly over the course of the median nerve as it passes under the flexor retinaculum between the flexor carpi radialis and palmaris longus. The examiner places gentle sustained pressure with the thumbs for 15 seconds to 2 minutes.

2 The pressure of the examiner's thumbs is removed and the examiner questions the patient on the relief of symptoms, which may take a few minutes.

3 A positive test is the reproduction of pain, paresthesia, or numbness distal to the site of compression in the distribution of the median nerve.

UTILITY SCORE 2

Study	Reliability	Sensitivity	Specificity	LR+	LR−	DOR	QUADAS Score (0–14)
Paley & McMurtry[56]	NT	NT	NT	NA	NA	NA	NT
*Williams et al.[77]	.92	100	97	33	0	NA	11
*Mondelli et al.[49]	NT	42	99	42	0.6	72	8
*Kaul et al.[39]	NT	55	68	1.7	0.7	2.6	10
*Yii & Elliot[78]	NT	81	100	NA	0.2	NA	8

Comments: This test differs from the carpal compression test in the location of pressure and in questioning the symptoms following the release of pressure.

*Indicates those studies using EMG/NCS as inclusion criteria.

TESTS FOR CARPAL TUNNEL SYNDROME

▶ Two-Point Discrimination

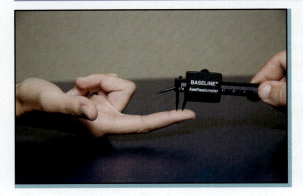

1 The examiner uses a two-point aesthesiometer on the index finger of the patient.

2 The smallest distance perceived as two separate points is recorded in millimeters.

3 A positive test is the inability of the patient to detect a distance of 6 mm or more.

UTILITY SCORE **2**

Study	Reliability	Sensitivity	Specificity	LR+	LR−	DOR	QUADAS Score (0–14)
*Buch-Jaeger & Foucher[8] (Static)	NT	06	99	6	0.9	6.3	9
*Katz et al.[36] (Moving)	NT	32	80	1.6	0.9	1.9	13
*Gerr & Letz[25] (Static)	NT	28	64	0.8	1.1	0.7	12
*Gellman et al.[23] (Static)	NT	33	100	NA	0.7	NA	9
Patel & Bassini[57] (Moving)	NT	30	92	3.8	0.8	4.9	3
*Szabo et al.[68] (Static)	NT	22	NT	NA	NA	NA	NT

Comments: Moving two-point discrimination was performed by Katz et al.[36] with electrocardiograph calipers set at 4 mm apart. The index and fifth finger were stroked five times. A positive test was the inability to identify the number of points on two of the five strokes. Two-point discrimination appears to be a much more specific test that may be useful for ruling in CTS.

*Indicates those studies using EMG/NCS as inclusion criteria.

TESTS FOR CARPAL TUNNEL SYNDROME

Semmes-Weinstein Monofilament Test

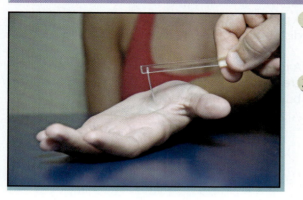

1. The examiner applies the monofilament perpendicular to the palmer digital surface and pressure is increased until the monofilament begins to bend.

2. A positive test is when the patient with eyes closed can verbally report which digit was receiving pressure at 2.83 milligrams.

UTILITY SCORE   2

Study	Reliability	Sensitivity	Specificity	LR+	LR−	DOR	QUADAS Score (0–14)
*Buch-Jaeger & Foucher[8]	NT	59	59	1.4	0.7	2.1	9
*Szabo et al.[69]	NT	65	88	5.4	0.4	14	9
Pagel et al.[55]	NT	98	15	1.2	0.1	8.6	10
*Gellman et al.[23]	NT	91	80	4.6	0.1	40	9
*MacDermid et al.[47]	0.22	86/85	60/32	2.2/1.3	0.2/0.5	9.2/2.7	9
Patel & Bassini[57]	NT	71	40	1.2	0.7	16	3
*Koris et al.[40]	NT	82	86	5.9	0.2	28	11
*Szabo et al.[68]	NT	83	NT	NA	NA	NA	NT
Borg & Lindblom[6]	NT	17	67	0.5	1.2	0.4	7

Comments: Koris et al.[40] assessed sensibility using Semmes-Weinstein Monofilament testing in combination with the wrist flexion test. Szabo et al.[69] also examined the combination of the wrist flexion test and Semmes-Weinstein Monofilament with similar results of sensitivity 83% and specificity 86%. MacDermid et al.[47] reported the diagnostic accuracy of both examiners used for the reliability studies.

*Indicates those studies using EMG/NCS as inclusion criteria.

TESTS FOR CARPAL TUNNEL SYNDROME

Hypoesthesia

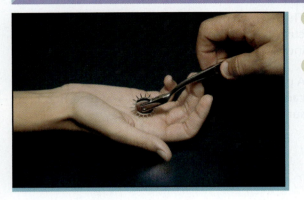

1. A pinwheel is rolled across the patient's hand in the distribution of the median nerve.

2. A positive test is the patient's ability to report a decrease in the ability to detect pain along the distribution of the median nerve.

UTILITY SCORE 2

Study	Reliability	Sensitivity	Specificity	LR+	LR−	DOR	QUADAS Score (0–14)
*de Krom et al.[14]	NT	46	48	0.9	1.1	0.8	10
*Kuhlman & Hennessey[41]	NT	51	85	3.4	0.6	5.9	10
*Golding et al.[27]	NT	15	93	2.1	0.9	2.3	7
Comments: * Indicates those studies using EMG/NCS as inclusion criteria.							

TESTS FOR CARPAL TUNNEL SYNDROME

Therapeutic Ultrasound

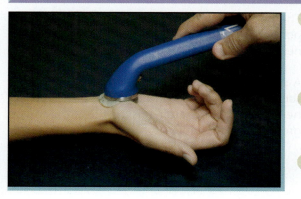

1 The examiner uses a 0.75 cm^2 sound head to apply 1 MHZ therapeutic ultrasound at intensity of 1.0 w/cm^2, 1.5 w/cm^2, and 2.0 w/cm^2 for a duration of 5 minutes.

2 The transducer is passed from the proximal wrist crease a distance of 5 cm distally in line with the ring finger in a slow movement.

3 A positive test is the experience of paresthesia, discomfort, or pain over the carpal tunnel or median nerve distribution.

UTILITY SCORE 2

Study	Reliability	Sensitivity	Specificity	LR+	LR−	DOR	QUADAS Score (0–14)
Molitor[48]	NT	89	94	14	0.11	127	9

Comments: Several biases exist in this study including recruitment bias, as it is unclear how many male and female patients comprised the study group. In addition, the same examiner interpreted the reference and index test. This study has not been replicated for diagnostic accuracy.

*Indicates those studies using EMG/NCS as inclusion criteria.

TESTS FOR CARPAL TUNNEL SYNDROME

Hand Elevation Test

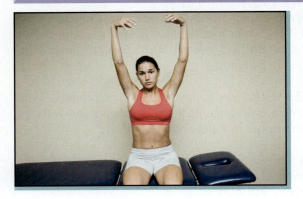

1 The patient raises both hands and maintains the position until the patient feels paresthesia or numbness in the distribution of the median nerve.

2 A positive test is the reproduction of symptoms such as tingling and numbness along the median nerve distribution after raising the arms for no greater than 2 minutes.

UTILITY SCORE 2

Study	Reliability	Sensitivity	Specificity	LR+	LR−	DOR	QUADAS Score (0–14)
*Ahn[1]	NT	76	99	76	.24	314	8
Amirfeyz et al.[3]	NT	88	98	44	.12	359	7

Comments: Although this clinical test has high diagnostic values there are numerous procedural biases in both study designs. The test may be positive in patients with thoracic outlet syndrome.

*Indicates those studies using EMG/NCS as inclusion criteria.

TESTS FOR CARPAL TUNNEL SYNDROME

Carpal Compression Test

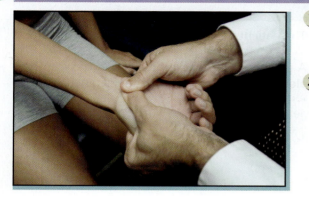

1 The examiner places even pressure with both thumbs directly over the patient's median nerve of the carpal tunnel for 30 seconds.

2 A positive test is the reproduction of pain, paresthesia, or numbness in the distribution of the median nerve distal to the carpal tunnel.

UTILITY SCORE 3

Study	Reliability	Sensitivity	Specificity	LR+	LR−	DOR	QUADAS Score (0–14)
*Kaul et al.[39]	NT	53	62	1.4	0.8	1.8	10
*Buch-Jaeger & Foucher[8]	NT	49	54	1.1	0.9	1.1	9
*Durkan[17]	NT	87	90	8.7	0.1	60	7
*Gonzalez del Pino et al.[28]	NT	87	95	17	0.1	127	10
**Szabo et al.[69]	NT	89	91	9.9	0.1	82	9
*Tetro et al.[70]	NT	82	99	11	0.3	40	9
*Fertl et al.[21]	NT	83	92	10	0.2	56	13
*Kuhlman & Hennessey[41]	NT	28	74	1.1	1.0	1.1	10
*Burke et al.[10]	NT	48	38	0.8	1.4	0.6	6
de Krom et al.[14]	NT	5	94	0.8	1.0	0.8	10
*Durkan[16]	NT	89	96	22	0.1	194	8
*Wainner et al.[72]	NT	36	57	0.8	1.1	0.7	11
*Wainner et al.[73]	0.77	64	30	0.9	1.2	0.8	12

Comments: There are some differences between studies in regard to time held for a positive test. Kuhlman & Hennessey[41] held this pressure for a total of 5 seconds. Tetro et al.[70] found the optimal cutoff to be 20 seconds of sustained pressure. Durkan[17] originally used a gauge to produce pressure over the median nerve at pressures of 11.94 pounds per square inch (psi) and 15.25 psi, which suggested would reproduce symptoms in patients with CTS.

*Indicates those studies using EMG/NCS as inclusion criteria.

Closed Fist/Lumbrical Provocation Test (Carpel Tunnel Syndrome from Lumbrical Excursion)

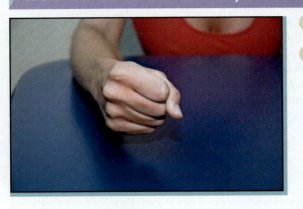

1 The patient is asked to make a fist for 1 minute.

2 A positive test is the reproduction of symptoms along the distribution of the median nerve.

UTILITY SCORE 3

Study	Reliability	Sensitivity	Specificity	LR+	LR−	DOR	QUADAS Score (0–14)
*Karl et al.[35]	NT	37	71	1.3	0.9	1.4	8
*Yii & Elliot[78]	NT	97	93	14	0.03	430	7

Comments: Studies do not indicate the amount of force needed to reproduce the symptoms of CTS during administration of the test. This test is based on the possibility of excursion of the lumbricals into the carpal tunnel, which may increase tunnel pressures.

*Indicates those studies using EMG/NCS as inclusion criteria.

TESTS FOR CARPAL TUNNEL SYNDROME

Wrist Extension (Reverse Phalen's)

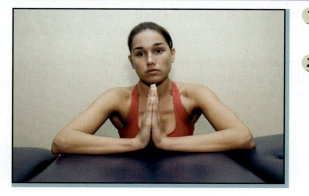

1) The patient is asked to keep both hands with the wrist in complete dorsal extension for 60 seconds.

2) A positive test is the reproduction of numbness or tingling in the distribution of the median nerve within 60 seconds.

UTILITY SCORE 3

Study	Reliability	Sensitivity	Specificity	LR+	LR−	DOR	QUADAS Score (0–14)
*Mondelli et al.[49]	NT	55	96	14	0.5	29	8
*MacDermid et al.[47]	0.72	65/75	96/85	16/5	0.4/0.3	45/17	9
*de Krom et al.[14]	NT	41	55	0.9	1.1	0.8	10

Comments: One of several variations of the original wrist flexion test described by Phalen. MacDermid et al.[47] described the diagnostic accuracy of both examiners used in the reliability study.

*Indicates those studies using EMG/NCS as inclusion criteria.

TESTS FOR CARPAL TUNNEL SYNDROME

▶ Tethered Stress Test

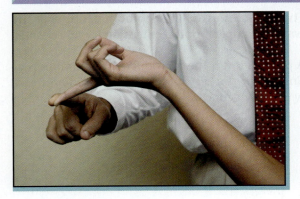

1 The examiner hyperextends the patient's supinated wrist by hyperextending the patient's index finger.

2 A positive test is the reproduction of dysesthesias in the hand with proximal radiation of pain to the volar forearm.

UTILITY SCORE 3

Study	Reliability	Sensitivity	Specificity	LR+	LR−	DOR	QUADAS Score (0–14)
*LaBan et al.[42]	NT	90	NT	NA	NA	NA	NT
*Kaul et al.[38]	NT	50	51	1.0	1.0	1.0	11
*MacDermid et al.[47]	0.49	52/36	92/95	6.5/7.2	0.5/0.7	12/11	9

Comments: LaBan et al.[42] reported that extension of the index finger with a supinated wrist may produce greater excursion of the median nerve and be responsible for the symptoms. MacDermid et al.[47] provided the sensitivity and specificity for both examiners used in the reliability study.

*Indicates those studies using EMG/NCS as inclusion criteria.

TESTS FOR CARPAL TUNNEL SYNDROME

Gilliat Tourniquet Test

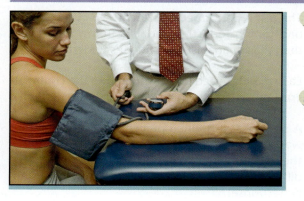

1. The examiner inflates a blood pressure cuff that has been placed over the patient's arm proximal to the elbow to a pressure above the patient's systolic pressure for 60 seconds.

2. A positive test is reproduction of paresthesia or numbness in the thumb or the index finger.

UTILITY SCORE 3

Study	Reliability	Sensitivity	Specificity	LR+	LR−	DOR	QUADAS Score (0–14)
*Buch-Jaeger & Foucher[8]	NT	52	36	0.8	1.3	0.6	9
*Golding et al.[27]	NT	21	87	1.6	0.9	1.8	7
*de Krom et al.[14]	NT	44	62	1.2	0.9	1.3	10
*Gellman et al.[23]	NT	65	60	1.6	0.6	2.8	9

Comments: There is little diagnostic accuracy to support the use of this particular test.
*Indicates those studies using EMG/NCS as inclusion criteria.

TESTS FOR CARPAL TUNNEL SYNDROME

Abnormal Vibration

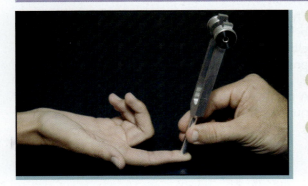

(1) The test is performed utilizing a 256-cycle per second tuning fork struck against a firm object and then placed against the patient's fingertip.

(2) Each digit is tested and compared to the contralateral limb.

(3) A positive test is when perception to the stimulus was considered altered when the patient stated that the two stimuli felt different and could qualify the difference as being lesser or greater or some similar response.

UTILITY SCORE 3

Study	Reliability	Sensitivity	Specificity	LR+	LR−	DOR	QUADAS Score (0–14)
*Buch-Jaeger & Foucher[8]	NT	20	81	1.1	1.0	1.1	9
*MacDermid et al.[47]	0.71	77	80/72	3.9/2.8	0.3/0.3	13/8.6	9
*Szabo et al.[69]	NT	87	NT	NA	NA	NA	NT
*Spindler & Dellon[66]	NT	78	NT	NA	NA	NA	NT
*Cherniack et al.[12]	NT	21	85	1.4	0.9	1.5	10
*Borg & Lindblom[6]	NT	52	NT	NA	NA	NA	NT
*Werner et al.[76]	NT	4	25	1	3.8	0.01	13
*Werner et al.[75]	NT	61	56	1.4	0.7	2.0	13
Gerr et al.[26]	NT	61	80	3.1	0.5	6.3	12
*Gerr & Letz[25]	NT	35	83	2.1	0.8	2.6	12

Comments: MacDermid et al.[47] calculated the sensitivity and specificity of both examiners used in determining the reliability. Werner et al.[75,76] used an electronic vibrometer in both studies in order to determine tolerance to vibration.

*Indicates those studies using EMG/NCS as inclusion criteria.

TESTS FOR CARPAL TUNNEL SYNDROME

Abductor Pollicis Brevis Weakness

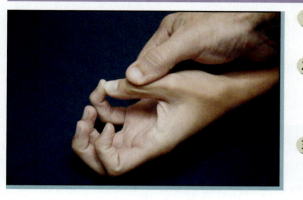

1 The examiner instructs the patient to touch the pads of the thumb and small finger together.

2 The examiner applies a strong force in order to resist thumb abduction and instructs the patient to keep the pads of the thumb and small finger together.

3 A positive test is weakness in thumb abduction with resisted testing.

UTILITY SCORE **3**

Study	Reliability	Sensitivity	Specificity	LR+	LR−	DOR	QUADAS Score (0–14)
*de Krom et al.[14]	NT	63	41	1.1	0.9	1.2	10
*Gerr & Letz[25]	NT	63	62	1.7	0.6	2.8	12
*Kuhlman & Hennessey[41]	NT	66	66	2.0	0.5	3.8	10

Comments: Studies performed to determine weakness in the abductor pollicis brevis are relatively consistent, demonstrating moderate diagnostic accuracy.

*Indicates those studies using EMG/NCS as inclusion criteria.

TESTS FOR CARPAL TUNNEL SYNDROME

Nocturnal Parasthesia

1 The patient is asked if he or she experiences paresthesia, which awakens him or her at night.

2 A positive test is the report of paresthesia along the median nerve distribution that awakens the patient at night from sleep.

UTILITY SCORE 3

Study	Reliability	Sensitivity	Specificity	LR+	LR−	DOR	QUADAS Score (0–14)
*Szabo et al.[69]	NT	96	100	NA	0.04	NA	9
*Buch-Jaeger & Foucher[8]	NT	51	68	1.6	0.7	2.2	9
*Katz et al.[36]	NT	77	27	1.1	0.9	1.2	13
Gupta & Benstead[30]	NT	84	33	1.3	0.5	2.6	11

Comments: Gupta & Benstead[30] reported nocturnal pain rather than paresthesia, which was a sensitive test. Interestingly, the study design of those patients with "exclusive" carpal tunnel only reported nocturnal pain and no patients reported daytime pain. Although this is considered a classic symptom of CTS in isolation, it does appear to have significant diagnostic accuracy.

*Indicates those studies using EMG/NCS as inclusion criteria.

Subjective Swelling

1 The patient is asked by the examiner if there is a feeling of swelling in the region of the carpal tunnel.

2 A positive test is the patient reporting symptoms of swelling in the region of the carpal tunnel.

UTILITY SCORE 3

Study	Reliability	Sensitivity	Specificity	LR+	LR−	DOR	QUADAS Score (0–14)
Burke et al.[10]	NT	49	32	0.8	1.3	0.6	6

Comments: No studies have been performed to replicate this clinical diagnostic test.

Key Points

1. Carpal tunnel syndrome has numerous diagnostic accuracy studies in part due to the high incidence and prevalence in the general and industrial population.

2. Very few clinical tests for the wrist and hand have been assessed for reliability.

3. A gap in the literature of diagnostic accuracy appears to be the low number of studies to determine diagnostic accuracy of clinical testing of wrist instability.

4. There exists a significant range of sensitivity and specificity with traditional testing of CTS, which may be indicative of procedural biases that are present.

5. A true reference standard for classifying CTS does not exist. Nerve conduction studies are considered the reference standard for having a moderate sensitivity. However, studies have demonstrated as much as 18% of the control group having positive NCS.

References

1. Ahn DS. Hand elevation: a new test for carpal tunnel syndrome. *Ann Plast Surg.* 2001;46: 120–124.

2. Alexander RD, Catalano LW, Barron OA, Glickel SZ. The extensor pollicis brevis entrapment test in the treatment of de Quervain's disease. *J Hand Surg [Am].* 2002;27:813–816.

3. Amirfeyz R, Gozzard C, Leslie IJ. Hand elevation test for assessment of carpal tunnel syndrome. *J Hand Surg [Br].* 2005;30:361–364.

4. Atroshi I, Breidenbach WC, McCabe SJ. Assessment of the carpal tunnel outcome instrument in patients with nerve-compression symptoms. *J Hand Surg [Am].* 1997;22:222–227.

5. Bland JD. The value of the history in the diagnosis of carpal tunnel syndrome. *J Hand Surg [Br].* 2000;25:445–450.

6. Borg K, Lindblom U. Diagnostic value of quantitative sensory testing (QST) in carpal tunnel syndrome. *Acta Neurol Scand.* 1988;78: 537–541.

7. Borg K, Lindblom U. Increase of vibration threshold during wrist flexion in patients with carpal tunnel syndrome. *Pain.* 1986;26:211–219.

8. Buch-Jaeger N, Foucher G. Correlation of clinical signs with nerve conduction tests in the diagnosis of carpal tunnel syndrome. *J Hand Surg [Br].* 1994;19:720–724.

9. Buehler MJ, Thayer DT. The elbow flexion test. A clinical test for the cubital tunnel syndrome. *Clin Orthop Relat Res.* 1988:213–216.

10. Burke DT, Burke MA, Bell R, Stewart GW, Mehdi RS, Kim HJ. Subjective swelling: a new sign for carpal tunnel syndrome. *Am J Phys Med Rehabil.* 1999;78:504–508.

11. Buterbaugh GA, Brown TR, Horn PC. Ulnar-sided wrist pain in athletes. *Clin Sports Med.* 1998;17:567–583.

12. Cherniack MG, Moalli D, Viscolli C. A comparison of traditional electrodiagnostic studies, electroneurometry, and vibrometry in the diagnosis of carpal tunnel syndrome. *J Hand Surg [Am].* 1996;21:122–131.

13. Cozen L. The painful elbow. *Ind Med Surg.* 1962;31:369–371.

14. de Krom MC, Knipschild PG, Kester AD, Spaans F. Efficacy of provocative tests for diagnosis of carpal tunnel syndrome. *Lancet.* 1990;335:393–395.

15. Docherty MA, Schwab RA, Ma OJ. Can elbow extension be used as a test of clinically significant injury? *South Med J.* 2002;95:539–541.

16. Durkan JA. The carpal-compression test: an instrumented device for diagnosing carpal tunnel syndrome. *Orthop Rev.* 1994;23:522–525.

17. Durkan JA. A new diagnostic test for carpal tunnel syndrome. *J Bone Joint Surg Am.* 1991; 73:535–538.

18. Easterling KJ, Wolfe SW. Scaphoid shift in the uninjured wrist. *J Hand Surg [Am].* 1994;19: 604–606.

19. Edwards A. Phalen's test with carpal compression: testing in diabetics for the diagnosis of carpal tunnel syndrome. *Orthopedics.* 2002;25: 519–520.

20. Elson RA. Rupture of the central slip of the extensor hood of the finger: a test for early diagnosis. *J Bone Joint Surg Br.* 1986;68:229–231.

21. Fertl E, Wober C, Zeitlhofer J. The serial use of two provocative tests in the clinical diagnosis of carpal tunnel syndrome. *Acta Neurol Scand.* 1998;98:328–332.

22. Finkelstein H. Stenosing tenovaginitis at the radial styloid process. *J Bone Joint Surg* 1930; 12:9–540.

23. Gellman H, Gelberman RH, Tan AM, Botte MJ. Carpal tunnel syndrome: an evaluation of the provocative diagnostic tests. *J Bone Joint Surg Am.* 1986;68:735–737.

24. Gelmers HJ. The significance of Tinel's sign in the diagnosis of carpal tunnel syndrome. *Acta Neurochir (Wien).* 1979;49:255–258.

25. Gerr F, Letz R. The sensitivity and specificity of tests for carpal tunnel syndrome vary with the comparison subjects. *J Hand Surg [Br].* 1998; 23:151–155.

26. Gerr F, Letz R, Harris-Abbott D, Hopkins LC. Sensitivity and specificity of vibrometry for detection of carpal tunnel syndrome. *J Occup Environ Med.* 1995;37:1108–1115.

27. Golding DN, Rose DM, Selvarajah K. Clinical tests for carpal tunnel syndrome: an evaluation. *Br J Rheumatol.* 1986;25:388–390.

28. Gonzalez del Pino J, Delgado-Martinez AD, Gonzalez I, Lovic A. Value of the carpal compression test in the diagnosis of carpal tunnel syndrome. *J Hand Surg [Br].* 1997;22:38–41.

29. Gunnarsson LG, Amilon A, Hellstrand P, Leissner P, Philipson L. The diagnosis of carpal tunnel syndrome: sensitivity and specificity of some clinical and electrophysiological tests. *J Hand Surg [Br].* 1997;22:34–37.

30. Gupta SK, Benstead TJ. Symptoms experienced by patients with carpal tunnel syndrome. *Can J Neurol Sci.* 1997;24:338–342.

31. Hansen PA, Micklesen P, Robinson LR. Clinical utility of the flick maneuver in diagnosing carpal tunnel syndrome. *Am J Phys Med Rehabil.* 2004;83:363–367.

32. Heller L, Ring H, Costeff H, Solzi P. Evaluation of Tinel's and Phalen's signs in diagnosis of the carpal tunnel syndrome. *Eur Neurol.* 1986;25: 40–42.

33. Heyman P, Gelberman RH, Duncan K, Hipp JA. Injuries of the ulnar collateral ligament of the thumb metacarpalphalangeal joint. Biomechanical and prospective clinical studies on the usefulness of valgus stress testing. *Clin Orthop Relat Res.* 1993:165–171.

34. Johnson RP, Carrera GF. Chronic capitolunate instability. *J Bone Joint Surg Am.* 1986;68: 1164–1176.

35. Karl AI, Carney ML, Kaul MP. The lumbrical provocation test in subjects with median inclusive paresthesia. *Arch Phys Med Rehabil.* 2001;82:935–937.

36. Katz JN, Larson MG, Sabra A, et al. The carpal tunnel syndrome: diagnostic utility of the history and physical examination findings. *Ann Intern Med.* 1990;112:321–327.

37. Katz JN, Stirrat CR. A self-administered hand diagram for the diagnosis of carpal tunnel syndrome. *J Hand Surg [Am].* 1990;15:360–363.

38. Kaul MP, Pagel KJ, Dryden JD. Lack of predictive power of the "tethered" median stress test in suspected carpal tunnel syndrome. *Arch Phys Med Rehabil.* 2000;81:348–350.

39. Kaul MP, Pagel KJ, Wheatley MJ, Dryden JD. Carpal compression test and pressure provocative test in veterans with median-distribution paresthesias. *Muscle Nerve.* 2001;24:107–111.

40. Koris M, Gelberman RH, Duncan K, Boublick M, Smith B. Carpal tunnel syndrome. Evaluation of a quantitative provocational diagnostic test. *Clin Orthop Relat Res.* 1990:157–161.

41. Kuhlman KA, Hennessey WJ. Sensitivity and specificity of carpal tunnel syndrome signs. *Am J Phys Med Rehabil.* 1997;76:451–457.

42. LaBan MM, Friedman NA, Zemenick GA. "Tethered" median nerve stress test in chronic carpal tunnel syndrome. *Arch Phys Med Rehabil.* 1986;67:803–804.

43. LaJoie AS, McCabe SJ, Thomas B, Edgell SE. Determining the sensitivity and specificity of common diagnostic tests for carpal tunnel syndrome using latent class analysis. *Plast Reconstr Surg.* 2005;116:502–507.

44. Lane LB. The scaphoid shift test. *J Hand Surg [Am].* 1993;18:366–368.

45. LaStayo P, Howell J. Clinical provocative tests used in evaluating wrist pain: a descriptive study. *J Hand Ther.* 1995;8:10–17.

46. Lester B, Halbrecht J, Levy IM, Gaudinez R. "Press test" for office diagnosis of triangular fibrocartilage complex tears of the wrist. *Ann Plast Surg.* 1995;35:41–45.

47. MacDermid JC, Kramer JF, Roth JH. Decision making in detecting abnormal Semmes-Weinstein monofilament thresholds in carpal tunnel syndrome. *J Hand Ther.* 1994;7:158–162.

48. Molitor PJ. A diagnostic test for carpal tunnel syndrome using ultrasound. *J Hand Surg [Br].* 1988;13:40–41.

49. Mondelli M, Passero S, Giannini F. Provocative tests in different stages of carpal tunnel syndrome. *Clin Neurol Neurosurg.* 2001;103:178–183.

50. Mossman SS, Blau JN. Tinel's sign and the carpal tunnel syndrome. *Br Med J (Clin Res Ed).* 1987;294:680.

51. Novak CB, Lee GW, Mackinnon SE, Lay L. Provocative testing for cubital tunnel syndrome. *J Hand Surg [Am].* 1994;19:817–820.

52. O'Driscoll SW, Bell DF, Morrey BF. Posterolateral rotatory instability of the elbow. *J Bone Joint Surg Am.* 1991;73:440–446.

53. O'Driscoll SW, Lawton RL, Smith AM. The "moving valgus stress test" for medial collateral ligament tears of the elbow. *Am J Sports Med.* 2005;33:231–239.

54. O'Gradaigh D, Merry P. A diagnostic algorithm for carpal tunnel syndrome based on Bayes's theorem. *Rheumatology (Oxford).* 2000;39:1040–1041.

55. Pagel KJ, Kaul MP, Dryden JD. Lack of utility of Semmes-Weinstein monofilament testing in suspected carpal tunnel syndrome. *Am J Phys Med Rehabil.* 2002;81:597–600.

56. Paley D, McMurtry R. Median nerve compression test in carpal tunnel syndrome diagnosis: reproduces signs and symptoms in affected wrist. *Orthop Rev.* 1985;14:41–45.

57. Patel MR, Bassini L. A comparison of five tests for determining hand sensibility. *J Reconstr Microsurg.* 1999;15:523–526.

58. Phalen GS. The carpal-tunnel syndrome: seventeen years' experience in diagnosis and treatment of six hundred fifty-four hands. *J Bone Joint Surg Am.* 1966;48:211–228.

59. Pryse-Phillips WE. Validation of a diagnostic sign in carpal tunnel syndrome. *J Neurol Neurosurg Psychiatry.* 1984;47:870–872.

60. Radecki P. A gender specific wrist ratio and the likelihood of a median nerve abnormality at the carpal tunnel. *Am J Phys Med Rehabil.* 1994;73:157–162.

61. Rayan GM, Jensen C, Duke J. Elbow flexion test in the normal population. *J Hand Surg [Am].* 1992;17:86–89.

62. Reagan DS, Linscheid RL, Dobyns JH. Lunotriquetral sprains. *J Hand Surg [Am].* 1984;9:502–514.

63. Ruland RT, Dunbar RP, Bowen JD. The Biceps squeeze test for diagnosis of distal Biceps tendon ruptures. *Clin Orthop Relat Res.* 2005:128–131.

64. Seror P. Phalen's test in the diagnosis of carpal tunnel syndrome. *J Hand Surg [Br].* 1988;13:383–385.

65. Seror P. Tinel's sign in the diagnosis of carpal tunnel syndrome. *J Hand Surg [Br].* 1987;12:364–365.

66. Spindler HA, Dellon AL. Nerve conduction studies and sensibility testing in carpal tunnel syndrome. *J Hand Surg [Am].* 1982;7:260–263.

67. Stewart JD, Eisen A. Tinel's sign and the carpal tunnel syndrome. *Br Med J.* 1978;2:1125–1126.

68. Szabo RM, Gelberman RH, Dimick MP. Sensibility testing in patients with carpal tunnel syndrome. *J Bone Joint Surg Am.* 1984;66:60–64.

69. Szabo RM, Slater RR, Jr., Farver TB, Stanton DB, Sharman WK. The value of diagnostic testing in carpal tunnel syndrome. *J Hand Surg [Am].* 1999;24:704–714.

70. Tetro AM, Evanoff BA, Hollstien SB, Gelberman RH. A new provocative test for carpal tunnel syndrome: assessment of wrist flexion and nerve compression. *J Bone Joint Surg Br.* 1998; 80:493–498.

71. Truong NP, Mann FA, Gilula LA, Kang SW. Wrist instability series: increased yield with clinical-radiologic screening criteria. *Radiology.* 1994;192:481–484.

72. Wainner RS, Boninger ML, Balu G, Burdett R, Helkowski W. Durkan gauge and carpal compression test: accuracy and diagnostic test properties. *J Orthop Sports Phys Ther.* 2000; 30:676–682.

73. Wainner RS, Fritz JM, Irrgang JJ, Delitto A, Allison S, Boninger ML. Development of a clinical prediction rule for the diagnosis of carpal tunnel syndrome. *Arch Phys Med Rehabil.* 2005; 86:609–618.

74. Walters C, Rice V. An evaluation of provocative testing in the diagnosis of carpal tunnel syndrome. *Mil Med.* 2002;167:647–652.

75. Werner RA, Franzblau A, Johnston E. Comparison of multiple frequency vibrometry testing and sensory nerve conduction measures in screening for carpal tunnel syndrome in an industrial setting. *Am J Phys Med Rehabil.* 1995; 74:101–106.

76. Werner RA, Franzblau A, Johnston E. Quantitative vibrometry and electrophysiological assessment in screening for carpal tunnel syndrome among industrial workers: a comparison. *Arch Phys Med Rehabil.* 1994;75:1228–1232.

77. Williams TM, Mackinnon SE, Novak CB, McCabe S, Kelly L. Verification of the pressure provocative test in carpal tunnel syndrome. *Ann Plast Surg.* 1992;29:8–11.

78. Yii NW, Elliot D. A study of the dynamic relationship of the lumbrical muscles and the carpal tunnel. *J Hand Surg [Br].* 1994;19:439–443.

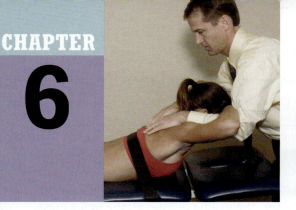

Physical Examination Tests for the Thoracic Spine

TESTS FOR THORACIC OUTLET SYNDROME

Hyperabduction Test

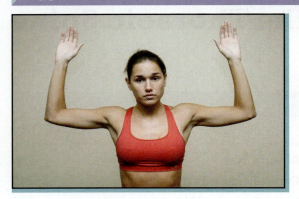

1 The patient sits very straight. Both arms are placed at the sides. The examiner assesses the radial pulse in this position.

2 The patient is instructed to place the arms above 90 degrees of abduction and in full external rotation. The head maintains a neutral position. The arms are held in this position for a full minute.

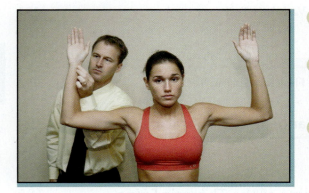

3 The examiner palpates the radial pulse in the hyperabducted position.

4 The radial pulse is recorded as no change, diminished or occluded. The patient is also queried for paresthesia.

5 A positive test is change in radial pulse and patient report of paresthesia.

TESTS FOR THORACIC OUTLET SYNDROME

UTILITY SCORE **2**

Study	Reliability	Sensitivity	Specificity	LR+	LR−	DOR	QUADAS Score (0–14)
Rayan & Jensen[8] (Vascular Changes)	NT	NT	43	NA	NA	NA	3
Rayan & Jensen[8] (Paresthesia)	NT	NT	90	NA	NA	NA	3
Plewa & Delinger[7] (Vascular Changes)	NT	NT	38	NA	NA	NA	9
Plewa & Delinger[7] (Pain)	NT	NT	79	NA	NA	NA	9
Plewa & Delinger[7] (Paresthesia)	NT	NT	64	NA	NA	NA	9

Comments: The test is also known as the elevated arm stress test (ESRT). Some texts have promoted the use of 2-minute holds. Because thoracic outlet syndrome is a controversial diagnosis, most tests examine specificity only.

Roos Test

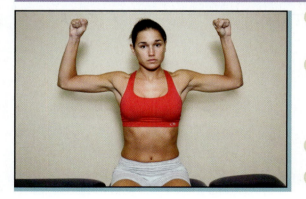

1. The patient sits straight with the arms at the side of his or her body.

2. The patient is instructed to abduct his or her arms and externally rotate to 90 degrees. The patient is then instructed to rapidly open and close his or her hands.

3. The activity is performed for a full minute.

4. A positive test is reproduction of concordant symptoms during opening and closing the fists.

UTILITY SCORE **2**

Study	Reliability	Sensitivity	Specificity	LR+	LR−	DOR	QUADAS Score (0–14)
Howard et al.[2]	NT	82	100	NA	NA	NA	5

Comments: Some have suggested pumping the hands for 2 minutes. It is likely that this test leads to a high amount of false positives. Note the very poor QUADAS score, suggesting bias.

TESTS FOR THORACIC OUTLET SYNDROME

Morley's Sign

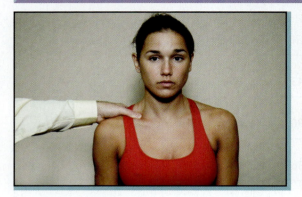

1 The patient sits straight with the arms at the side of his or her body.

2 The examiner palpates the supraclavicular fossa with his or her thumb.

3 Tenderness in the supraclavicular fossa is considered a positive finding for thoracic outlet syndrome.

UTILITY SCORE 3

Study	Reliability	Sensitivity	Specificity	LR+	LR−	DOR	QUADAS Score (0–14)
Matsuyama et al.[6]	NT	NT	NT	NA	NA	NA	NT

Comments: This test will likely also be painful with patients with cervical radiculopathy. To increase the specificity, referral of symptoms along the lower brachial plexus should be targeted.

TESTS FOR THORACIC OUTLET SYNDROME

Supraclavicular Pressure Test

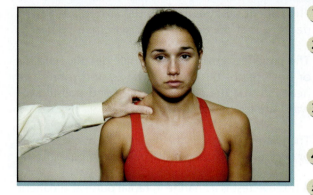

1 The patient sits straight with the arms at the sides.

2 The examiner places his or her fingers on the upper trapezius and the thumbs contacting the lowest portion of the anterior scalene muscle near the first ribs.

3 The examiner squeezes the fingers and thumbs together for 30 seconds.

4 The patient is queried for changes in paresthesia.

5 A positive test is a report of paresthesia by the patient.

UTILITY SCORE 3

Study	Reliability	Sensitivity	Specificity	LR+	LR−	DOR	QUADAS Score (0–14)
Plewa & Delinger[7] (Vascular Changes)	NT	NT	79	NA	NA	NA	9
Plewa & Delinger[7] (Pain)	NT	NT	98	NA	NA	NA	9
Plewa & Delinger[7] (Paresthesia)	NT	NT	85	NA	NA	NA	9

Comments: The test differs from Morley's sign only in the compression of both thumb and forefinger. This test will likely also be painful with patients with cervical radiculopathy.

TESTS FOR THORACIC OUTLET SYNDROME

▶ Adson's Test

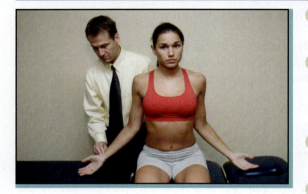

1 The patient sits straight with the arms placed at 15 degrees of abduction. The radial pulse is palpated.

2 The patient is instructed to inhale deeply, hold his or her breath, tilt the head back, and rotate the head, so that the chin is elevated and pointed toward the examined side.

3 The examiner records the radial pulse as diminished or occluded and queries the patient for paresthesia.

4 A positive test is a change in radial pulse and patient report of paresthesia.

UTILITY SCORE **3**

Study	Reliability	Sensitivity	Specificity	LR+	LR−	DOR	QUADAS Score (0–14)
Rayan & Jensen[8] (Vascular Changes)	NT	NT	87	NA	NA	NA	3
Rayan & Jensen[8] (Paresthesia)	NT	NT	74	NA	NA	NA	3
Plewa & Delinger[7] (Vascular Changes)	NT	NT	89	NA	NA	NA	9
Plewa & Delinger[7] (Pain)	NT	NT	100	NA	NA	NA	9
Plewa & Delinger[7] (Paresthesia)	NT	NT	89	NA	NA	NA	9
Lee et al.[3]	NT	50	NT	NA	NA	NA	4

Comments: Lee et al.[3] used Doppler imaging to classify a positive test. Because vascular problems associated with thoracic outlet are less prevalent, it is likely that neurological changes will be missed using this test.

TESTS FOR THORACIC OUTLET SYNDROME

Cyriax Release Test

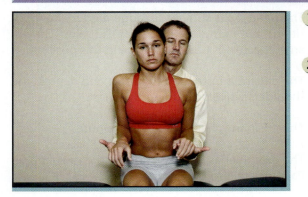

1. The patient can assume either a sitting or standing position.

2. The examiner stands behind the patient and grasps under the forearms holding the elbows at approximately 80–90 degrees while maintaining the forearms, wrists, and hands in neutral.

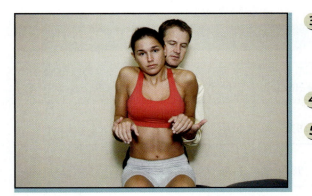

3. The examiner should lean the patient's trunk posteriorly, approximately 15 degrees from vertical, and elevate the patient's shoulder girdle close to end range (lifted).

4. This position is held up to 3 minutes.

5. The patient is queried for reproduction of the patient's symptoms or a release phenomenon.

UTILITY SCORE 3

Study	Reliability	Sensitivity	Specificity	LR+	LR−	DOR	QUADAS Score (0–14)
Brismee et al.[1] (1-minute hold)	NT	NT	97	NA	NA	NA	7
Brismee et al.[1] (15-minute hold)	NT	NT	77	NA	NA	NA	7

Comments: Hold times have varied between 1 minute and several minutes. The examiner may use a chair to "prop" the arms in position if a longer hold time is selected. A release phenomenon occurs when symptoms abate with positioning. True test value is questionable.

TESTS FOR THORACIC OUTLET SYNDROME

Costoclavicular Maneuver

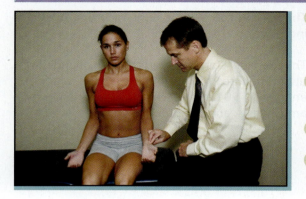

1. The patient sits straight (exaggerated military position). Both arms are placed at the sides. The examiner assesses the radial pulse in this position.

2. The patient is instructed to retract and depress the shoulders while protruding the chest.

3. The position is held for one full minute.

4. The examiner assesses changes in the radial pulse. Patients are also queried for paresthesia.

UTILITY SCORE 3

Study	Reliability	Sensitivity	Specificity	LR+	LR−	DOR	QUADAS Score (0–14)
Rayan & Jensen[8] (Vascular Changes)	NT	NT	53	NA	NA	NA	3
Rayan & Jensen[8] (Paresthesia)	NT	NT	98	NA	NA	NA	3
Plewa & Delinger[7] (Vascular Changes)	NT	NT	89	NA	NA	NA	9
Plewa & Delinger[7] (Pain)	NT	NT	100	NA	NA	NA	9
Plewa & Delinger[7] (Paresthesia)	NT	NT	85	NA	NA	NA	9

Comments: The test appears to be specific, although study design is lacking on both reported findings and nearly all tests have methodological biases.

TESTS FOR THORACIC OUTLET SYNDROME

Wright's Test

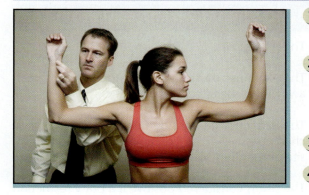

1 The patient assumes a sitting position. The examiner palpates the radial pulse.

2 The patient is instructed to hyperabduct his or her shoulders and flex his or her elbows to 90 degrees. The head should be turned toward the unaffected side.

3 The position is held for 1 to 2 minutes.

4 A positive test includes reproduction of paresthesia or a decrease in the radial pulse.

UTILITY SCORE ?

Study	Reliability	Sensitivity	Specificity	LR+	LR−	DOR	QUADAS Score (0–14)
Not tested	NT	NT	NT	NA	NA	NA	NA
Comments: The test is similar to the Hyperabduction Test but adds rotation away from the affected side.							

TESTS FOR RESTRICTED FIRST RIB

Cervical Rotation Lateral Flexion Test (Associated with Brachialgia)

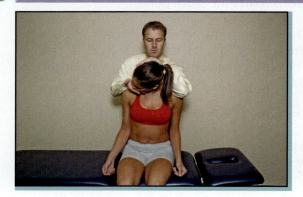

1 The patient sits.

2 The examiner passively rotates the patient's head away from the affected side.

3 The examiner gently side flexes the head (ear to chest) passively. The side flexion should be opposite of rotation.

4 The test is considered positive if a bony restriction blocks the lateral flexion.

UTILITY SCORE ?

Study	Reliability	Sensitivity	Specificity	LR+	LR−	DOR	QUADAS Score (0–14)
Lindgren et al.[4]	1.0 Kappa	NT	NT	NA	NA	NA	NA

Comments: A number of additional factors may influence the finding, including thoracic outlet syndrome, cervical radiculopathy, and upper thoracic pain. Lindgren did show validity with radiographic measures of first rib elevation.

TESTS FOR RESTRICTED FIRST RIB

First Rib Spring Test

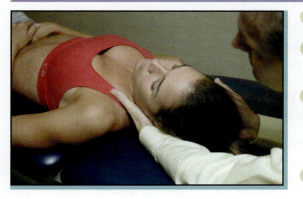

1 The patient lies in a supine position.

2 The examiner passively rotates the patient's head toward the rib that is assessed.

3 The examiner places his or her hand posterior to the first rib. The examiner presses downward in a ventral and caudal direction (toward the opposite hip or opposite shoulder).

4 The opposite side is assessed for comparison. The test is considered positive if the rib is considered stiff as compared with the other side.

UTILITY SCORE ?

Study	Reliability	Sensitivity	Specificity	LR+	LR−	DOR	QUADAS Score (0–14)
Smedmark et al.[9] (C2-3 Rotation)	.43 kappa	NT	NT	NA	NA	NA	NA
Comments: By pushing toward the opposite hip or shoulder, the examiner targets the movement of the first rib.								

TEST TO DETERMINE POTENTIAL OF MOBILITY CHANGE IN THE THORACIC SPINE

Structural versus Flexible Kyphosis Test

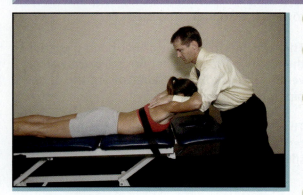

1. The patient assumes a prone position.

2. The examiner uses a stabilization belt to block the patient near T8 or the thoracic apex of kyphosis.

3. The patient either actively or is passively lifted into extension of the thoracic spine by either pulling the patient from the shoulder girdle while standing caudally, or by looping the arms through the patient's hands (pictured).

4. Failure to progress toward thoracic extension is considered a structural kyphosis.

UTILITY SCORE ?

Study	Reliability	Sensitivity	Specificity	LR+	LR−	DOR	QUADAS Score (0–14)
Not tested	NT	NT	NT	NA	NA	NA	NA

Comments: The test is considered useful during assessment of postural deformities and to determine if an extension-based program for the thoracic spine may be useful.

TEST FOR DISCOGENIC OR SYMPATHETIC SYMPTOMS OF THE THORACIC SPINE

Thoracic Slump Test (Sympathetic Slump Test)

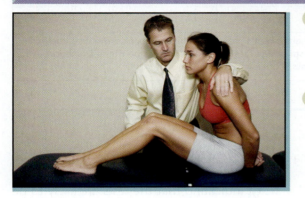

1 The patient assumes a long sitting position with the knees bent approximately 45 degrees. The hands are placed behind the back to allow examiner maneuvering. Resting symptoms are assessed.

2 The examiner loads the patient over the shoulders. Resting symptoms are assessed.

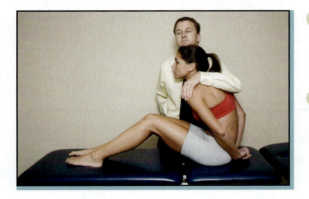

3 The patient is instructed to flex the lower cervical spine and extend the upper cervical spine. The examiner may add overpressure to the movement. Resting symptoms are assessed.

4 The examiner can then add side flexion to the right or left and/or rotation to the right or left to further engage the dural tissue (not pictured). Symptoms are further assessed to determine the concordant nature.

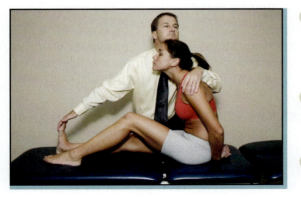

5 The examiner then passively moves the lower extremity on the concordant side into extension and the ankle into dorsiflexion. Resting symptoms are again assessed.

6 In addition, the patient may extend both knees or perform upper limb tension movements during this examination.

7 A positive test is characterized by (1) asymmetry, (2) reproduction of the concordant pain, and (3) sensitization. All three must be present for a positive test.

(continued)

TEST FOR DISCOGENIC OR SYMPATHETIC SYMPTOMS OF THE THORACIC SPINE

UTILITY SCORE ?

Study	Reliability	Sensitivity	Specificity	LR+	LR−	DOR	QUADAS Score (0–14)
Maitland et al.[5]	NT	NT	NT	NA	NA	NA	NA

Comments: The test is unexamined for diagnostic accuracy. Furthermore, if a patient exhibits low back symptoms, the position of the slump sit will be too painful to examine the thoracic spine separately. Some may describe the examination with initiation of the knee movements followed by thoracic movements.

Key Points

1. Nearly all of the thoracic clinical special tests exhibit high levels of procedural bias.

2. Thoracic clinical special tests are significantly understudied.

3. The lack of a common accepted reference standard has resulted in few studies that have investigated the sensitivity of clinical special tests of thoracic outlet syndrome.

4. The majority of thoracic outlet syndrome special tests demonstrate moderate to poor specificity, indicating that the tests are likely to be positive for patients with conditions outside TOS. Nearly all have not been measured for sensitivity.

References

1. Brismee JM, Gilbert K, Isom K, Hall R, Leathers B, Sheppard N, Sawyer S, Sizer P. Rate of false positive using the Cyriax Release test for thoracic outlet syndrome in an asymptomatic population. *J Man Manipulative Ther.* 2004; 12:73–81.

2. Howard M, Lee C, Dellon AL. Documentation of brachial plexus compression (in the thoracic inlet) utilizing provocative neurosensory and muscular testing. *J Reconstr Microsurg.* 2003; 19(5):303–312.

3. Lee AD, Agarwal S, Sadhu D. Doppler Adson's test: predictor of outcome of surgery in non-specific thoracic outlet syndrome. *World J Surg.* 2006;30(3):291–292.

4. Lindgren KA, Leino E, Manninen H. Cervical rotation lateral flexion test in brachialgia. *Arch Phys Med Rehabil.* 1992;73(8):735–737.

5. Maitland GD. *Maitland's vertebral manipulation.* 6th ed. London; Butterworth-Heinemann: 2001.

6. Matsuyama T, Okuchi K, Goda K. Upper plexus thoracic outlet syndrome—case report. *Neurol Med Chir (Tokyo).* 2002;42(5):237–241.

7. Plewa MC, Delinger M. The false-positive rate of thoracic outlet syndrome shoulder maneuvers in healthy patients. *Acad Emerg Med.* 1998;5(4):337–342.

8. Rayan GM, Jensen C. Thoracic outlet syndrome: provocative examination maneuvers in a typical population. *J Shoulder Elbow Surg.* 1995;4(2):113–117.

9. Smedmark V, Wallin M, Arvidsson I. Inter-examiner reliability in assessing passive intervertebral motion of the cervical spine. *Man Ther.* 2000;5:97–101.

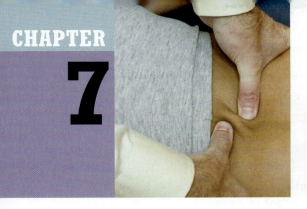

Physical Examination Tests for the Lumbar Spine

TESTS FOR DISCOGENIC SYMPTOMS

Centralization

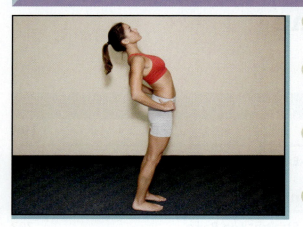

1 The patient either stands or lies prone depending on the intent of a loaded or unloaded assessment.

2 Multiple directions of repeated end-range lumbar testing is targeted. Movements may include extension, flexion, or side flexion.

3 Movements are repeated generally for 5–20 attempts until a definite centralization or peripheralization occurs.

4 Centralization of symptoms is considered a positive finding.

UTILITY SCORE 1

Study	Reliability	Sensitivity	Specificity	LR+	LR−	DOR	QUADAS Score (0–14)
Laslett et al.[18]	NT	40	94	6.7	0.63	10.6	13
Donelson et al.[8]	NT	92	64	2.6	0.12	21.6	12

Comments: Centralization is defined as the progressive retreat of referred pain toward the midline of the back in response to standardized movement testing during evaluation of the effect of repeated movements on pain location and intensity. Centralization is commonly associated with discogenic symptoms.

TESTS FOR DISCOGENIC SYMPTOMS

Extension Loss

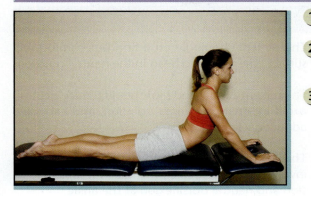

1 The patient is instructed to lie prone.

2 The patient is instructed to extend his or her lumbar spine while keeping pelvis in contact with the plinth.

3 A positive test is moderate or major loss of extension.

UTILITY SCORE 3

Study	Reliability	Sensitivity	Specificity	LR+	LR−	DOR	QUADAS Score (0–14)
Laslett et al.[17]	NT	27	87	2.01	0.84	2.4	10
Comments: The test is scored using visual observation only.							

TESTS FOR HERNIATED NUCLEUS PULPOSIS OR LUMBAR RADICULOPATHY

Well Leg Raise

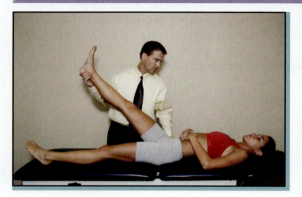

1 The patient should lie on a firm but comfortable surface, the neck and head in the neutral position.

2 The patient's trunk and hips should remain neutral; avoid internal or external rotation, and excessive adduction or abduction.

3 The examiner then supports the patient's non-involved leg at the heel, maintaining knee extension and neutral dorsiflexion at the ankle.

4 Raise to the point of symptom reproduction of the opposite, comparable leg.

5 A positive test is identified by reproduction of the patient's concordant pain during the raising of the opposite extremity.

UTILITY SCORE   1

Study	Reliability	Sensitivity	Specificity	LR+	LR−	DOR	QUADAS Score (0–14)
Knuttson[13]	NT	25	95	5	0.79	6.3	3
Hakelius & Hindmarsh[11]	NT	28	88	2.33	0.82	2.8	3
Spangfort[25]	NT	23	88	1.91	0.86	2.2	5
Kosteljanetz et al.[14]	NT	24	100	NA	NA	NA	7
Kerr et al.[12]	NT	43	97	14.3	0.59	24.2	7

Comments: The test is highly specific and is not sensitive. The test is inappropriate for use as a screen and best functions as a diagnostic test.

TESTS FOR HERNIATED NUCLEUS PULPOSIS OR LUMBAR RADICULOPATHY

Slump Sit Test

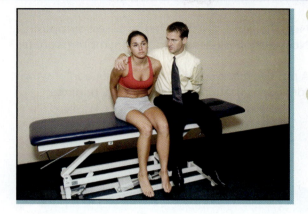

1 The patient sits straight with the arms behind the back, the legs together, and the posterior aspect of the knees against the edge of the treatment table.

2 The patient slumps as far as possible, producing full trunk flexion; the examiner applies firm over-pressure into flexion to the patient's back, being careful to keep the sacrum vertical.

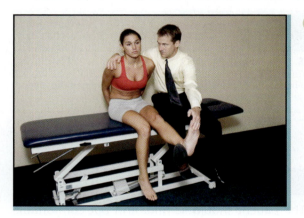

3 While maintaining full spinal flexion with overpressure, the examiner asks the patient to extend the knee, or passively extends the knee.

(continued)

TESTS FOR HERNIATED NUCLEUS PULPOSIS OR LUMBAR RADICULOPATHY

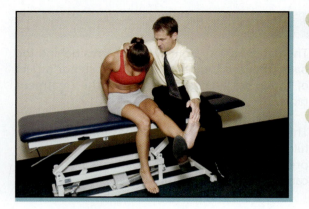

4. The examiner then moves the foot into dorsiflexion while maintaining knee extension.

5. Neck flexion is then added to assess symptoms. Neck flexion is released to see if symptoms abate.

6. A positive test is concordant reproduction of symptoms, sensitization, and asymmetry findings.

| | UTILITY SCORE | **2** |

Study	Reliability	Sensitivity	Specificity	LR+	LR−	DOR	QUADAS Score (0–14)
Stankovic et al.[26]	NT	83	55	1.82	0.32	5.7	11

Comments: The slump has been described as distal and proximal initiation. At present, no studies have examined the differences in diagnostic values of each.

Straight Leg Raise

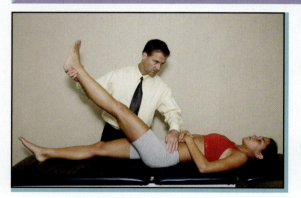

1. The patient should lie on a firm but comfortable surface, the neck and head in the neutral position.

2. The examiner then supports the patient's leg at the heel, maintaining knee extension and neutral dorsiflexion at the ankle. The clinician raises the leg to the point of symptom reproduction.

3. The patient's trunk and hips should remain neutral, avoiding internal or external rotation of the leg or adduction or abduction of the hip.

4. A positive test is concordant reproduction of symptoms, sensitization, and asymmetry findings.

TESTS FOR HERNIATED NUCLEUS PULPOSIS OR LUMBAR RADICULOPATHY

UTILITY SCORE 2

Study	Reliability	Sensitivity	Specificity	LR+	LR−	DOR	QUADAS Score (0–14)
Bertilson et al.[3]	.92 kappa	NT	NT	NA	NA	NA	NA
Charnley[5]	NT	78	64	2.16	0.34	6.4	5
Knuttson[13]	NT	96	10	1.06	0.40	2.7	3
Hakelius & Hindmarsh[11]	NT	96	17	1.15	0.24	4.8	3
Spangfort[26]	NT	97	11	1.08	0.27	4	5
Kosteljanetz et al.[14]	NT	76	45	1.38	0.53	2.6	9
Kosteljanetz et al.[15]	NT	89	14	1.03	0.78	1.3	7
Lauder et al.[19] (Used EMG as Reference Standard)	NT	19	84	1.61	0.90	1.8	6
Albeck[2]	NT	82	21	1.03	0.86	1.2	7
Gurdjian et al.[10]	NT	81	52	1.68	0.36	4.7	4
Kerr et al.[12]	NT	98	44	1.75	0.05	35	7
Vroomen et al.[27]	NT	97	57	2.23	0.05	44.6	10
Lyle et al.[20] (For Degenerative Spine)	NT	16	NT	NT	NT	NT	9
Porchet et al.[24] (Extreme Lateral Disc Herniation)	NT	83	NT	NT	NT	NT	5

Comments: In many cases, the procedure and the reference for a positive test was variable. Traditionally, the foot should be held in neutral dorsiflexion for testing.

TEST FOR FAR LATERAL LUMBAR DISC HERNIATION

Femoral Nerve Tension Test

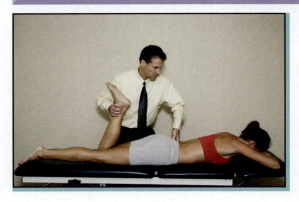

1 The patient lies prone in a symmetric pain-free posture.

2 The examiner places one hand on the PSIS, the same side of the knee that the examiner will bend into flexion.

3 The examiner then gently moves the lower extremity into knee flexion, bending the knee until the onset of symptoms.

4 Once symptoms are engaged, the examiner slightly backs the leg out of the painful position.

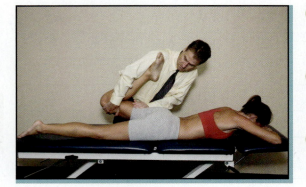

5 At this point, the examiner may use plantarflexion, dorsiflexion, or head movements to sensitize the findings.

6 Further sensitization can be elicited by implementing hip extension. The examiner can repeat on the opposite side if desired.

7 A positive test is reproduction of pain in the affected extremity.

UTILITY SCORE 3

Study	Reliability	Sensitivity	Specificity	LR+	LR−	DOR	QUADAS Score (0–14)
Porchet et al.[24]	NT	84	NT	NA	NA	NA	5

Comments: All cases in the Porchet et al.[24] study were associated with extreme lateral disc herniations. The test is sometimes described as an upper lumbar disc assessment and frequently as a femoral nerve tension test. Only the far lateral disc herniation patient pool has been investigated.

TEST FOR UPPER LUMBAR HERNIATION

Crossed Femoral Nerve Tension Test

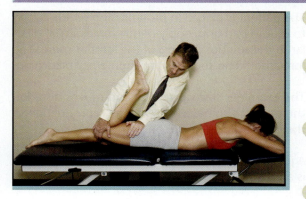

1 The patient lies prone in a symmetric pain-free posture.

2 The examiner places one hand on the PSIS, the same side of the knee that the examiner will bend into flexion.

3 The examiner then gently moves the noninvolved lower extremity into knee flexion, bending the knee until the onset of symptoms.

4 Once symptoms are engaged, the examiner slightly backs out of the painful position. At this point, the examiner may use plantarflexion, dorsiflexion, or head movements to sensitize the findings.

5 Further sensitization can be elicited by implementing hip extension.

6 A positive test is reproduction of concordant pain in the opposite extremity.

UTILITY SCORE ?

Study	Reliability	Sensitivity	Specificity	LR+	LR−	DOR	QUADAS Score (0–14)
Kreitz et al.[16]	NT	NT	NT	NA	NA	NA	NT

Comments: The test is sometimes described as a far lateral disc herniation assessment and frequently as a femoral nerve tension test when performed unilaterally on the affected side.

TESTS FOR LEVEL OF PATHOLOGY OR RADIOGRAPHIC INSTABILITY OF THE SPINE

Posterior-Anterior (PA)

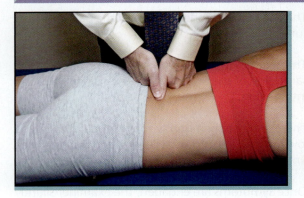

(1) The patient is placed in prone. Using a thumb pad to thumb pad grip, apply gentle force perpendicular to the spinous process of the lumbar spine. The force should be about 4kg or thumb nail blanching.

(2) The examiner starts proximal and moves distal on the patient's spine, asking for the reproduction of the concordant sign of the patient.

(3) A joint is cleared if a significant amount of PA force is applied and no pain is present.

(4) A dysfunctional joint will elicit the concordant sign during the mobilization, and may reproduce radicular or referred symptoms. Repeated movement or sustained holds help determine the appropriateness of the technique.

(5) A positive test is identified by reproduction of the patient's concordant pain or presence of linear displacement during assessment.

UTILITY SCORE 2

Study	Reliability	Sensitivity	Specificity	LR+	LR−	DOR	QUADAS Score (0–14)
Bertilson et al.[3] (For Identification of Pain)	.44 Kappa	NT	NT	NA	NA	NA	NA
Matyas & Bach[22]	0.09–0.46r	NT	NT	NA	NA	NA	NA
Maher & Adams[21] (L1-5) (For Identification of Pain)	.67–.73 ICC	NT	NT	NA	NA	NA	NA
Maher & Adams[21] (L1-5) (For Identification of Stiffness)	.03–.37 ICC	NT	NT	NA	NA	NA	NA
Binkley & Stratford[4] (Identification of Proper Level to Treat)	.30 Kappa	NT	NT	NA	NA	NA	NA

TESTS FOR LEVEL OF PATHOLOGY OR RADIOGRAPHIC INSTABILITY OF THE SPINE

Study	Reliability	Sensitivity	Specificity	LR+	LR−	DOR	QUADAS Score (0–14)
Binkley & Stratford[4] (Assessment of Mobility)	.09 Kappa	NT	NT	NA	NA	NA	NA
Chiradejnant et al.[6]	.78 ICC	NT	NT	NA	NA	NA	9
Phillips & Twomey[23] (Tissue Response Agreement for Transverse Glides [TG], Central PAs [CPA], and Unilateral PAs [UPA])	−0.16–0.22 (TG) −0.15–0.19 (CPA) −0.09–0.28 (UPA)	NT	NT	NA	NA	NA	9
Phillips & Twomey[23] (Verbal Response Combined to Identify the Painful Segment)	NA	75	90	7.5	0.27	27.8	9
Phillips & Twomey[23] (Nonverbal Response Combined to Identify the Painful Segment)	NA	50	78	2.24	0.64	3.5	9
Abbott et al.[1] (Rotational PAs to Diagnose Radiographic Instability)	NT	33	88	2.75	0.75	3.7	11
Abbott et al.[1] (Transitional PAs to Diagnose Radiographic Instability)	NT	29	89	2.63	0.79	3.3	11
Fritz, Piva, & Childs[9] (Lack of Hypomobility to Diagnose Radiographic Instability)	NT	43	95	8.6	0.60	14.3	12
Fritz, Piva, & Childs[9] (Presence of Hypermobility to Diagnose Radiographic Instability)	.48 kappa	46	81	2.42	0.66	3.7	12
Fritz, Piva, & Childs[9] (Presence of Pain to Diagnose Radiographic Instability)	.57 kappa	43	81	2.26	0.70	3.21	12

Comments: Unfortunately, the procedure and positive identifier for each study was variable. The test is likely not diagnostic, but is a useful tool to identify the impaired segment.

TESTS FOR RADIOGRAPHIC INSTABILITY OF THE SPINE

Passive Physiological Intervertebral Movements (PPIVMs) Extension

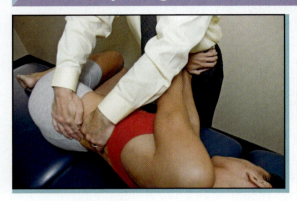

1 The patient is placed in a sidelying position. The patient's elbows are locked in extension and his or her hands are placed on the ASIS of the assessing examiner.

2 The examiner applies a posterior to anterior (PA) force at the caudal level (i.e., at L5 when assessing L4-L5 mobility).

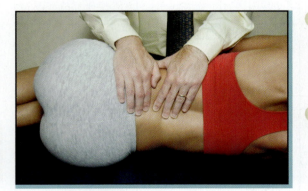

3 The cephalic segment is palpated just inferior at the interspinous space (i.e., during L4-L5 assessment, the interspinous space is palpated to assess movement). One may repeat on the other side, although most likely results are similar.

4 A positive test is identified by detection of excessive movement during examination.

UTILITY SCORE **2**

Study	Reliability	Sensitivity	Specificity	LR+	LR−	DOR	QUADAS Score (0–14)
Abbott et al.[1] (Extension Rotational PPIVMs)	NT	22	97	7.3	0.80	9.1	11
Abbott et al.[1] (Extension Transitional PPIVMSs)	NT	16	98	8	0.85	9.4	11
Comments: Abbott et al.[1] used very specific criteria in identifying a positive finding, which explains the low sensitivity values.							

TESTS FOR RADIOGRAPHIC INSTABILITY OF THE SPINE

Passive Physiological Intervertebral Movements (PPIVMs) Flexion

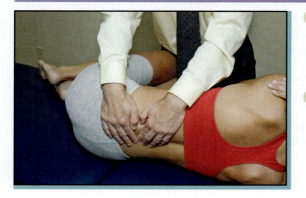

1 The patient is placed in a sidelying position. The hips of the patient are flexed to 90 degrees and the patient's knees are placed against the ASIS of the examiner.

2 The examiner stabilizes the superior segments by pulling posterior to anterior on the patient's spine. The examiner applies an anterior to posterior force at the caudal level (i.e., at L5 when assessing L4-L5 mobility) by applying a force through the flexed femurs.

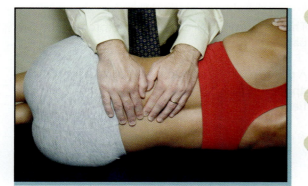

3 The cephalic segment is palpated just inferior at the interspinous space (i.e., during L4-L5 assessment, the interspinous space is palpated to assess movement.

4 One may repeat on the other side, although most likely results are similar.

5 A positive test is identified by detection of excessive movement during examination.

UTILITY SCORE 2

Study	Reliability	Sensitivity	Specificity	LR+	LR−	DOR	QUADAS Score (0–14)
Abbott et al.[1] (Flexion Rotational PPIVMs)	NT	05	99	5	0.96	5.2	11
Abbott et al.[1] (Flexion Transitional PPVIMs)	NT	05	99	10	0.95	10.5	11
Comments: Abbott et al.[1] used very specific criteria in identifying a positive finding, which explains the low sensitivity values.							

TESTS FOR RADIOGRAPHIC INSTABILITY OF THE SPINE

Prone Instability Test

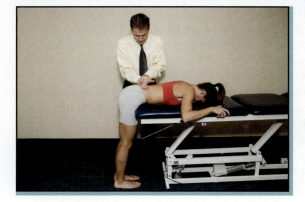

1 The patient is prone with the torso on the examining table and the legs over the edge of the plinth and the feet resting on the floor.

2 The examiner performs a PA spring on the low back to elicit back pain using the pisiform grip.

3 The patient is requested to lift his or her legs off the floor by using a back contraction.

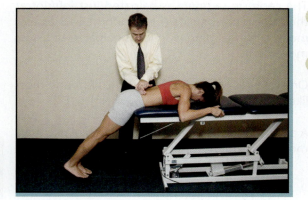

4 The examiner maintains the PA force to the low back.

5 A positive test is reduction of painful symptoms (as applied during the PA) during raising of the patient's legs.

UTILITY SCORE 3

Study	Reliability	Sensitivity	Specificity	LR+	LR−	DOR	QUADAS Score (0–14)
Fritz, Piva, & Childs[9]	.69 kappa	61	57	1.41	0.69	2.0	12
Comments: The test has poor diagnostic value but has been used in a clinical prediction rule for detecting lumbar instability.							

TESTS FOR RADIOGRAPHIC INSTABILITY OF THE SPINE

Specific Spine Torsion Test

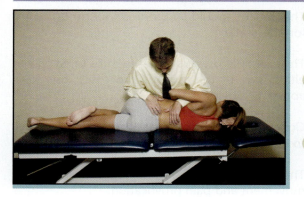

1. The patient is asked to lie on his or her side and is positioned at 60 degrees of hip flexion and approximately 90 degrees of knee flexion (top leg).

2. The examiner uses his or her forearm to take up the slack in the hip and his or her finger to loop underneath the spinous process of S1.

3. Using a force of the examiner's forearm placed on the side of the rib cage and by gently applying a force on L5 toward the treatment table with his or her thumb, the examiner applies a distraction moment at the L5-S1 facet.

4. The force is in a diagonal to emphasize the direction of the facets.

5. Excessive movement, pain, or gapping should be noted since ideally, rotation is minimal in nature.

6. Progress cephalically and perform the same procedure for L4-L5.

7. A positive test is reproduction of the patient's pain and/or hypermobility during torsion testing.

UTILITY SCORE ?

Study	Reliability	Sensitivity	Specificity	LR+	LR−	DOR	QUADAS Score (0–14)
Cook et al.[7]	NT	NT	NT	NA	NA	NA	NT
Comments: The Specific Spine Torsion test is untested.							

TESTS FOR RADIOGRAPHIC INSTABILITY OF THE SPINE

Prone Torsion Instability Test

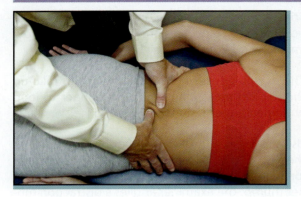

1 The patient should lie prone on a firm but comfortable surface.

2 The examiner uses his or her thumbs to palpate at either side of the spinous processes: one level above, one below.

3 Concurrently, the examiner applies a medial force to both spinous processes.

4 The examiner assesses multiple levels, feeling for movement and pain provocation.

5 A positive test is reproduction of the patient's pain and/or hypermobility during torsion testing.

UTILITY SCORE ?

Study	Reliability	Sensitivity	Specificity	LR+	LR−	DOR	QUADAS Score (0–14)
None	NT	NT	NT	NA	NA	NA	NT

Comments: The Prone Torsion test is untested. Because so little rotation is available at the lumbar spine, one should feel very little movement during testing.

TEST FOR DEGENERATIVE CHANGES IN THE SPINE

Extension Quadrant Test

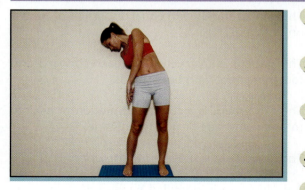

1. The patient stands with equal dispersion of weight on both legs.

2. The patient is instructed to lean back, rotate, and side-flex toward one side.

3. The movement is a combined motion of extension, rotation, and side flexion.

4. The movement is repeated to the opposite side.

5. A positive test is identified by reproduction of the patient's concordant pain.

UTILITY SCORE 3

Study	Reliability	Sensitivity	Specificity	LR+	LR−	DOR	QUADAS Score (0–14)
Lyle et al.[20]	NT	70	NT	NA	NA	NA	9

Comments: The test is commonly used to rule out the lumbar spine when differentiating between hip and lumbar spine. It is questionable whether this test is appropriate as a screen.

TEST FOR LUMBAR FLEXION DYSFUNCTION

Flexion Quadrant Test

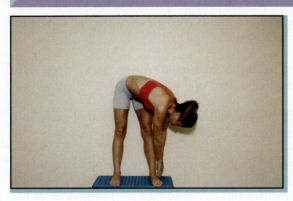

1. The patient stands with equal dispersion of weight on both legs.

2. The patient is instructed to reach forward and touch one foot with both hands.

3. The movement is a combined motion of flexion, rotation, and side flexion to one side.

4. The movement is repeated to the opposite side.

5. A positive test is identified by reproduction of the patient's concordant pain.

UTILITY SCORE ?

Study	Reliability	Sensitivity	Specificity	LR+	LR−	DOR	QUADAS Score (0–14)
None	NT	NT	NT	NA	NA	NA	NA
Comments: The test is often used to rule out a disc herniation.							

Key Points

1. The majority of clinical special tests of the lumbar spine have demonstrated poor diagnostic value.

2. Tests such as the SLR and slump are somewhat sensitive but lack specificity. They are not conclusive tests for herniation of the lumbar spine.

3. Centralization is a moderately strong predictor of discogenic dysfunction.

4. Clinical special tests designed to measure instability are understudied and often lack a common reference for instability.

5. Posterior-anterior and passive physiological tests lack a common procedural standard for the index test, resulting in a variety of potential outcomes for these tests.

References

1. Abbott JH, McCane B, Herbison P, Moginie G, Chapple C, Hogarty T. Lumbar segmental instability: a criterion-related validity study of manual therapy assessment. *BMC Musculoskelet Disord.* 2005;6:56.

2. Albeck M. A critical assessment of clinical diagnosis of disc herniation in patients with monoradicular sciatica. *Acta Neurochir.* 1996;138:40.

3. Bertilson BC, Bring J, Sjoblom A, Sundell K, Strender LE. Inter-examiner reliability in the assessment of low back pain (LBP) using the Kirkaldy-Willis classification (KWC). *Eur Spine J.* 2006;1–9.

4. Binkley J, Stratford PW, Gill C. Interrater reliability of lumbar accessory motion mobility testing. *Phys Ther.* 1995;75(9):786–792.

5. Charnley J. Orthopaedic signs in the diagnosis of disc protrusion with special reference to the straight-leg raising test. *Lancet.* 1951;1: 186–192.

6. Chiradejnant A, Maher CG, Latimer J. Objective manual assessment of lumbar posteroanterior stiffness is now possible. *J Manipulative Physiol Ther.* 2003;26(1):34–39.

7. Cook C, Cook A, Fleming R. Rehabilitation for clinical lumbar instability in an adolescent diver with spondylolisthesis. *J Man Manipulative Ther.* 2004;12(2):91–99.

8. Donelson R, Aprill C, Medcalf R, Grant W. A prospective study of centralization of lumbar and referred pain. A predictor of symptomatic discs and anular competence. *Spine.* 1997;22 (10):1115–1122.

9. Fritz JM, Piva S, Childs J. Accuracy of the clinical examination to predict radiographic instability of the lumbar spine. *Eur Spine J.* 2005; 14(8):743–50.

10. Gurdijan E, Webster J, Ostrowski AZ, Hardy W, Lindner D, Thomas L. Herniated lumbar intervertebral discs: an analysis of 1176 operated cases. *J Trauma.* 1961;1:158–176.

11. Hakelius A, Hindmarsh J. The comparative reliability of preoperative diagnostic methods in lumbar disc surgery. *Acta Orthop Scand.* 1972; 43:234–238.

12. Kerr RSC, Cadoux-Hudson TA, Adams CBT. The value of accurate clinical assessment in the surgical management of the lumbar disc protrusion. *J Neurol Neurosurg Psychiatr.* 1988;51: 169–173.

13. Knuttson B. Comparative value of electromyographic, myelographic, and clinical-neurological examinations in diagnosis of lumbar root compression syndrome. *Acta Ortho Scand.* 1961;(Suppl 49):19–49.

14. Kosteljanetz M, Bang F, Schmidt-Olsen S. The clinical significance of straight leg raising (Lasegue's sign) in the diagnosis of prolapsed lumbar disc. *Spine.* 1988;13:393–395.

15. Kosteljanetz M, Espersen O, Halaburt H, Miletic T. Predictive value of clinical and surgical findings in patients with lumbago-sciatica: a prospective study (part 1). *Acta Neurochirugiica.* 1984;73:67–76.

16. Kreitz BG, Cote P, Yong-Hing K. Crossed femoral stretching test: a case report. *Spine.* 1996;21(13):1584–1586.

17. Laslett M, Aprill CN, McDonald B, Oberg B. Clinical predictors of lumbar provocation discography: a study of clinical predictors of lumbar provocation discography. *Eur Spine J.* 2006;1–12.

18. Laslett M, Oberg B, Aprill CN, McDonald B. Centralization as a predictor of provocation discography results in chronic low back pain, and the influence of disability and distress on diagnostic power. *Spine J.* 2005;5(4):370–380.

19. Lauder TD, Dillingham TR, Andary MT, Kumar S, Pezzin LE, Stephens RT. Effect of history and exam in predicting electrodiagnostic outcome among patients with suspected lumbosacral radiculopathy. *Am J Phys Med Rehabil.* 2000;79: 60–68.

20. Lyle MA, Manes S, McGuinness M, Ziaei S, Iversen MD. Relationship of physical examination findings and self-reported symptom sever-

ity and physical function in patients with degenerative lumbar conditions. *Phys Ther.* 2005;85(2):120–133.

21. Maher C, Adams R. Reliability of pain and stiffness assessments in clinical manual lumbar spine examination. *Phys Ther.* 1994;74(9): 801–809.

22. Matyas T, Bach T. The reliability of selected techniques in clinical arthrometrics. *Aust J Physio.* 1985;31:175–199.

23. Phillips DR, Twomey LT. A comparison of manual diagnosis with a diagnosis established by a uni-level lumbar spinal block procedure. *Man Ther.* 1996;1(2):82–87.

24. Porchet F, Fankhauser H, de Tribolet N. Extreme lateral lumbar disc herniation: clinical presentation in 178 patients. *Acta Neurochir (Wien).* 1994;127(3-4):203–209.

25. Spangfort EV. The lumbar disc herniation: a computer aided analysis of 2504 operations. *Acta Orthop Scand.* 1972;11(Supl 142):1–93.

26. Stankovic R, Johnell O, Maly P, Willner S. Use of lumbar extension, slump test, physical and neurological examination in the evaluation of patients with suspected herniated nucleus pulposus: a prospective clinical study. *Man Ther.* 1999;4(1):25–32.

27. Vroomen PC, de Krom MC, Wilmink JT, Kester AD, Knottnerus JA. Diagnostic value of history and physical examination in patients suspected of lumbosacral nerve root compression. *J Neurol Neurosurg Psychiatry.* 2002;72(5):630–634.

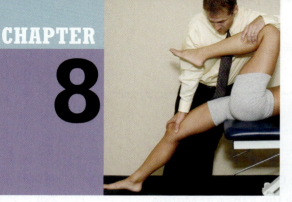

Physical Examination Tests for the Sacroiliac Joint and Pelvis

TESTS FOR SACROILIAC PAIN ORIGIN

Combinations of Tests

Thigh Thrust, Distraction Test, Sacral Thrust, and Compression Test

UTILITY SCORE 1

Study	Reliability	Sensitivity	Specificity	LR+	LR−	DOR	QUADAS Score (0–14)
Laslett et al.[18] (2 of 4)	NT	88	78	4.00	0.16	25	12

Distraction Test, Compression Test, Thigh Thrust, Patrick Sign, Gaenslen's Test

UTILITY SCORE 1

Study	Reliability	Sensitivity	Specificity	LR+	LR−	DOR	QUADAS Score (0–14)
Van der Wuff et al.[37] (3 of 5)	NT	85	79	4.02	0.19	21.2	12

Distraction Test, Thigh Thrust, Gaenslen's Test, Compression Test, and Sacral Thrust

UTILITY SCORE 1

Study	Reliability	Sensitivity	Specificity	LR+	LR−	DOR	QUADAS Score (0–14)
Laslett et al.[20] (3 of 5)	NT	91	87	4.16	0.11	37.8	13

Standing Flexion, Sitting Posterior Superior Iliac Spine (PSIS) Palpation, Supine to Sit Test, Prone Knee Flexion Test

UTILITY SCORE 3

Study	Reliability	Sensitivity	Specificity	LR+	LR−	DOR	QUADAS Score (0–14)
Cibulka & Koldehoff[7] (4 of 4)	NT	82	88	6.83	0.20	34.2	5

(continued)

TESTS FOR SACROILIAC PAIN ORIGIN

Standing Flexion, Prone Knee Flexion, Supine Long Sitting Test, Sitting PSIS Test

UTILITY SCORE ?

Study	Reliability	Sensitivity	Specificity	LR+	LR−	DOR	QUADAS Score (0–14)
Riddle & Freburger[32] (3 of 4)	0.11–0.23	NT	NT	NA	NA	NA	NA

Gapping, Compression Test, Gaenslen's Test, Thigh Thrust, and Patrick's Test

UTILITY SCORE ?

Study	Reliability	Sensitivity	Specificity	LR+	LR−	DOR	QUADAS Score (0–14)
Kokmeyer et al.[17] (3 of 5)	0.71	NT	NT	NA	NA	NA	NA

Supine to Sit Test and Sitting Flexion Test

UTILITY SCORE ?

Study	Reliability	Sensitivity	Specificity	LR+	LR−	DOR	QUADAS Score (0–14)
Levangie[23] (2 of 2)	NT	NT	NT	NA	NA	NA	NA

Comments: Studies that involved combinations of pain provocation tests yielded the highest quality and best outcomes. The findings from Cibulka and Koldehoff[7] were associated with potential bias.

Thigh Thrust (also known as the Oostagard Test, 4 P Test, Sacrotuberous Stress Test, and POSH Test)

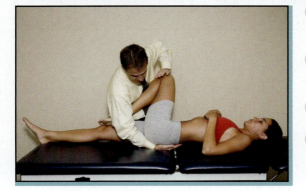

1) The patient is positioned in supine. Resting symptoms are assessed.

2) The examiner stands opposite the painful side of the patient.

3) The hip on the painful side is flexed to 90 degrees.

4) The examiner places his or her hand under the sacrum to form a stable "bridge" for the sacrum.

TESTS FOR SACROILIAC PAIN ORIGIN

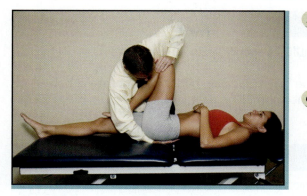

5 A downward pressure is applied through the femur to force a posterior translation of the innominate. The patient's symptoms are assessed to determine if they are concordant.

6 A positive test is concordant pain that is posterior to the hip or near the sacroiliac joint. A positive test requires reproduction of pain on the thrust side (the side of the loaded femur).

UTILITY SCORE | 2

Study	Reliability	Sensitivity	Specificity	LR+	LR−	DOR	QUADAS Score (0–14)
Laslett & Williams[19]	0.82	NT	NT	NA	NA	NA	NA
Dreyfuss et al.[11]	0.64	36	50	0.72	1.28	0.56	10
Kokmeyer et al.[17]	0.67	NT	NT	NA	NA	NA	NA
Damen et al.[9]	NT	62	72	2.2	0.53	4.2	8
Ostgaard & Andersson[30]	NT	80	81	4.21	0.25	16.8	5
Broadhurst & Bond[5]	NT	80	100	NA	NA	NA	9
Albert et al.[1]	0.70	84–93*	98	46.5	0.07–0.16	290–664	7
Laslett et al.[18]	NT	88	69	2.8	0.17	16.3	12

Comments: One of the few sacroiliac tests that exhibits fair sensitivity. To accurately perform the test, make sure the thigh is held in neutral adduction and at 90 degrees of flexion.

TESTS FOR SACROILIAC PAIN ORIGIN

Pain Mapping

1 During the patient history, the patient identifies a specific pain referral pattern.

2 A positive test is representative of pain in the "sacroiliac pain pattern" of unilateral buttock pain below the level of L5, in the absence of midline pain.

UTILITY SCORE 3

Study	Reliability	Sensitivity	Specificity	LR+	LR−	DOR	QUADAS Score (0–14)
Slipman et al.[35] (Lower Lumbar and Buttock)	NT	30	NT	NA	NA	NA	6
Slipman et al.[35] (Buttock Alone)	NT	12	NT	NA	NA	NA	6
Slipman et al.[35] (Lower Lumbar, Buttock, and Thigh)	NT	10	NT	NA	NA	NA	6
Slipman et al.[35] (Lower Lumbar, Buttock, Thigh, and Leg)	NT	10	NT	NA	NA	NA	6
Slipman et al.[35] (Lower Lumbar Alone)	NT	6	NT	NA	NA	NA	6
Slipman et al.[35] (Buttock and Thigh)	NT	4	NT	NA	NA	NA	6
Slipman et al.[35] (Buttock, Groin, and Thigh)	NT	4	NT	NA	NA	NA	6
Slipman et al.[35] (Buttock, Thigh, Leg, Ankle, and Foot)	NT	4	NT	NA	NA	NA	6
Slipman et al.[35] (Buttock and Leg)	NT	2	NT	NA	NA	NA	6
Slipman et al.[35] (Lower Lumbar, Buttock, and Groin)	NT	2	NT	NA	NA	NA	6

Comments: It appears the referral pattern of sacroiliac pain is variable and lacks sensitivity and should never be used in isolation.

TESTS FOR SACROILIAC PAIN ORIGIN

Groin Pain

(1) During the patient interview, the patient identifies a referred pain pattern that includes the groin.

(2) A positive test is identified by pain reported in the groin.

UTILITY SCORE | **3**

Study	Reliability	Sensitivity	Specificity	LR+	LR−	DOR	QUADAS Score (0–14)
Dreyfuss et al.[11]	.70	19	63	.09	1.3	0.07	10
Slipman et al.[35] (Any Variation of Groin Pain)	NT	14	NT	NA	NA	NA	6
Comments: This finding appears to be neither sensitive nor specific for sacroiliac pain.							

Distraction Test (Gapping Test)

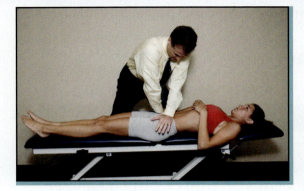

1) The patient assumes a supine position. Resting symptoms are assessed.

2) The medial aspect of both anterior superior iliac spines are palpated by the examiner. The examiner crosses his or her arms, creating an X at the forearms, and a force is applied in a lateral-posterior direction. For comfort, it is often required that the examiner relocate his or her hands on the anterior superior iliac spine (ASIS) several times.

3) The examiner holds the position for 30 seconds, then applies a vigorous force repeatedly in an attempt to reproduce the concordant sign of the patient.

4) A positive test is reproduction of the concordant sign of the patient.

UTILITY SCORE 3

Study	Reliability	Sensitivity	Specificity	LR−	LR−	DOR	QUADAS Score (0–14)
Blower & Griffen[3]	63% agreement	NT	89	NA	NA	NA	5
Russell et al.[34]	NT	11	90	1.1	0.98	1.1	5
Laslett & Williams[19]	0.69	NT	NT	NA	NA	NA	NA
McCombe et al.[25]	0.36	NT	NT	NA	NA	NA	NA
Kokmeyer et al.[17]	0.46	NT	NT	NA	NA	NA	NA
Albert et al.[1]	0.84	04–14	100	NA	NA	NA	7
Laslett et al.[18]	NT	60	81	3.2	0.5	6.4	12
Ham et al.[15]*	NT	50	74	1.9	0.67	2.8	10
Potter & Rothstein[31]	94% agreement	NT	NT	NA	NA	NA	NA

Comments: Of the many sacroiliac tests, the Distraction test is considered to have fair reliability and moderate specificity.
*Ham et al.[15] used the Distraction test as a measure for pelvis fracture.

TESTS FOR SACROILIAC PAIN ORIGIN

Compression Test

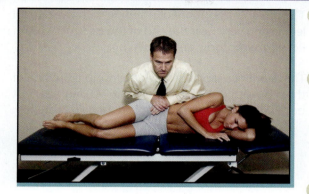

1. The patient assumes a sidelying position with his or her painful side up superior to the plinth. Resting symptoms are assessed.

2. The examiner then cups the iliac crest of the painful side and applies a downward force through the ilium. This position is held fo 30 seconds. As with the other sacroiliac tests, considerable vigor is required to reproduce the symptoms; in some cases, repeated force is necessary.

3. A positive test is reproduction of the concordant sign of the patient.

UTILITY SCORE 3

Study	Reliability	Sensitivity	Specificity	LR+	LR−	DOR	QUADAS Score (0–14)
Blower & Griffen[3]	64% agreement	NT	100	NA	NA	NA	5
Russell et al.[34]	NT	7	90	0.7	1.03	0.68	5
Kokmeyer et al.[17]	0.57	NT	NT	NA	NA	NA	NA
Strender et al.[36]	0.26	NT	NT	NA	NA	NA	NA
Laslett and Williams[19]	0.77	NT	NT	NA	NA	NA	NA
McCombe et al.[25]	0.16	NT	NT	NA	NA	NA	NA
Albert et al.[1]	0.79	25–38	100	NA	NA	NA	7
Laslett et al.[18]	NT	69	69	2.2	0.4	4.9	12
Ham et al.[15*]	NT	60	63	1.6	.63	2.5	10
Potter & Rothstein[31]	76% agreement	NT	NT	NA	NA	NA	NA

Comments: The test has fair reliability and fair specificity. However, the sensitivity is low to fair and the test should not be considered a screen.

*Ham et al.[15] used the test as a measure of pelvis fracture.

TESTS FOR SACROILIAC PAIN ORIGIN

Gaenslen's Test

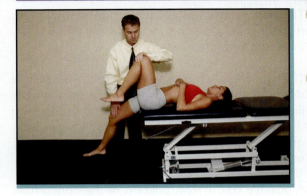

1 The patient is positioned in supine with the painful leg resting very near the end of the treatment table. Resting symptoms are assessed.

2 The examiner sagitally raises the nonpainful side of the hip (with the knee bent) up to 90 degrees. Test both sides if the patient complains of pain bilaterally.

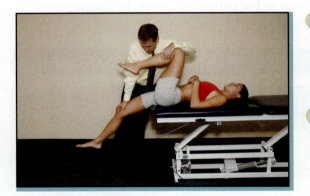

3 A downward force (up to 6 bouts) is applied to the lower leg (painful side) while a flexion-based counterforce is applied to the flexed leg (pushing the leg in the opposite direction). The effect causes a torque to the pelvis. Concordant symptoms are assessed.

4 The test is positive if the torque reproduces pain of the concordant sign.

UTILITY SCORE 3

Study	Reliability	Sensitivity	Specificity	LR+	LR−	DOR	QUADAS Score (0–14)
Laslett & Williams[19]	0.72	NT	NT	NA	NA	NA	NA
Dreyfuss et al.[11]	0.61	71	26	1.02	1.11	0.92	10
Kokmeyer et al.[17]	0.60	NT	NT	NA	NA	NA	NA
Laslett et al.[18] (Right)	NT	53	71	1.8	0.66	2.76	12
Laslett et al.[18] (Left)	NT	50	77	2.2	0.65	3.3	12

Comments: Occasionally, the test is required on both sides to determine pain. This test demonstrates poor diagnostic value secondary to poor to fair specificity.

TESTS FOR SACROILIAC PAIN ORIGIN

Sacral Thrust

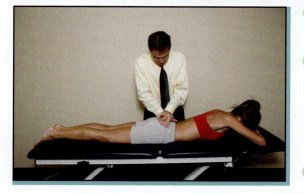

1. The patient lies in a prone position. Resting symptoms are assessed.

2. The examiner palpates the second or third spinous process of the sacrum. Using the pisiform the examiner places a downward pressure on the sacrum at S3. By targeting the midpoint of the sacrum, the examiner is less likely to force the lumbar spine into hyperextension.

3. Vigorously and repeatedly (up to 6 thrusts), the examiner applies a strong downward force to the sacrum in an attempt to reproduce the concordant sign of the patient.

4. A positive test is a reproduction of the concordant sign during downward pressure.

UTILITY SCORE   3

Study	Reliability	Sensitivity	Specificity	LR+	LR−	DOR	QUADAS Score (0–14)
Laslett & Williams[19]	0.32	NT	NT	NA	NA	NA	NA
Dreyfuss et al.[11]	0.30	53	29	0.74	1.62	0.46	10
Laslett et al.[18]	NT	63	75	2.5	.49	5.1	12
Blower & Griffen[3]	64% agreement	NT	86	NA	NA	NA	5

Comments: It is imperative not to push the lumbar spine into extension; otherwise, the test specificity will be artificially reduced. In isolation, the test provides only marginal diagnostic value.

Patrick's Test (also known as the FABER Test)

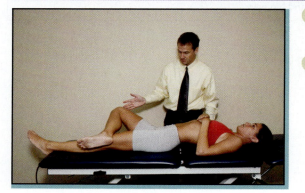

1. The patient is positioned in supine. Resting symptoms are assessed.

2. The painful side leg is placed in a "figure four" position. The ankle is placed just above the knee of the other leg.

(continued)

TESTS FOR SACROILIAC PAIN ORIGIN

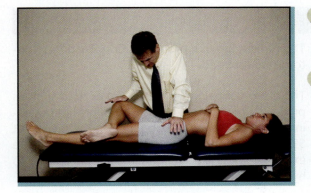

3) The examiner provides a gentle downward pressure on both the knee of the painful side and the ASIS of the nonpainful side.

4) Concordant pain is assessed, specifically the location and type of pain.

UTILITY SCORE 3

Study	Reliability	Sensitivity	Specificity	LR+	LR−	DOR	QUADAS Score (0–14)
Dreyfuss et al.[11]	0.62	69	16	0.82	1.94	0.42	10
Van Deursen et al.[38]	0.38	NT	NT	NA	NA	NA	NA
Broadhurst & Bond[5]	NT	77	100	NA	NA	NA	9
Albert et al.[1]	0.54	40–70	99	41	0.58–0.60	68–71	7
Hansen et al.[16] (Piriformis)	NT	48	77	2.1	0.68	3.1	7
Rost et al.[33] (One-Side Positive) (PPPP)	NT	36	NT	NA	NA	NA	7
Rost et al.[33] (Two-Sides Positive) (PPPP)	NT	36	NT	NA	NA	NA	7

Comments: The wide range of values are likely reflective of the variety of patients used in each study and the bias that results. For sacroiliac pain, the chief complaint is typically posterior. The test is also used to assess hip dysfunction, although the location of pain is different between sacroiliac dysfunction and hip pain.

TESTS FOR SACROILIAC PAIN ORIGIN

Menell's Test

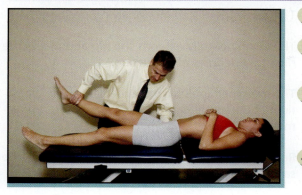

1. The patient is supine.

2. The patient moves one leg into 30 degrees abduction and 10 degrees of flexion of the hip joint.

3. The examiner pushes the lower leg into and then away from the pelvis in a sagittal motion (extension then flexion).

4. A positive test is reproduction of concordant symptoms.

UTILITY SCORE 3

Study	Reliability	Sensitivity	Specificity	LR+	LR−	DOR	QUADAS Score (0–14)
Albert et al.[1]	.87	.54–.70	100	NA	NA	NA	7
Comments: Weakness is not considered a positive finding.							

Resisted Hip Abduction

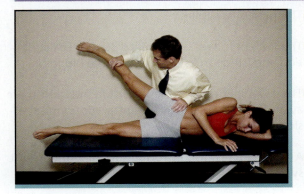

1 The patient is placed in a sidelying position.

2 The examiner fully extends the hip and places the hip at 30 degrees of abduction.

3 The examiner applies a force medially while the patient counters the force by lateral pressure (movement into abduction).

4 Reproduction of pain in the cephalic aspect of the sacroiliac joint is considered positive.

UTILITY SCORE **3**

Study	Reliability	Sensitivity	Specificity	LR+	LR−	DOR	QUADAS Score (0–14)
Broadhurst & Bond[5]	NT	87	100	NA	NA	NA	9
Comments: Weakness is not considered a positive finding.							

TESTS FOR SACROILIAC PAIN ORIGIN

Fortin Finger Test

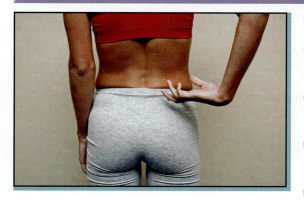

1. The patient completes a pain diagram.

2. The patient is instructed to point to the region of pain with one finger.

3. The examiner reviews the area of pain and the pain diagram for consistency.

4. The patient is requested to repeat the procedure of pointing to his or her pain.

5. A positive test is identified by (1) the patient could localize the pain with one finger, (2) the area pointed to was within 1 cm of and immediately inferomedial to the posterior superior iliac spine, and (3) the patient consistently pointed to the same area over at least two trials.

UTILITY SCORE 3

Study	Reliability	Sensitivity	Specificity	LR+	LR−	DOR	QUADAS Score (0–14)
Fortin & Falco[13]	NT	100	NT	NA	NA	NA	5
Dreyfuss et al.[11]	.81% agreement	76	47	.09	1.3	0.07	10

Comments: This test was poorly performed by Fortin and Falco, and no mention of referred pain is made for the Fortin Finger Test.

TESTS FOR SACROILIAC PAIN ORIGIN

Standing ASIS Asymmetry

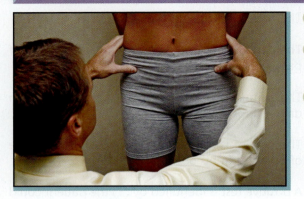

1 The patient is placed in standing.

2 Using the iliac crests as a guide, the examiner measures the symmetry of the iliac crests then the ASIS.

3 A positive test is characterized by asymmetry.

UTILITY SCORE **3**

Study	Reliability	Sensitivity	Specificity	LR+	LR−	DOR	QUADAS Score (0–14)
Levangie[22]	.75	74	21	.94	1.24	0.76	11
Potter & Rothstein[31]	37.5% agreement	NT	NT	NA	NA	NA	NA
Comments: Based on Levangie's findings, this test actually provides bias and no value during the examination.							

TESTS FOR SACROILIAC PAIN ORIGIN

Seated ASIS Asymmetry

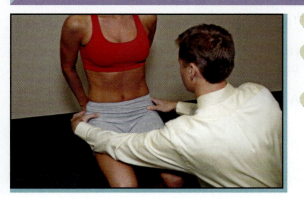

1. The patient sits in front of the examiner.

2. Using the iliac crests as a guide, the examiner evaluates the symmetry of the ASIS.

3. A positive test is characterized by asymmetry.

UTILITY SCORE   3

Study	Reliability	Sensitivity	Specificity	LR+	LR−	DOR	QUADAS Score (0–14)
Potter & Rothstein[31]	43.7% agreement	NT	NT	NA	NA	NA	NA
Comments: The test appears to lack reliability. Agreement is not chance corrected, meaning that the findings could be related to luck versus skill of the examination.							

TESTS FOR SACROILIAC PAIN ORIGIN

Standing PSIS Asymmetry

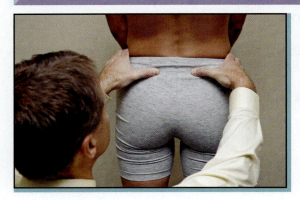

1. The patient is placed in standing.

2. Using the iliac crests as a guide, the examiner measures the symmetry of the iliac crests, then the PSIS.

3. A positive test is characterized by asymmetry.

UTILITY SCORE   3

Study	Reliability	Sensitivity	Specificity	LR+	LR−	DOR	QUADAS Score (0–14)
Levangie[23]	.70	79	29	1.11	0.72	1.5	11
Rost et al.[33]	NT	55.8	NT	NA	NA	NA	7
Potter & Rothstein[31]	35.2% agreement	NT	NT	NA	NA	NA	NA

Comments: Based on Levangie's[23] findings, this test actually provides little value during the examination and certainly does not qualify as a screening tool.

TESTS FOR SACROILIAC PAIN ORIGIN

Seated PSIS Asymmetry

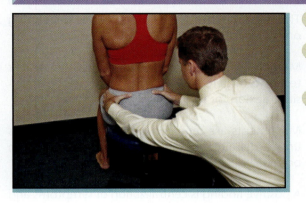

1 The patient sits in front of the examiner.

2 Using the iliac crests as a guide, the examiner evaluates the symmetry of the PSIS.

3 A positive test is characterized by asymmetry.

UTILITY SCORE 3

Study	Reliability	Sensitivity	Specificity	LR+	LR−	DOR	QUADAS Score (0–14)
Levangie[22]	.63	69	22	.88	1.4	0.62	11
Potter & Rothstein[31]	35.2% agreement	NT	NT	NA	NA	NA	NA

Comments: Based on Levangie's[22] findings, this test actually provides little value during the examination and certainly does not qualify as a screening tool.

TESTS FOR SACROILIAC PAIN ORIGIN

Centralization

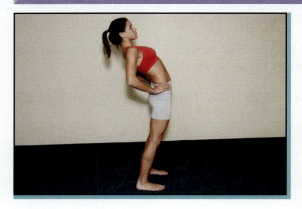

1. The patient either stands or lies prone depending on the intent of a loaded or unloaded assessment.

2. Multiple directions of repeated end-range lumbar testing is targeted. Movements may include extension, flexion, or side flexion.

3. Movements are repeated up to 5 to 20 attempts until a definite centralization or peripheralization occurs.

4. A positive finding is centralization of symptoms and is generally considered a low back dysfunction.

UTILITY SCORE 3

Study	Reliability	Sensitivity	Specificity	LR+	LR−	DOR	QUADAS Score (0–14)
Young et al.[40]	NT	9	79	.42	1.2	0.37	10

Comments: Centralization is defined as the progressive retreat of referred pain toward the midline of the back in response to standardized movement testing during evaluation of the effect of repeated movements on pain location and intensity. The test is sometimes used to rule out the presence of SIJ dysfunction, since the test exhibits strong diagnostic value for lumbar spine dysfunction.

TESTS FOR SACROILIAC PAIN ORIGIN

Piedallus Test

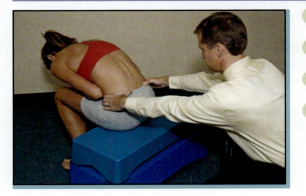

1. The patient sits on a hard surface.

2. The examiner palpates the levels of the PSIS.

3. The patient is instructed to flex forward.

4. Asymmetry in the PSIS is considered a positive finding.

UTILITY SCORE 3

Study	Reliability	Sensitivity	Specificity	LR+	LR−	DOR	QUADAS Score (0–14)
Albert et al.[1]	.0 kappa	14–69	98	35	0.9–0.87	7.9–109	7

Comments: This test differs from the Sitting Bend Over Test in that the surface used for sitting is hard instead of soft. Like other palpatory tests, this examination lacks reliability.

TESTS FOR SACROILIAC PAIN ORIGIN

Sacroiliac Joint Palpation

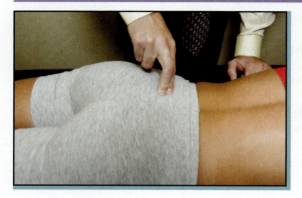

1) The patient is placed in a prone position.

2) The examiner carefully palpates the sacrum, bilateral sacroiliac joints, and surrounding ligaments and muscles.

3) A positive test is associated with local tenderness with moderately deep palpation.

UTILITY SCORE 3

Study	Reliability	Sensitivity	Specificity	LR+	LR−	DOR	QUADAS Score (0–14)
Hansen et al.[16] (Sacroiliac Joint)	NT	86	92	10.8	0.15	72	7
Hansen et al.[16] (Sacrotuberous Ligament)	NT	33	86	2.4	0.78	3.1	7
Hansen et al.[16] (Piriformis)	NT	62	97	20.7	0.39	53.1	7
Hansen et al.[16] (Paravertebral Muscles)	NT	43	84	2.7	0.68	3.9	7
Hansen et al.[16] (Glutei Muscles)	NT	33	97	11	0.69	15.9	7
Hansen et al.[16] (Iliopsoas)	NT	43	81	2.26	0.7	3.2	7
Albert et al.[1] (Long Dorsal Ligament)	.34 Kappa	11 to 49	100	NA	NA	NA	7
Dreyfuss et al.[17]	NT	95	9	1.04	.55	1.88	10

Comments: A positive test is identified by reproduction of the patient's concordant pain during palpation of the long dorsal ligament, surrounding sacroiliac ligaments, or other related structures. Regarding Dreyfuss et al.[17] findings, the test may be useful as an initial screen. This test deserves further study and better designs.

TESTS FOR SACROILIAC PAIN ORIGIN

Laguere's Sign

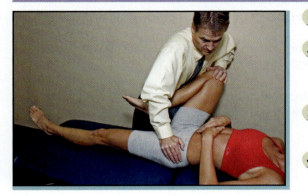

1 The patient is placed in a supine position.

2 The examiner applies a passive force into flexion, abduction, and external rotation at the hip. Overpressure is applied in this position.

3 The examiner stabilizes the opposite side by applying a downward force on the pelvis.

4 A positive test was replication of concordant symptoms during the testing.

UTILITY SCORE ?

Study	Reliability	Sensitivity	Specificity	LR+	LR−	DOR	QUADAS Score (0–14)
Magee[24]	NT	NT	NT	NA	NA	NA	NA
Comments: Expect to see many false positives in patients with hip pathology.							

Mazion's Pelvic Maneuver (Standing Lunge Test)

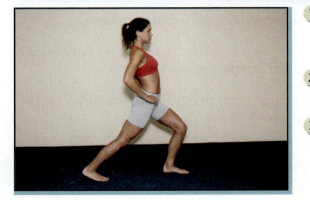

1 The patient stands in a straddle position with the unaffected side forward. The feet need to be 2–3 feet apart (pictured).

2 The patient bends forward in an attempt to touch the floor until the heel of the rear foot rises.

3 If pain is reproduced on the affected side, the test is considered positive.

UTILITY SCORE ?

Study	Reliability	Sensitivity	Specificity	LR+	LR−	DOR	QUADAS Score (0–14)
Evans[12]	NT	NT	NT	NA	NA	NA	NA
Comments: Essentially, this is a test of torque on the affected (rear) side.							

TESTS FOR SACROILIAC PAIN ORIGIN

Prone Distraction Test

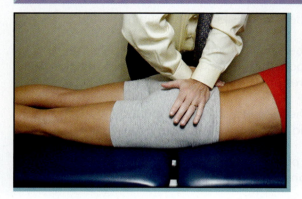

1 The patient assumes a prone position.

2 The examiner applies a compressive force over the PSIS of the patient.

3 Reproduction of concordant symptoms is considered a positive test.

UTILITY SCORE **?**

Study	Reliability	Sensitivity	Specificity	LR+	LR−	DOR	QUADAS Score (0–14)
Not tested	NT	NT	NT	NA	NA	NA	NA
Comments: An uninvestigated test.							

Torsion Stress Test

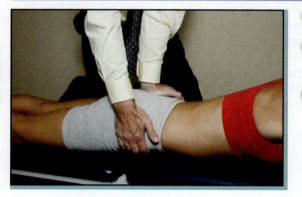

1 The patient assumes a prone position.

2 The examiner applies a downward force on the sacrum and pulls upward on the ASIS.

3 A positive test is pain reproduction during the torsion movement.

UTILITY SCORE **?**

Study	Reliability	Sensitivity	Specificity	LR+	LR−	DOR	QUADAS Score (0–14)
Not tested	NT	NT	NT	NA	NA	NA	NA
Comments: The position is sometimes used for manipulation of the sacroiliac joint.							

Squish Test

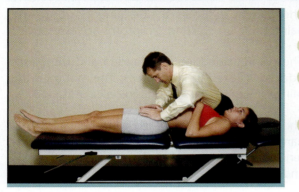

① The patient assumes a supine position.

② The examiner places both hands on the ASIS.

③ The examiner applies a downward and medial force on the ASIS.

④ Reproduction of concordant pain is considered a positive sign.

UTILITY SCORE ?

Study	Reliability	Sensitivity	Specificity	LR+	LR−	DOR	QUADAS Score (0–14)
Magee[24]	NT	NT	NT	NA	NA	NA	NA
Comments: The test position is sometimes used during mobilization of the ilium on the sacrum.							

TESTS FOR SACROILIAC PAIN ORIGIN

Passive Physiological Counternutation

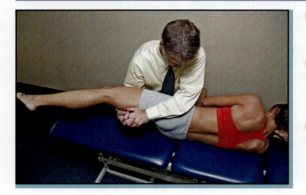

1 The patient assumes a side-lying position, the painful side up. Resting symptoms are assessed.

2 The painful sided leg is extended and the plinth side leg is flexed to 90 degrees. The motion is the mirror image of passive physiological nutation.

3 The examiner cradles the leg with the caudal side hand and encourages further movement into hip extension. The cranial side arm is placed on the PSIS and promotes anterior rotation of the innominate.

4 The patient's pelvis is passively moved to the first sign of concordant pain.

5 The examiner then moves the patient beyond the first point of pain toward end range. The patient's symptoms are reassessed for concordance.

6 If concordant pain is bilateral, the process is repeated on the opposite side.

UTILITY SCORE **?**

Study	Reliability	Sensitivity	Specificity	LR+	LR−	DOR	QUADAS Score (0–14)
Cook[8]	NT	NT	NT	NA	NA	NA	NA

Comments: The test position is also sometimes used as a treatment if pain recedes during movement.

Passive Physiological Nutation

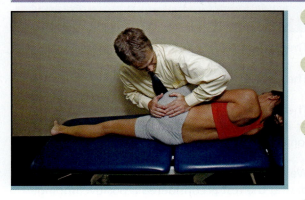

1. The patient assumes a side-lying position, the painful side up. Resting symptoms are assessed.

2. The painful-sided leg is flexed beyond 90 degrees to engage the pelvis and to promote passive physiological flexion.

3. The examiner then situates his or her body into the popliteal fold of the painful-sided leg to "snug up" the position. The plinth-sided leg remains in an extended position.

4. The examiner then places his or her hands on the ischial tuberosity and the ASIS to promote further physiological rotation. The patient's pelvis is passively moved to the first sign of concordant pain.

5. The examiner then moves the patient beyond the first point of pain toward end range. The patient's symptoms are reassessed for concordance.

6. If concordant pain is bilateral, the process is repeated on the opposite side.

UTILITY SCORE ?

Study	Reliability	Sensitivity	Specificity	LR+	LR−	DOR	QUADAS Score (0–14)
Cook[8]	NT	NT	NT	NA	NA	NA	NA
Comments: The test position is also sometimes used as a treatment if pain recedes during movement.								

TEST FOR SACROILIAC PAIN OR PUBIS SYMPHYSIS ORIGIN

Resisted Hip Adduction

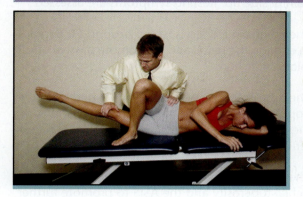

(1) The patient is placed in a sidelying position.

(2) The patient is instructed to lift the lower leg.

(3) The patient is instructed to push medially with his or her knee while the instructor applies a lateral force.

(4) Weakness of the hip adductors secondary to pain during the test is considered a positive finding.

UTILITY SCORE 3

Study	Reliability	Sensitivity	Specificity	LR+	LR−	DOR	QUADAS Score (0–14)
Mens et al.[29]	0.79 ICC	NT	NT	NA	NA	NA	NA
Rost et al.[33] (PPPP) (For Pain Reproduction)	NT	54	NT	NA	NA	NA	7
Blower & Griffen[3]	53% agreement	NT	92	NA	NA	NA	5
Comments: PPPP is pregnancy-related posterior pelvic pain. This test suffers from poor designs.							

TESTS FOR SACROILIAC DYSFUNCTION

Standing or Unilateral Standing

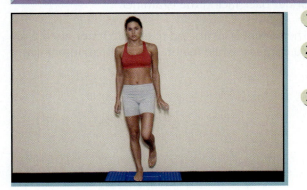

1 The patient assumes a standing position.

2 The patient is instructed to stand unilaterally on one leg.

3 Reproduction of pain at the pubis symphysis or the sacroiliac joint is considered a positive test.

UTILITY SCORE 2

Study	Reliability	Sensitivity	Specificity	LR+	LR−	DOR	QUADAS Score (0–14)
Hansen et al.[16] (Unilateral Standing)	NT	19	100	NA	NA	NA	7
Dreyfuss et al.[11] (Bilateral Standing)	NT	7	98	3.5	.95	3.7	10
Comments: Unilateral standing as a measure of sacroiliac pain lacks sensitivity and should not be used during screening.							

TESTS FOR SACROILIAC DYSFUNCTION

Gillet Test (Marching Test)

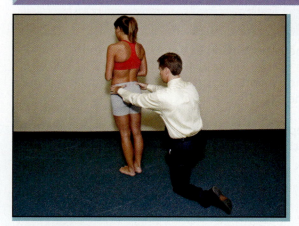

1 The patient stands in front of the examiners with his or her back facing the examiner.

2 The patient is instructed to elevate his or her hip to 90 degrees, while maintaining stance on one leg.

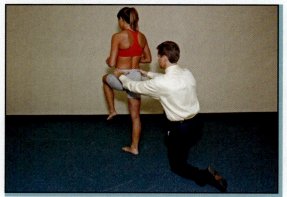

3 The examiner palpates both PSIS and evaluates whether the same-sided PSIS drops during hip flexion (a normal response) or rotates anteriorly (or superior in respect to the weight-bearing side).

4 If the PSIS does not drop or slides superiorly, the test is considered positive for that side.

UTILITY SCORE **3**

Study	Reliability	Sensitivity	Specificity	LR+	LR−	DOR	QUADAS Score (0–14)
Dreyfuss et al.[11]	.22	43	68	1.34	0.84	1.6	10
Carmichael et al.[6]	0.02	NT	NT	NA	NA	NA	NA
Levangie[23]	NT	8	93	1.07	0.99	1.1	10
Dreyfuss et al.[10]	NT	NT	84	NA	NA	NA	7
Meijne et al.[27]	0.08 kappa	NT	NT	NA	NA	NA	NA
Potter & Rothstein[31]	46.7% agreement	NT	NT	NA	NA	NA	NA

Comments: This test is purported to be a screen for sacroiliac dysfunction, but demonstrates poor reliability and has a very poor sensitivity.

TESTS FOR SACROILIAC DYSFUNCTION

Sitting Bend Over Test (Sitting Forward Flexion Test)

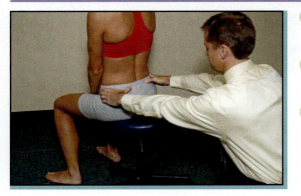

(1) The patient assumes a sitting position on a soft surface.

(2) The examiner palpates both PSIS (inferiorly) of the patient.

(3) The patient is instructed to bend forward toward the midline. Midline movement ensures equity of movement on the left and right.

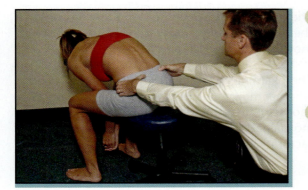

(4) The examiner palpates both PSIS and evaluates whether movements are symmetrical (a normal response) or asymmetrical. The test is repeated during palpation of the inferior lateral angle of the sacrum.

(5) A positive finding is asymmetry or palpable differences between PSIS and sacral movements.

UTILITY SCORE   3

Study	Reliability	Sensitivity	Specificity	LR+	LR−	DOR	QUADAS Score (0–14)
Riddle & Freburger[32]	.37	NT	NT	NA	NA	NA	NA
Dreyfuss et al.[10]	.22	3	90	0.3	1.08	0.3	10
Levangie[23]	NT	9	93	1.01	0.98	1.03	11
Dreyfuss et al.[10]	NT	NT	92	NA	NA	NA	7
Potter & Rothstein[31]	50% agreement	NT	NT	NA	NA	NA	NA
Comments: This test is purported to be a screen for sacroiliac dysfunction, but demonstrates poor sensitivity, poor reliability, and has a very poor diagnostic value. The test differs from the Piedallus test based on surface selection.							

TESTS FOR SACROILIAC DYSFUNCTION

Standing Bend Over Test (Standing Flexion Test)

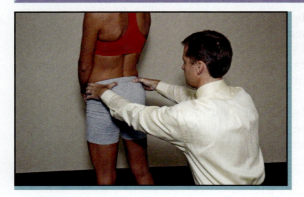

1 The patient assumes a standing position.

2 The examiner palpates both PSIS of the patient.

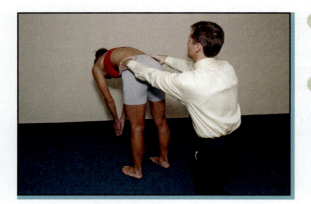

3 The patient is instructed to bend forward toward the midline. Midline movement ensures equity of movement on the left and right.

4 The examiner palpates both PSIS and evaluates whether movements are symmetrical (a normal response) or asymmetrical. The test is repeated during palpation of the inferior lateral angle of the sacrum.

UTILITY SCORE 3

Study	Reliability	Sensitivity	Specificity	LR+	LR−	DOR	QUADAS Score (0–14)
Vincent-Smith et al.[39]	0.05 kappa	NT	NT	NA	NA	NA	NA
Bowman and Gribbe[4]	0.23 kappa	NT	NT	NA	NA	NA	NA
Riddle & Freburger[32]	0.32 kappa	NT	NT	NA	NA	NA	NT
Levangie[23]	NT	17	79	0.81	1.05	0.77	11
Dreyfuss et al.[10]	NT	NT	87	NA	NA	NA	7
Potter & Rothstein[31]	43.7% agreement	NT	NT	NA	NA	NA	NA

Comments: This test is purported to be a screen for sacroiliac dysfunction, but demonstrates poor sensitivity and reliability, and has a very poor diagnostic value.

Long Sit Test (Leg Length Test)

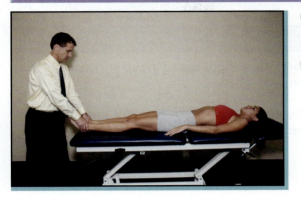

1 The patient is instructed to lie supine in a hooklying position.

2 The patient is instructed to bridge and return to hooklying. The examiner passively moves the knees into extension.

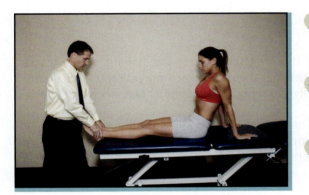

3 The examiner evaluates the leg length differences by assessing the comparative levels of the medial malleoli.

4 The patient is directed to sit up and the examiner again measures the comparative length of the malleoli.

5 If one leg moves further than another, the patient is considered to have a pelvic rotation.

UTILITY SCORE 3

Study	Reliability	Sensitivity	Specificity	LR+	LR−	DOR	QUADAS Score (0–14)
Riddle & Freburger[32]	0.19	NT	NT	NA	NA	NA	NA
Albert et al.[1]	0.06	NT	NT	NA	NA	NA	7
Levangie[23] (LS)	NT	44	64	1.37	0.88	1.56	10
Potter & Rothstein[31]	40% agreement	NT	NT	NA	NA	NA	NA
Bemis & Daniel[2]	NT	62	83	3.6	.46	7.9	7

Comments: Supine to sit of one malleolus from short to long is indicative of a posterior rotation of the innominate. Supine to sit of one malleolus from long to short is indicative of an anterior rotation of the innominate. Nonetheless, the test demonstrates poor reliability, questionable validity, and may not yield useful results. Bemis and Daniel[2] used a reference standard that does not reflect sacroiliac dysfunction.

TESTS FOR SACROILIAC PAIN ASSOCIATED WITH PREGNANCY-RELATED POSTERIOR PELVIC PAIN

Active Straight Leg Raise

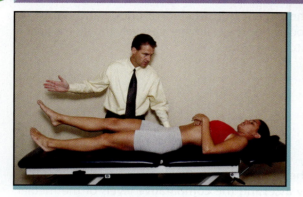

1. The patient is positioned in supine. Resting symptoms are assessed.

2. The patient is asked to raise the affected leg approximately 6 inches. Pain is queried.

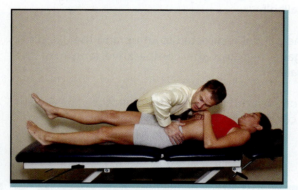

3. If the previous request was painful, the examiner stabilizes the pelvis by compressing the ASIS medially, or by placing a sacroiliac belt around the pelvis.

4. The patient is again asked to raise the affected leg approximately 6 inches. If the movement is no longer painful, the test is considered positive.

UTILITY SCORE 2

Study	Reliability	Sensitivity	Specificity	LR+	LR−	DOR	QUADAS Score (0–14)
Mens et al.[28]	0.82 ICC	87	94	14.5	0.13	111.5	8
Damen et al.[9]	NT	77	55	1.7	0.42	4.1	8
Rost et al.[33] (PPPP) (One-Sided Positive)	NT	51	NT	NA	NA	NA	7
Rost et al.[33] (PPPP) (Two-Sided Positive)	NT	15	NT	NA	NA	NA	7

Comments: PPPP is pregnancy-related posterior pelvic pain. The test appears to be useful with PPPP and is often graded in degrees of impairment. Past studies have shown that higher degrees of impairment (inability to perform) are associated with higher disability scores. As a whole, the studies that have examined this test are mediocre.

Prone Active Straight Leg Raise

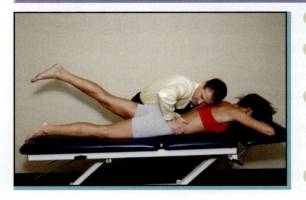

1 The patient assumes a prone position.

2 The patient performs hip extension and is queried for pain provocation.

3 The examiner compresses the innominates with his or hands or a belt and instructs the patient to repeat hip extension. If pain subsides, the test is considered positive.

4 The examiner may repeat the test by adding resistance to hip extension.

5 A positive test is pain during hip extension that decreases with stabilization of the innominate.

UTILITY SCORE ?

Study	Reliability	Sensitivity	Specificity	LR+	LR−	DOR	QUADAS Score (0–14)
Lee[21]	NT	NT	NT	NA	NA	NA	NA
Comments: Although described by Lee,[21] the examination procedure is untested.							

TEST FOR SYMPHYSIOLYSIS

Pubic Symphysis Palpation

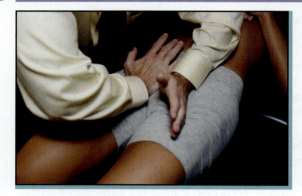

1 The patient is placed in a supine position.

2 The examiner palpates the pubic symphysis near midline.

3 An alternative involves a pubic shear force to the superior and inferior pubis bones (pictured).

4 A positive test is identified by reproduction of the patient's concordant pain.

UTILITY SCORE 1

Study	Reliability	Sensitivity	Specificity	LR+	LR−	DOR	QUADAS Score (0–14)
Albert et al.[1]	.89	81	99	4.68	0.19	24.6	7
Hansen et al.[16]	NT	76	94	12.7	0.26	48.8	7
Comments: This test appears useful in the diagnosis of symphysiolysis.							

TESTS FOR PELVIC RING FRACTURE

Posterior Pelvic Palpation

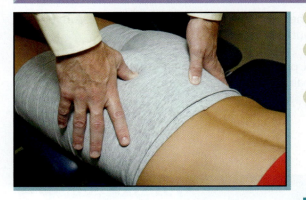

1 The patient is placed in a sitting or prone position.

2 The examiner carefully palpates the sacrum and bilateral sacroiliac joints.

3 A positive test is associated with local tenderness with moderately deep palpation.

UTILITY SCORE 1

Study	Reliability	Sensitivity	Specificity	LR+	LR−	DOR	QUADAS Score (0–14)
McCormick et al.[26]	NT	98	94	16.3	0.02	815	7

Comments: The test should only be considered positive if pain is concordant and if the patient exhibits historical information synonymous with a pelvis fracture. This finding is more compelling if swelling is also present.

Hip Flexon Test

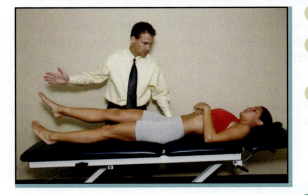

1 The patient is placed in a supine position.

2 The examiner instructs the patient to raise his or her leg actively (straight leg raise).

3 A positive test is associated with reproduction of pain during active movement or inability to raise the leg.

UTILITY SCORE 1

Study	Reliability	Sensitivity	Specificity	LR+	LR−	DOR	QUADAS Score (0–14)
Ham et al.[15]	NT	90	95	18	0.10	171	10

Comments: The test may be useful if the patient history suggests a pelvis fracture.

TESTS FOR PELVIC RING FRACTURE

Pubic Compression Test

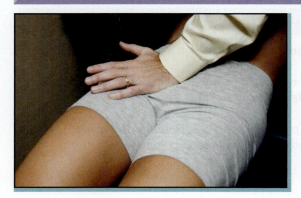

1. The patient is placed in a supine position.

2. The examiner applies a downward pressure on the pubic bones.

3. A positive test is associated with reproduction of pain during compression.

UTILITY SCORE 2

Study	Reliability	Sensitivity	Specificity	LR+	LR−	DOR	QUADAS Score (0–14)
Ham et al.[15]	NT	55	84	3.4	0.53	6.4	10

Comments: The test value was significantly associated with diagnosis. This test may be useful if patient history suggests a fracture.

Active Hip Range of Motion

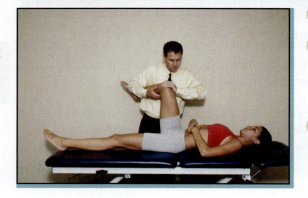

1. The patient is placed in a supine position.

2. The examiner performs a straight leg raise on each side, followed by passive hip flexion, abduction, adduction, internal rotation (pictured), and external rotation.

3. A positive test is associated with reproduction of pain during passive movement.

UTILITY SCORE 3

Study	Reliability	Sensitivity	Specificity	LR+	LR−	DOR	QUADAS Score (0–14)
McCormick et al.[26]	NT	53	76	2.2	0.62	3.5	7

Comments: The test value was significantly associated with diagnosis.

TEST FOR BURSITIS, TUMOR, OR ABSCESS OF THE BUTTOCK REGION

Sign of the Buttock

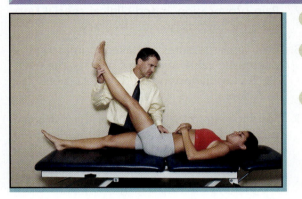

1. The patient lies supine.

2. The examiner passively performs a straight leg raise to the point of pain or restriction.

3. The examiner flexes the knee while holding the thigh in the same angle at the hip.

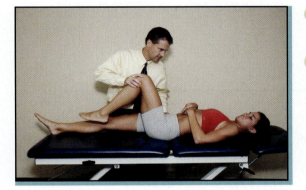

4. The examiner then applies further flexion to the hip.

5. If hip flexion is still restricted or results in the same pain as with the SLR, the finding is positive.

UTILITY SCORE ?

Study	Reliability	Sensitivity	Specificity	LR+	LR−	DOR	QUADAS Score (0–14)
Greenwood et al.[14]	NT	NT	NT	NA	NA	NA	NT
Comments: A positive finding is a red flag that suggests further workup is essential.							

Key Points

1. Clinical special tests of the sacroiliac joint as a whole demonstrate poor diagnostic accuracy and poor reliability.

2. Movement-based clinical special tests suffer from very poor reliability.

3. The movement-based clinical special tests that have demonstrated good diagnostic value were performed poorly.

4. Clusters of tests, once low back pain and other contributing disorders have been ruled out, appear to be more accurate than performing tests in singular fashion.

5. Almost all of the sacroiliac tests demonstrate poor sensitivity.

6. Tests that have not used double-blinded double injections as the reference standard have questionable validity. However, it is likely that extraarticular disorders of SIJ are missed with injections.

7. Pain provocation–based clinical special tests have the best diagnostic accuracy.

8. Even after measures are taken to improve the diagnostic value of clusters of tests, the overall LR+ for diagnosing SIJ disorders is only fair to moderate.

9. Tests to determine fractures of the pelvis are more accurate compared to those designed to measure pain of SIJ origin. Patient history should always be considered.

10. Pregnancy-related pelvic girdle pain is often diagnosed by using index tests, thus reducing the validity of the reference standard.

References

1. Albert H, Godskesen M, Westergaard J. Evaluation of clinical tests used in classification procedures in pregnancy-related pelvic joint pain. *Eur Spine J.* 2000;9(2):161–166.

2. Bemis T, Daniel M. Validation of the long sitting test on patients with iliosacral dysfunction. *J Orthop Sports Phys Ther.* 1987;8:336–343.

3. Blower P, Griffin A. (abstract). Clinical sacroiliac tests in ankylosing spondylitis and other causes of low back pain—2 studies. *Annales of Rheumatic Disorders.* 1984;43:192–195.

4. Bowman C, Gribbe R. The value of the forward flexion test and three tests of leg length changes in the clinical assessment of the movement of the sacroiliac joint. *J Orthopaedic Med.* 1995;17:66–67.

5. Broadhurst NA, Bond MJ. Pain provocation tests for the assessment of sacroiliac joint dysfunction. *J Spinal Disord.* 1998;11(4):341–345.

6. Carmichael J. Inter- and intra-examiner reliability of palpation for sacroiliac joint dysfunction. *J Manipulative Physiol Therapeutics.* 1987;10:164–171.

7. Cibulka MT, Koldehoff R. Clinical usefulness of a cluster of sacroiliac joint tests in patients with and without low back pain. *J Orthop Sports Phys Ther.* 1999;29(2):83–89.

8. Cook C. *Orthopedic manual therapy: An evidence based approach.* Upper Saddle River, NJ: Prentice Hall Publishing; 2007.

9. Damen L, Buyruk HM, Guler-Uysal F, Lotgering FK, Snijders CJ, Stam HJ. The prognostic value of asymmetric laxity of the sacroiliac joints in pregnancy-related pelvic pain. *Spine.* 2002;27(24):2820–2824.

10. Dreyfuss P, Dreyer S, Griffin J, Hoffman J, Walsh N. Positive sacroiliac screening tests in asymptomatic adults. *Spine.* 1994;19(10):1138–1143.

11. Dreyfuss P, Michaelsen M, Pauza K, McLarty J, Bogduk N. The value of medical history and physical examination in diagnosing sacroiliac joint pain. *Spine*. 1996;21(22):2594–2602.

12. Evans RC. *Illustrated essentials in orthopedic physical assessment*. St. Louis, MO: Mosby Publishing; 1994.

13. Fortin FJ, Falco JD. The Fortin finger test: an indicator of sacroiliac pain. *Am J Orthop*. 1997; 26(7):477–480.

14. Greenwood MJ, Erhard RE, Jones DL. Differential diagnosis of the hip vs. lumbar spine: five case reports. *J Orthop Sports Phys Ther*. 1998; 27(4):308–315.

15. Ham SJ, van Walsum DP, Vierhout PAM. Predictive value of the hip flexion test for fractures of the pelvis. *Injury*. 1996;27:543–544.

16. Hansen A, Jensen DV, Larsen EC, Wilken-Jensen C, Kaae BE, Frolich S, Thomsen JS, Hansen TM. Postpartum pelvic pain—the "pelvic joint syndrome": a follow-up study with special reference to diagnostic methods. *Acta Obstet Gynecol Scand*. 2005;84(2):170–176.

17. Kokmeyer DJ, Van der Wurff P, Aufdemkampe G, Fickenscher TC. The reliability of multitest regimens with sacroiliac pain provocation tests. *J Manipulative Physiol Ther*. 2002;25(1): 42–48.

18. Laslett M, Aprill C, McDonald B, Young S. Diagnosis of sacroiliac joint pain: validity of individual provocation tests and composites of tests. *Man Ther*. 2005;10:207–218.

19. Laslett M, Williams M. The reliability of selected pain provocation tests for sacroiliac joint pathology. *Spine*. 1994;19(11):1243–1249.

20. Laslett M, Young SB, Aprill CN, McDonald B. Diagnosing painful sacroiliac joints: A validity study of a McKenzie evaluation and sacroiliac provocation tests. *Aust J Physiotherapy*. 2003; 49:89–97.

21. Lee D. *The pelvic girdle*. 2nd ed. Edinburgh, UK: Churchill Livingston; 1999.

22. Levangie PK. The association between static pelvic asymmetry and low back pain. *Spine*. 1999;24(12):1234–1242.

23. Levangie PK. Four clinical tests of sacroiliac joint dysfunction: the association of test results with innominate torsion among patients with and without low back pain. *Phys Ther*. 1999; 79(11):1043–1057.

24. Magee D. *Orthopedic physical assessment*. 4th edition. Philadelphia: Saunders; 2002.

25. McCombe P, Fairbank J, Cockersole B, Pynesent P. Reproducibility of physical signs in low back pain. *Spine*. 1989;14:908–917.

26. McCormick JP, Morgan SJ, Smith WR. Clinical effectiveness of the physical examination in diagnosis of posterior pelvic ring injuries. *J Orthop Trauma*. 2003;17(4):257–261.

27. Meijne W, van Neerbos K, Aufdemkampe G, van der Wurff P. Intraexaminer and interexaminer reliability of the Gillet test. *J Manipulative Physiol Ther*. 1999;22:4–9.

28. Mens JM, Vleeming A, Snijders CJ, Koes BW, Stam HJ. Validity of the active straight leg raise test for measuring disease severity in patients with posterior pelvic pain after pregnancy. *Spine*. 2002a;27(2):196–200.

29. Mens JM, Vleeming A, Snijders CJ, Ronchetti I, Stam HJ. Reliability and validity of hip adduction strength to measure disease severity in posterior pelvic pain since pregnancy. *Spine*. 2002b;27(15):1674–1679.

30. Ostgaard H, Andersson G. Previous back pain and risk of developing back pain in future pregnancy. *Spine*. 1991;16:432–436.

31. Potter NA, Rothstein JM. Intertester reliability for selected clinical tests of the sacroiliac joint. *Phys Ther*. 1985;65(11):1671–1675.

32. Riddle DL, Freburger JK. Evaluation of the presence of sacroiliac joint region dysfunction using a combination of tests: a multicenter intertester reliability study. *Phys Ther*. 2002; 82(8):772–781.

33. Rost CC, Jacqueline J, Kaiser A, Verhagen AP, Koes BW. Pelvic pain during pregnancy: a descriptive study of signs and symptoms of 870 patients in primary care. *Spine*. 2004;29(22): 2567–2572.

34. Russell A, Maksymovich W, LeClerq S. Clinical examination of the sacroiliac joints: a prospective study. *Arthritis Rheumatism.* 1981;24: 1575–1577.

35. Slipman C, Jackson H, Lipetz J. Sacroiliac joint pain referral zones. *Arch Phys Med Rehab.* 2000;81:334–338.

36. Strender L, Sjoblom A, Sundell K, Ludwig R, Taube A. Interexaminer reliability in physical examination of patients with low back pain. *Spine.* 1997;22:814–820.

37. van der Wurff P, Buijs EJ, Groen GJ. A multitest regimen of pain provocation tests as an aid to reduce unnecessary minimally invasive sacroiliac joint procedures. *Arch Phys Med Rehabil.* 2006;87(1):10–14.

38. van Deursen L, Oatijn J, Ockhuysen A, Vortman B. The value of some clinical tests of the sacroiliac joint. *Man Med.* 1990;5:96–99.

39. Vincent-Smith B, Gibbons P. Inter-examiner and intra-examiner reliability of the standing flexion test. *Man Ther.* 1999;4(2):87–93.

40. Young S, Aprill C, Laslett M. Correlation of clinical examination characteristics with three sources of chronic low back pain. *Spine J.* 2003; 3(6):460–465.

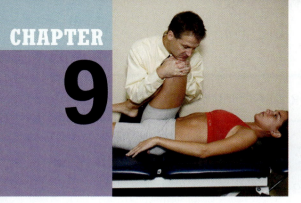

Physical Examination Tests for the Hip

TESTS FOR HIP LABRUM TEAR OR DEGENERATION

Patient History—Clicking or Locking

(1) The patient is queried regarding pain during sitting.

(2) The patient is queried regarding clicking or popping during gait, squatting, or other activities.

(3) A positive test is present if a click is present during active or passive motion of the hip.

UTILITY SCORE 3

Study	Reliability	Sensitivity	Specificity	LR+	LR−	DOR	QUADAS Score (0–14)
Dorrell & Catterall[8]	NT	50	NT	NA	NA	NA	6
Narvani et al.[16]	NT	100	85	NA	NA	NA	7

Comments: Most authors use click and catch synonymously. Essentially, the study designs were so poor one cannot extrapolate the benefits of these findings.

Posterior Hip Labrum Test

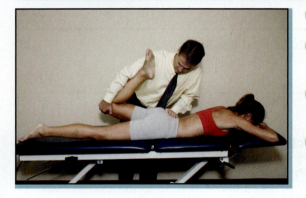

(1) The patient lies in a prone position.

(2) The examiner slowly moves the hip on the painful side near full extension and moderate abduction.

(3) The examiner then applies a concurrent external hip rotation while completing the full extension.

(4) A positive test is identified by reproduction of the patient's concordant pain.

UTILITY SCORE 3

Study	Reliability	Sensitivity	Specificity	LR+	LR−	DOR	QUADAS Score (0–14)
Leuning et al.[11]	NT	22	NT	NA	NA	NA	8

Comments: Leuning et al.[11] only investigated patients with known hip labrum tears, thus the specificity of this test is unknown. It is likely that patients with tight anterior hip flexors will experience false positives with this test.

TESTS FOR HIP LABRUM, CAPSULITIS, OSTEOARTHRITIS, AND FEMORAL ACETABULAR IMPINGEMENT SYNDROME

Hip Scour

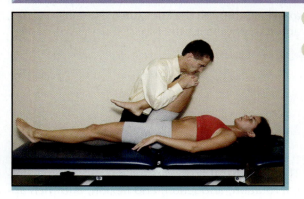

1 The patient assumes a supine position.

2 The examiner flexes the patient's knee and provides an axial load through the femur.

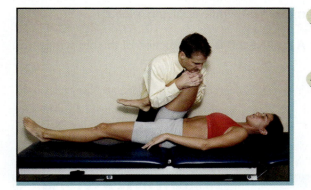

3 The examiner performs a sweeping compression and rotation movement from external rotation to internal rotation.

4 A positive test is pain or apprehension at a given point during the examination.

UTILITY SCORE 2

Study	Reliability	Sensitivity	Specificity	LR+	LR−	DOR	QUADAS Score (0–14)
Narvani et al.[16]	NT	75	43	1.3	0.58	2.24	7
Klaue et al.[10]	NT	NT	NT	NA	NA	NA	7
Leuning et al.[11]	NT	91	NT	NA	NA	NA	8
Mitchell et al.[15]	NT	NT	NT	NA	NA	NA	7
Comments: Many other studies used this test as a screening tool to identify potential cases of hip labrum tears. The sensitivity values of this test are higher than the Hip Quadrant test (page 262), although the study designs are poor.							

TESTS FOR HIP, LABRUM, CAPSULITIS, OSTEOARTHRITIS, AND FEMORAL ACETABULAR IMPINGEMENT SYNDROME

Hip Quadrant

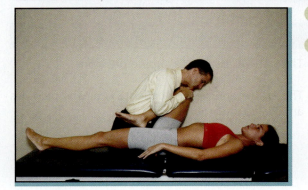

1. The patient assumes a supine position.

2. The examiner flexes the patient's knee, provides an axial load through the knee, then externally rotates, abducts, and flexes the hip.

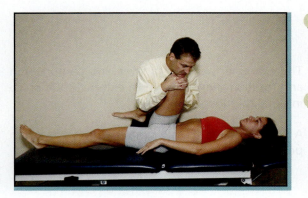

3. The examiner then lowers the hip away from external rotation, abduction, and flexion, and then applies an internal rotation, adduction, and flexion movement, while applying a load.

4. A positive test is reproduction of the hip symptoms.

UTILITY SCORE 3

Study	Reliability	Sensitivity	Specificity	LR+	LR−	DOR	QUADAS Score (0–14)
Suenaga et al.[17]	NT	79	50	1.6	0.42	3.81	6

Comments: The Hip Quadrant differs from the Hip Scour in that the quadrant does not compress the acetabular rim during movement from abduction to adduction. Suenaga et al.[17] indicated that a partial tear of the labrum was the only positive finding.

TESTS FOR A TEAR OF THE GLUTEUS MEDIUS OF THE HIP

Trendelenburg's Sign

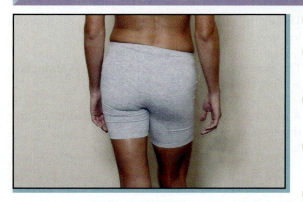

1. The patient stands in front of the examiner.

2. The examiner instructs the patient to stand on one leg.

3. The examiner evaluates the degree of drop of the contralateral pelvis once the leg is lifted.

4. Confirmation of abnormal pelvic drop is required during gait.

5. A positive test is identified by an asymmetric drop of one hip compared to the other during single stance.

UTILITY SCORE 2

Study	Reliability	Sensitivity	Specificity	LR+	LR−	DOR	QUADAS Score (0–14)
Bird et al.[4]	.676 kappa	73	77	3.15	.355	8.86	11

Comments: The test is performed in standing and confirmed during gait observation. In essence, the study is neither sensitive nor specific, although the likelihood ratio is fair. It is likely that significant weakness of the gluteus medius will present similiar to a tear.

TESTS FOR A TEAR OF THE GLUTEUS MEDIUS OF THE HIP

Resisted Hip Abduction

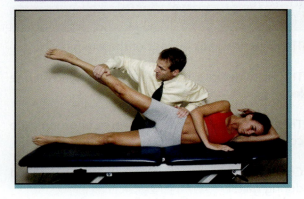

1. The patient is placed in a sidelying position.

2. The examiner instructs the patient to abduct the leg to 45 degrees.

3. The examiner applies force, resisting hip abduction against the leg.

4. A positive test is replication of symptoms during the testing.

UTILITY SCORE 3

Study	Reliability	Sensitivity	Specificity	LR+	LR−	DOR	QUADAS Score (0–14)
Bird et al.[4]	.625 kappa	73	46	1.35	0.59	2.29	11

Comments: Weakness is not a positive finding for the test. The poor specificity may be related to the myriad of other disorders such as hip bursitis or abductor tendonitis that would also be painful during this procedure.

TESTS FOR A TEAR OF THE GLUTEUS MEDIUS OF THE HIP

Passive Internal Rotation

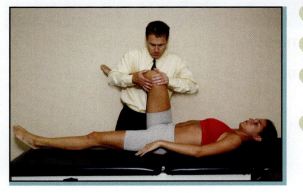

1. The patient lies in a supine position.

2. The hip is passively flexed to 90 degrees.

3. The examiner passively moves the hip into internal rotation.

4. A positive test is identified by reproduction of the patient's concordant pain (for a tear) or substantial limitation of internal rotation (for osteoarthritis).

UTILITY SCORE 3

Study	Reliability	Sensitivity	Specificity	LR+	LR−	DOR	QUADAS Score (0–14)
Bird et al.[4]	.027 kappa	55	69	1.77	0.66	2.69	11
Brown et al.[6] (Pain during IR)	NT	61	NT	NA	NA	NA	11
Brown et al.[6] (Limitation during IR)	NT	72	NT	NA	NA	NA	11
Comments: Note the only fair sensitivity, suggesting that this test is not appropriate as a screen. A tear is typically associated with pain, whereas limitations are associated with osteoarthritis.							

TESTS FOR OSTEOARTHRITIS

Range of Motion Planes

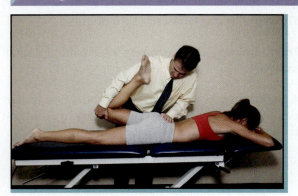

1. The patient lies in a prone position.

2. The examiner passively moves the hip into extension.

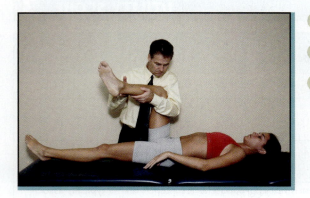

1. The patient lies in a supine position.

2. The hip is passively flexed to 90 degrees.

3. The examiner passively moves the hip into external rotation.

TESTS FOR OSTEOARTHRITIS

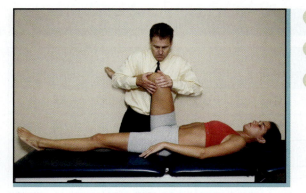

1 The patient lies in a supine position.

2 The hip is passively flexed to 90 degrees.

3 The examiner passively moves the hip into internal rotation.

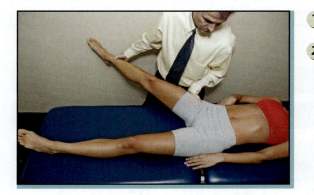

1 The patient lies in a supine position.

2 The examiner passively moves the hip into abduction.

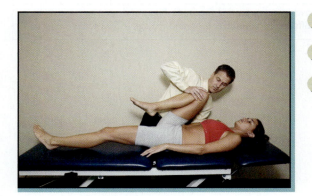

1 The patient lies in a supine position.

2 The examiner passively moves the hip into flexion.

3 A positive test is identified by reproduction of the patient's concordant pain concurrently during documented range of motion loss in comparison to the opposite extremity.

(*continued*)

TESTS FOR OSTEOARTHRITIS

UTILITY SCORE 2

Study	Reliability	Sensitivity	Specificity	LR+	LR−	DOR	QUADAS Score (0–14)
Birrell et al.[5] (0 planes)	NT	100	0	NA	NA	NA	8
Birrell et al.[5] (1 plane)	NT	100	42	NA	NA	NA	8
Birrell et al.[5] (2 planes)	NT	81	69	2.61	0.28	9.49	8
Birrell et al.[5] (3 planes)	NT	54	88	4.5	0.52	8.6	8

Comments: Specificity only increases to a good value if three planes or more are restricted. Note that a capsular pattern is not used as it has not shown predictability in patients with osteoarthritis.

Combined Results

UTILITY SCORE 2

Study	Reliability	Sensitivity	Specificity	LR+	LR−	DOR	QUADAS Score (0–14)
Altman et al.[2]	NT	86	75	3.4	0.19	18.4	8

Comments: Clinical diagnosis was used, which included the following index testing methods. Signs and symptoms involve (1) hip pain, (2) IR < 15 degrees, (3) pain with IR, (4) morning stiffness up to 60 minutes, and (5) age > 50 years.

TEST FOR ILIOTIBIAL BAND RESTRICTION

Ober Test

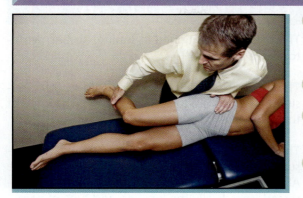

(1) The patient lies sidelying. The symptomatic leg is placed upward; the asymptomatic leg is placed on the plinth side.

(2) The examiner prepositions the knee into flexion.

(3) The examiner then stabilizes the pelvis at the iliac crest.

(4) The examiner then guides the lower extremity (at the hip) into extension and slight abduction.

(5) Using a goniometer or inclinometer, the examiner then measures the degree of abduction or adduction.

(6) A comparison of both sides is warranted.

(7) A positive test is failure of the knee to drop to the plinth and is indicative of tightness of structures.

UTILITY SCORE ?

Study	Reliability	Sensitivity	Specificity	LR+	LR−	DOR	QUADAS Score (0–14)
Melchione & Sullivan[13]	.94 ICC	NT	NT	NA	NA	NA	NT

Comments: This extremely common technique is untested for diagnostic value. Melchione and Sullivan[12] improve the reliability by attaching a level to the spine to maintain pelvis position. They used a goniometer to measure the angle at the hip. The test can be repeated with the knee in extension or slight flexion.

TESTS FOR ANTERIOR OR LATERAL CAPSULAR RESTRICTION OR HIP FLEXOR TIGHTNESS

Flexion Abduction External Rotation (FABER) Test (Patrick Test)

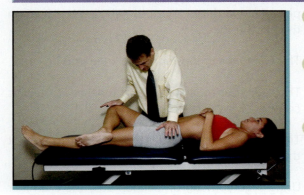

(1) The patient is positioned in supine. Resting symptoms are assessed.

(2) The painful side leg is placed in a "figure four" position. The ankle is placed just above the knee of the other leg.

(3) The examiner provides a gentle downward pressure on both the knee of the painful side and the ASIS of the nonpainful side. Concordant pain is assessed, specifically the location and type of pain.

(4) A positive test is concordant pain near the anterior or lateral capsule of the hip.

UTILITY SCORE 2

Study	Reliability	Sensitivity	Specificity	LR+	LR−	DOR	QUADAS Score (0–14)
Mitchell et al.[15]	NT	88	NT	NA	NA	NA	7

Comments: The FABER test is also a test for sacroiliac pain. Pain posteriorly is associated with sacroiliac dysfunction. The high sensitivity is suggestive of a screen, although the current study has demonstrated poor design.

TESTS FOR ANTERIOR OR LATERAL CAPSULAR RESTRICTION OR HIP FLEXOR TIGHTNESS

Thomas Test

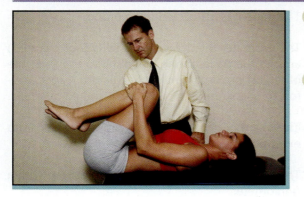

1 The patient sits at the edge of the plinth. The patient is then instructed to lie back, pulling both knees to his or her chest.

2 One knee (the asymptomatic side) is held to the chest and the other is slowly lowered into extension of the hip. The knee is allowed to extend.

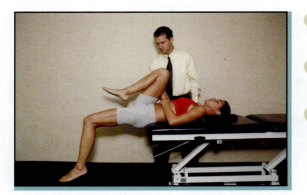

3 The patient is instructed to pull his or her pelvis into posterior rotation.

4 The examiner then uses a goniometer to measure the extension angle of the hip and/or the knee.

5 A positive test is significant tightness of the hip flexors of the extended leg.

UTILITY SCORE   3

Study	Reliability	Sensitivity	Specificity	LR+	LR−	DOR	QUADAS Score (0–14)
Narvani et al.[16]	NT	NT	NT	NA	NA	NA	7

Comments: This popular test is untested for diagnostic value. There are multiple suggested iterations of the test, none of which has been substantiated.

TESTS FOR ANTERIOR OR LATERAL CAPSULAR RESTRICTION OR HIP FLEXOR TIGHTNESS

Prone Hip Extension Test

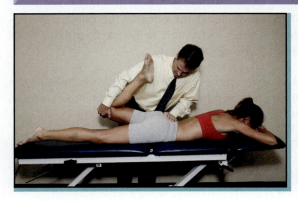

1. The patient is instructed to lie prone.

2. The examiner then places two belts (not pictured) around the patient: one just distal to the PSIS, the other just proximal to the gluteal fold. A special effort to unencumber hip extension should be made.

3. The examiner then passively moves the hip into extension.

4. The extension angle at the hip is measured with a goniometer.

5. A positive test is significant tightness of the hip flexors of the extended hip.

UTILITY SCORE ?

Study	Reliability	Sensitivity	Specificity	LR+	LR−	DOR	QUADAS Score (0–14)
None	NT	NT	NT	NA	NA	NA	NA

Comments: It is likely that other conditions (i.e., labral tear) that would also be positive in this position may hamper the test's specificity.

TESTS FOR EARLY SIGNS OF HIP DYSPLASIA

Passive Hip Abduction Test

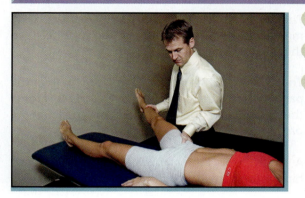

1 The patient assumes a supine position.

2 The examiner passively moves the hip into abduction.

3 A restriction of abduction as compared to the opposite side is considered a positive finding.

UTILITY SCORE 2

Study	Reliability	Sensitivity	Specificity	LR+	LR−	DOR	QUADAS Score (0–14)
Jari et al.[9]	NT	70	90	7.0	0.33	21	7
Castelein & Korte[7]	NT	69	54	1.5	0.57	2.61	5
Comments: Although the test designs were poor, this test does not appear overly sensitive but may be specific.							

TESTS FOR EARLY SIGNS OF HIP DYSPLASIA

Flexion Adduction Test

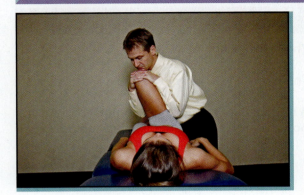

1 The patient assumes a supine position.

2 The examiner flexes the knee to 90 degrees while maintaining the contact of the patient's pelvis to the plinth.

3 The examiner attempts to adduct the thigh of the patient toward the opposite hip. Inability to adduct the hip passively beyond midline is considered a precursor to early hip disease.

4 A positive test is the inability to adduct the flexed hip past midline toward the opposite hip.

UTILITY SCORE 3

Study	Reliability	Sensitivity	Specificity	LR+	LR−	DOR	QUADAS Score (0–14)
Woods and Macnicol[19]	NT	100	NT	NA	NA	NA	3
Comments: The test was performed on adolescents and demonstrated many design flaws.							

TEST FOR FRACTURE OF THE HIP OR FEMUR

Patellar-Pubic Percussion Test

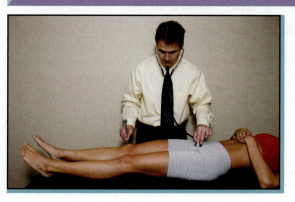

1 The patient assumes a supine position.

2 The examiner places a stethoscope over the pubic symphysis of the patient.

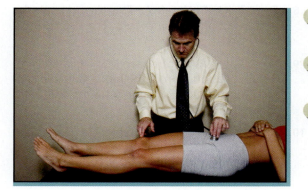

3 The examiner taps the patella of the patient's affected side and qualitatively reports the sound.

4 The examiner repeats the process on the opposite side to determine a difference in auscultation.

5 A positive test is a diminished percussion note on the side of pain and a negative test is no difference in percussion note. A tuning fork can be used in place of tapping.

UTILITY SCORE **1**

Study	Reliability	Sensitivity	Specificity	LR+	LR−	DOR	QUADAS Score (0–14)
Tiru et al.[18]	NT	96	86	6.73	.75	8.97	8
Adams & Yarnold[1]	89.2% agreement	94	95	20.4	.06	313.8	9
Bache & Cross[3]	NT	91	82	5.1	.11	46.1	8
Misurya et al.[14]	NT	89	NT	NA	NA	NA	5
Comments: Although the designs are not superb, this test does appear to have diagnostic value as a screening tool and as a diagnostic tool. The vibration testing appeared to demonstrate better results.							

Key Points

1. Clinical special tests of the hip are exceedingly understudied.

2. Most of the clinical special tests of the hip have been performed poorly and are hampered by internal bias.

3. The patellar-percussion test appears to be an effective screen and diagnostic tool for hip-related fractures.

4. The majority of hip labrum tests lack specificity and only display moderate to good sensitivity.

5. While assessment of loss of range of motion planes is an effective screen for osteoarthritis, the finding is not specific enough in absence of radiographic findings.

6. Clinical special tests such as the hip scour (quadrant) could potentially be positive for conditions such as hip labrum, capsulitis, osteoarthritis, and femoral acetabular impingement syndrome.

References

1. Adams S, Yarnold P. Clinical use of the patellar-pubic percussion sign in hip trauma. *Am J Emerg Med.* 1997;15:173–175.

2. Altman R, Alarcon G, Appelrouth D, Bloch D, Borenstein D, Brandt K, Brown C, Cooke TD, Daniel W, Feldman D, et al. The American College of Rheumatology criteria for the classification and reporting of osteoarthritis of the hip. *Arthritis Rheum.* 1991;34(5):505–514.

3. Bache JB, Cross AB. The Barford test: a useful diagnostic sign in fractures of the femoral neck. *Practitioner.* 1984;228(1389):305–308.

4. Bird PA, Oakley SP, Shnier R, Kirham BW. Prospective evaluation of magnetic resonance imaging and physical examination findings in patients with greater trochanteric pain syndrome. *Arthritis Rheumatism.* 2001;44: 2138–2145.

5. Birrell F, Croft P, Cooper C, Hosie G, Macfarlane G, Silman A. Predicting radiographic hip osteoarthritis from range of movement. *Rheumatology.* 2001;40:506–512.

6. Brown M, Gomez-Martin O, Brookfield K, Stokes P. Differential diagnosis of hip disease versus spine disease. *Clin Orthop.* 2004;419: 280–284.

7. Castelein RM, Korte J. Limited hip abduction in the infant. *J Ped Orthoped.* 2001;21:668–670.

8. Dorrell JH, Catterall A. The torn acetabular labrum. *J Bone Joint Surg Br.* 1986;68(3): 400–403.

9. Jari S, Paton RW, Srinivasan MS. Unilateral limitation of abduction of the hip: a valuable clinical sign for DDH? *J Bone Jnt Surg.* 2002;84: 104–107.

10. Klaue K, Durnin CW, Ganz R. The acetabular rim syndrome: a clinical presentation of dysplasia of the hip. *J Bone Jnt Surg.* 1991;73: 423–429.

11. Leuning M, Werlen S, Ungersbock A, Ito K, Ganz R. Evaluation of the acetabular labrum by MR arthrography. *J Bone Joint Surg Br.* 1997; 79(2):230–234.

12. Margo K, Drezner J, Motzkin D. Evaluation and management of hip pain: an algorithmic approach. *J Fam Pract.* 2003;52(8):607–617.

13. Melchione W, Sullivan S. Reliability of measurements obtained by use of an instrument designed to measure iliotibial band length indirectly. *J Orthop Sports Phys Ther.* 1993;18: 511–515.

14. Misurya RK, Khare A, Mallick A, Sural A, Vishwakarma GK. Use of tuning fork in diagnostic auscultation of fractures. *Injury.* 1987;18(1): 63–64.

15. Mitchell B, McCrory P, Burkner P, O'Donnell J, Colson E, Howells R. Hip joint pathology: clinical presentation and correlation between magnetic resonance arthrography, ultrasound, and arthroscopic findings. *Clin J Sport Med.* 2003;13:152–156.

16. Narvani A, Tsiridis E, Kendall S, Chaudhuri R, Thomas P. A preliminary report on prevalence of acetabular labrum tears in sports patients with groin pain. *Knee Surg Traumatol Arthrosc.* 2003;11:403–408.

17. Suenaga E, Noguchi Y, Jingushi S, Shuto T, Nakashima Y, Miyanishi K, Iwamoto Y. Relationship between the maximum flexion-internal rotation test and the torn acetabular labrum of a dysplastic hip. *J Orthop Sci.* 2002; 7:26–32.

18. Tiru M, Goh S, Low B. Use of percussion as a screening tool in the diagnosis of occult hip fractures. *Signapore Med J.* 2002;43:467–469.

19. Woods D, Macnicol M. The flexion-adduction test: an early sign of hip disease. *J Ped Orthop.* 2001:10:180–185.

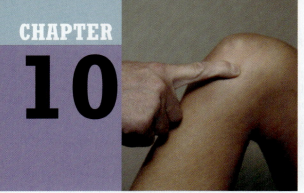

10

Physical Examination Tests for the Knee

Tests for Torn Posterior Cruciate Ligament (PCL) and Posterior Rotary Instability 313

Tests for Torn Collateral Ligament 332

Tests for Patellofemoral Dysfunction 335

Tests for Plica Syndrome 350

Tests for Proximal Tibiofibular Joint Instability 356

TESTS FOR FRACTURE AT THE KNEE

Ottawa Knee Decision Rule

Criteria
1. Age ≥ 55 years
2. Tenderness at the head of the fibula
3. Isolated tenderness of the patella
4. Inability to flex the knee to at least 90 degrees
5. Inability by the patient to bear weight both immediately and in the emergency department for four steps

1 A positive test is the presence of any one of the four characteristics and is an indication for referral for an x-ray to confirm fracture.

UTILITY SCORE **1**

Study	Reliability	Sensitivity	Specificity	LR+	LR−	DOR	QUADAS Score (0–14)
Jackson et al.[41]	NT	100	49	1.9	.11	NT	NA
Richman et al.[81]	NT	85	50	1.7	.30	5.7	12

Comments: The Jackson et al.[41] study reported diagnostic values based on the compilation of seven studies. Richman et al.[81] compared the Bauer et al.[12] criteria with the Ottawa[97,98,99] criteria in two hospitals: a community hospital and a tertiary care center. The Ottawa Knee Rule[97,98,99] is a valuable tool in the primary care setting to rule out a knee fracture.

TESTS FOR FRACTURE AT THE KNEE

Pittsburgh Knee Decision Rule

Criteria
1. Patient history of blunt trauma or a fall
2. Inability by the patient to bear weight both immediately and in the emergency department for four steps
3. Age younger than 12 or older than 50 years

(1) A positive test is a patient history of blunt trauma or fall and one of either the 2nd or 3rd criterion.

(2) A positive test is an indication to refer for an x-ray to confirm a fracture at the knee.

UTILITY SCORE 1

Study	Reliability	Sensitivity	Specificity	LR+	LR−	DOR	QUADAS Score (0–14)
Seaberg & Jackson[86]	NT	100	79	NA	NA	NA	11
Seaberg et al.[87]	NT	99	60	2.5	.02	125	11

Comments: The Pittsburgh Knee Rule[86] appears to be a valuable tool in the primary care setting to rule out a knee fracture but more research is needed.

TESTS FOR FRACTURE AT THE KNEE

Knee Decision Rule of Bauer

Criteria
1. Inability by the patient to bear weight both immediately and in the emergency department for four steps
2. Presence of knee effusion
3. Presence of ecchymosis

(1) A positive test is the presence of any one of the three characteristics and is an indication for referral for an x-ray to confirm fracture.

UTILITY SCORE 2

Study	Reliability	Sensitivity	Specificity	LR+	LR−	DOR	QUADAS Score (0–14)
Bauer et al.[12]	NT	100	63	NA	NA	NA	11
Richman et al.[81]	NT	85	49	1.7	.31	5.5	12

Comments: Not enough research has been performed to validate the decision rule of Bauer et al.,[12] the values of which are slightly lower than the two more established decision rules.

TESTS FOR A TORN TIBIAL MENISCUS

Composite Physical Exam

UTILITY SCORE 2

Study	Reliability	Sensitivity	Specificity	LR+	LR−	DOR	QUADAS Score (0–14)
Dervin et al.[21] (Fellows)	κ = .24	87	21	1.1	.62	1.8	11
(Orthopedic Staff)		88	20	1.5	.60	2.5	11
Rose & Gold[82] (Medial)	NT	92	60	2.3	.13	17.7	10
(Lateral)	NT	67	90	6.7	.37	18.1	10
Kocabey et al.[47] (Medial)	NT	87	68	2.7	.19	14.2	10
(Lateral)	NT	75	95	15.0	.26	57.7	10
Kocher et al.[48] (Medial)	NT	62	81	3.3	.47	7.0	11
(Lateral)	NT	50	89	4.5	.56	8.0	11
O'Shea et al.[77] (Medial)	NT	88	77	3.8	.16	23.8	9
(Lateral)	NT	51	90	5.1	.54	9.4	9
Jackson et al.[41] (Medial)	NT	86	72	3.1	.19	NT	NA
(Lateral)	NT	88	92	11.0	.13	NT	NA

Comments: The study by Dervin et al.[21] combined history, physical findings, special tests, and radiographic findings and although the level of agreement was fair, likelihood ratios would indicate that a composite physical examination is not an accurate predictor of an unstable torn meniscus in those with primary osteoarthritis of the knee. This article can make no conclusions about those with meniscus tears not related to chronic degeneration. The Kocher et al.[48] study would seem to indicate that there is small value in composite physical examination for meniscus tears in athletic children. The O'Shea et al.[77] study was performed only on male military personnel. Apparently, none of the physical examinations were performed in the acute stage of injury. The Jackson et al.[41] study is a meta-analysis and combines the data of 19 studies for the medial meniscus and 17 studies for the lateral meniscus. The data supplied by these authors would seem to suggest that in nonarthritis-related meniscus injuries, composite physical exam (including radiographs) for the lateral meniscus improves the posttest probability of detecting a torn lateral meniscus by a large amount and for the medial meniscus, a small amount.

TESTS FOR A TORN TIBIAL MENISCUS

McMurray's Test

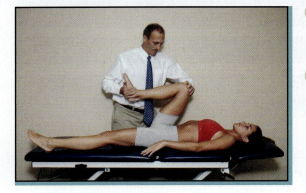

1 The patient assumes a supine position. The examiner stands to the side of the patient's involved knee.

2 The examiner grasps the patient's heel and flexes the knee to end range with one hand while using the thumb and index finger of the other hand to palpate the medial and lateral tibiofemoral joint line.

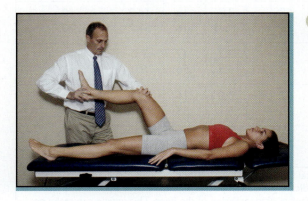

3 To test the medial meniscus, the examiner rotates the tibia into external rotation, then slowly extends the knee.

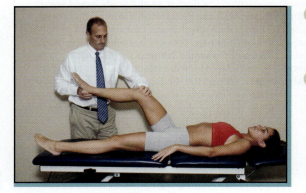

4 To test the lateral meniscus, the examiner reflexes the knee but now internally rotates the patient's tibia and slowly extends the knee.

5 A positive test traditionally is indicated by an audible or palpable "thud" or "click."

TESTS FOR A TORN TIBIAL MENISCUS

UTILITY SCORE 2

Study	Reliability	Sensitivity	Specificity	LR+	LR−	DOR	QUADAS Score (0–14)
Karachalios et al.[45] (Medial)	.95	48	94	8.0	.55	14.5	9
(Lateral)	.95	65	86	4.6	.41	11.2	9
Akseki et al.[2] (Medial)	NT	67	69	2.2	.48	4.6	11
(Lateral)	NT	53	88	4.4	.53	8.3	11
Kurosaka et al.[50] (Combined)	NT	37	77	1.6	.86	1.9	10
Corea et al.[18] (Medial)	NT	65	93	9.3	.38	24.5	7
(Lateral)	NT	52	94	8.7	.51	17.1	7
(Combined)	NT	59	93	8.4	.44	19.1	7
Evans et al.[24] (Medial)	κ = .35	16	98	8.0	.86	9.3	10
Dervin et al.[21]	κ = .16	NT	NT	NA	NA	NA	NA
Pookarnjanamorakot et al.[79] (Combined)	NT	28	92	3.5	.78	4.5	11
Saengnipanthkul et al.[84] (Medial)	NT	47	94	7.8	.56	13.9	8
Boeree & Ackroyd[13] (Medial)	NT	29	87	2.2	.82	2.7	9
(Lateral)	NT	25	90	2.5	.83	3.0	9
Fowler & Lubliner[28] (Combined)	κ = .25	29	96	7.3	.74	9.9	10
Anderson & Lipscomb[6] (Combined)	NT	58	29	.82	1.45	.57	9
Noble & Erat[74] (Combined)	NT	63	57	1.5	.65	2.3	9

Comments: McMurray's Test[68] has changed over the years and many examiners have added varus/valgus stress and used reproduction of joint line pain as another positive sign of meniscus tear. Generally speaking, whether trying to detect a torn medial meniscus, lateral meniscus, or a tear of either meniscus, McMurray's Test has some value as a specific test where a positive test would rule in the disease. However, the more recently performed studies have design flaws that make this conclusion tentative. Interobserver agreement in regard to the interpretation of McMurray's Test is generally fair.

TESTS FOR A TORN TIBIAL MENISCUS

Apley's Test

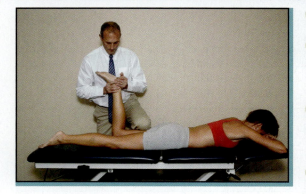

1. The patient lies prone.

2. The examiner half-kneels, placing his or her knee on the hamstring of the patient and flexes the knee to 90 degrees.

3. The examiner grasps the patient's foot with both hands, distracts the tibia, and rotates the tibia, noting whether or not pain is reproduced.

4. A positive test is indicated by worse pain with rotation and is indicative of a "rotation sprain" of soft tissue.

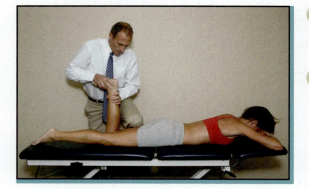

5. The examiner then leans on the patient's foot, providing a compressive force to the tibia and again rotates the tibia.

6. A positive test for a meniscus tear is indicated by more pain in compression than with distraction.

TESTS FOR A TORN TIBIAL MENISCUS

UTILITY SCORE **2**

Study	Reliability	Sensitivity	Specificity	LR+	LR−	DOR	QUADAS Score (0–14)
Karachalios et al.[45]							
(Medial)	.95	41	93	5.9	.63	9.4	9
(Lateral)	.95	41	86	2.9	.69	4.2	9
Kurosaka et al.[50] (Combined)	NT	13	90	1.3	.97	1.3	10
Fowler & Lubliner[28] (Combined)	NT	16	80	.80	1.1	.73	10
Pookarnjanamorakot et al.[79] (Combined)	NT	16	100	NA	NA	NA	11

Comments: The original description of Apley's[8] Test is a bit confusing with the narrative being different from the illustrations of the test. However, as originally described, distraction was the first force applied followed by compression force. Pain reproduced with distraction and rotation was diagnosed as a "rotation sprain" of soft tissue including collateral ligaments and/or capsule. The Karachalios et al.[45] study employs a case-control design, which dramatically overstates the diagnostic accuracy of a test. The remaining three studies seem to show, according to the likelihood ratios, that there is no value in Apley's Test to detect a torn meniscus. Some may find value in Apley's Test as a specific test to rule in a meniscus tear when positive.

TESTS FOR A TORN TIBIAL MENISCUS

Thessaly Test at 20 Degrees/Disco Test

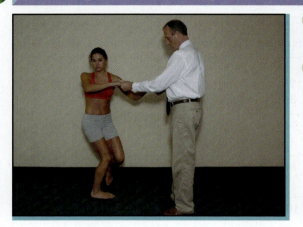

1 The patient stands on one leg facing the examiner and grasps the examiner's hands.

2 The patient flexes the knee to 20 degrees (partial squat) and rotates his or her body, first to the left and then to the right.

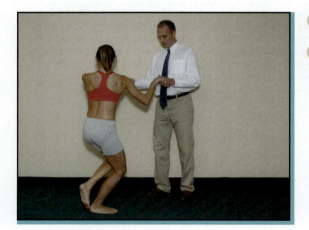

3 Step 2 is repeated three times in each direction.

4 A positive test for meniscus tear is indicated by joint-line discomfort and possibly a sense of locking or catching.

UTILITY SCORE **2**

Study	Reliability	Sensitivity	Specificity	LR+	LR−	DOR	QUADAS Score (0–14)
Karachalios et al.[45] (Medial)	.95	89	97	29.7	.11	270	9
(Lateral)	.95	92	96	23	.08	287.5	9

Comments: The Karachalios et al.[45] study employs a case-control design, which dramatically overstates the diagnostic accuracy of a test. Furthermore, the use in that study of MRI and not arthroscopy as a criterion standard may bias the results. More research needs to be performed to corroborate the statistics of the original authors. Losee[61] reported the use of this test (calling it the "Disco Test") to reproduce apprehension of the patient with a torn anterior cruciate ligament. No data is available on the Disco Test.

TESTS FOR A TORN TIBIAL MENISCUS

Thessaly Test at 5 Degrees

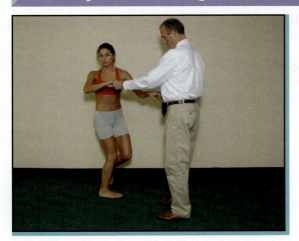

1 The patient stands on one leg facing the examiner and grasps the examiner's hands.

2 The patient flexes the knee to 5 degrees (partial squat) and rotates his or her body, first to the left and then to the right.

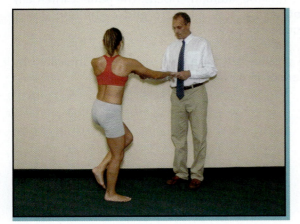

3 Step 2 is repeated three times in each direction.

4 A positive test for meniscus tear is indicated by joint-line discomfort and possibly a sense of locking or catching.

UTILITY SCORE 2

Study	Reliability	Sensitivity	Specificity	LR+	LR−	DOR	QUADAS Score (0–14)
Karachalios et al.[45] (Medial)	.95	66	96	16.5	.35	47.1	9
(Lateral)	.95	81	91	9.0	.21	42.9	9
Pookarnjanamorakot et al.[79] (Merke's—Combined)	NT	27	96	6.8	.76	8.9	11

Comments: The Karachalios et al.[45] study employs a case-control design, which dramatically overstates the diagnostic accuracy of a test. Furthermore, the use in that study of MRI and not arthroscopy as a criterion standard may bias the results. More research needs to be performed to corroborate the statistics of the original authors. This test, when performed in full knee extension, is sometimes referred to as Merke's Sign.

TESTS FOR A TORN TIBIAL MENISCUS

Ege's Test

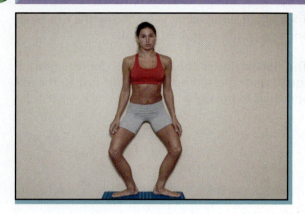

1 The patient stands with feet 30–40 cm from each other and knees in full extension.

2 To test the medial meniscus, the patient externally rotates the lower legs to end range and slowly squats then stands up.

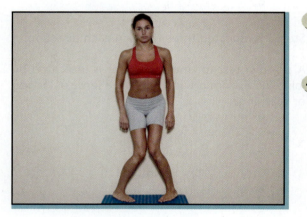

3 To test the lateral meniscus, the patient internally rotates the lower legs to end range and slowly squats then stands up.

4 A positive test for a torn meniscus is indicated by concordant pain and/or a click.

UTILITY SCORE 2

Study	Reliability	Sensitivity	Specificity	LR+	LR−	DOR	QUADAS Score (0–14)
Akseki et al.[2] (Medial)	NT	67	81	3.5	.41	8.5	11
(Lateral)	NT	64	90	6.4	.40	16	11

Comments: Ege's Test improves the posttest probability of detecting a torn meniscus by a small to moderate amount. Further research needs to be performed to corroborate the statistics reported in this study.

TESTS FOR A TORN TIBIAL MENISCUS

Axial Pivot-Shift Test

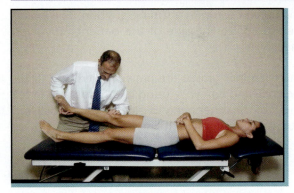

1 The patient is supine with the knee in full extension.

2 The examiner cradles the patient's leg and applies a valgus and internal rotation force to the proximal tibia.

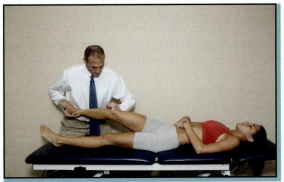

3 Axial compression is applied and the knee flexed to 30 and 45 degress of flexion.

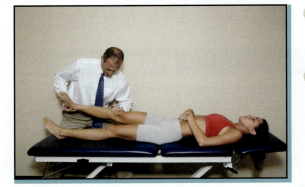

4 The valgus, internal rotation, and axial compression forces are maintained as the knee is returned to full extension.

5 A positive test for a torn meniscus is indicated by concordant joint line pain and/or a click felt by the examiner.

UTILITY SCORE 2

Study	Reliability	Sensitivity	Specificity	LR+	LR−	DOR	QUADAS Score (0–14)
Kurosaka et al.[50] (Combined)	NT	71	83	4.2	.35	12	10

Comments: The Axial Pivot-Shift Test improves the posttest probability of detecting a torn meniscus by a small amount in patients who have symptoms for longer than 8 weeks. More research is needed to confirm this conclusion.

TESTS FOR A TORN TIBIAL MENISCUS

Steinmann I Sign

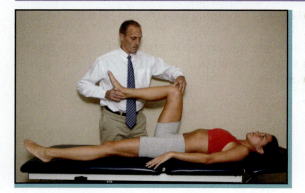

1. The patient assumes a supine position. The examiner stands to the side of the patient's involved knee.

2. The examiner grasps the patient's heel and flexes the knee and hip while using the thumb and index finger of the other hand to palpate the medial and lateral tibiofemoral joint line.

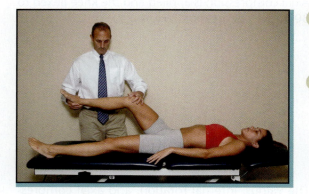

3. The examiner internally and externally rotates the tibia at various degrees of knee flexion but the knee should not be moving with any part of the test.

4. A positive test for a meniscus tear is indicated by joint-line pain.

UTILITY SCORE 2

Study	Reliability	Sensitivity	Specificity	LR+	LR−	DOR	QUADAS Score (0–14)
Dervin et al.[21]	κ = .05	NT	NT	NA	NA	NA	NA
Pookarnjanamorakot et al.[79]	NT	29	100	NA	NA	NA	11

Comments: The one study to examine the diagnostic accuracy of the Steinmann I Sign indicates a perfectly specific test that would rule in a meniscus tear if positive. However, the lack of interobserver agreement of this test and the fact that only one study has examined this test make any conclusions about diagnostic accuracy tentative.

TESTS FOR A TORN TIBIAL MENISCUS

 Dynamic Test

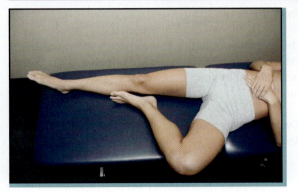

1 The patient is supine with the hip abducted 60 degrees, flexed, and externally rotated 45 degrees; the knee is flexed to 90 degrees, the lateral border of the foot resting on the examination table.

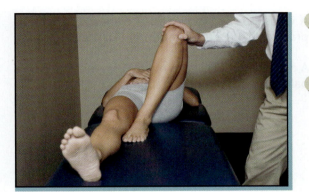

2 The examiner palpates the lateral joint-line then slowly adducts the hip while maintaining the knee in 90 degrees of flexion.

3 A positive test for a torn lateral meniscus is indicated by either an increase of pain above that elicited by lateral joint-line palpation or a sharp pain at the end of hip adduction.

UTILITY SCORE 2

Study	Reliability	Sensitivity	Specificity	LR+	LR−	DOR	QUADAS Score (0–14)
Mariani et al.[64] (Lateral)	κ = .61–.85	85	90	8.5	.17	50	9

Comments: The Dynamic Test has moderate diagnostic accuracy and the interobserver agreement is substantial. Further research needs to be performed to corroborate the statistics reported in this study.

TESTS FOR A TORN TIBIAL MENISCUS

Medial-Lateral Grind Test

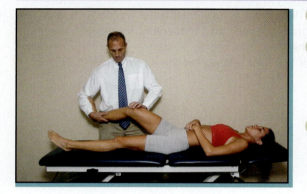

1 The patient is supine.

2 The examiner cradles the patient's affected lower extremity in one hand and, using the thumb and index finger, palpates the anterior tibiofemoral joint line.

3 A valgus stress is applied as the knee is flexed to 45 degrees.

4 A varus stress is applied as the knee is extended, producing a circular motion of the knee.

5 A positive test for a torn meniscus is indicated by a palpable "grinding" sensation.

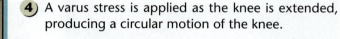

UTILITY SCORE 3

Study	Reliability	Sensitivity	Specificity	LR+	LR−	DOR	QUADAS Score (0–14)
Anderson & Lipscomb[6] (Combined)	NT	70	67	2.12	.45	51.8	9

Comments: The Medial-Lateral Grind Test improves the posttest probability of detecting a torn meniscus by a small amount. Further research needs to be performed to corroborate the statistics reported in this study since it possesses some design bias.

TESTS FOR A TORN TIBIAL MENISCUS

Joint-Line Tenderness

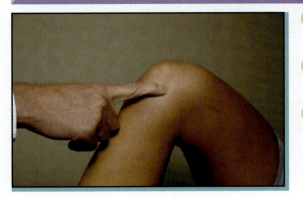

1 The patient is supine with the affected knee flexed to 90 degrees.

2 The examiner palpates the medial and lateral tibiofemoral joint-line.

3 A positive test for meniscus tear is indicated by re-production of the patient's pain (concordant sign).

UTILITY SCORE 3

Study	Reliability	Sensitivity	Specificity	LR+	LR−	DOR	QUADAS Score (0–14)
Karachalios et al.[45] (Medial)	.95	71	87	5.5	.33	16.7	9
(Lateral)	.95	78	90	7.8	.24	32.5	9
Akseki et al.[2] (Medial)	NT	88	44	1.6	.27	5.9	11
(Lateral)	NT	67	80	3.4	.41	8.3	11
Eren[23] (Medial)	NT	86	67	2.6	.21	12.4	9
(Lateral)	NT	93	97	31.0	.07	442.9	9
Kurosaka et al.[50] (Combined)	NT	55	67	1.7	.67	2.5	10
Shelbourne et al.[90] (Medial)	NT	58	53	1.2	.79	1.5	9
(Lateral)	NT	38	71	1.3	.87	1.5	9
Saengnipanthkul et al.[84] (Medial)	NT	58	74	2.2	.57	3.9	8
Boeree & Ackroyd[13] (Medial)	NT	64	69	2.1	.52	4.1	8
(Lateral)	NT	28	87	2.2	.83	2.7	8
Abdon et al.[1] (Medial)	NT	78	54	1.7	.41	4.1	8
(Lateral)	NT	78	92	9.8	.24	40.1	8
Fowler & Lubliner[28] (Combined)	$\kappa = .15$	85	30	1.2	.50	2.4	10

(continued)

TESTS FOR A TORN TIBIAL MENISCUS

Study	Reliability	Sensitivity	Specificity	LR+	LR−	DOR	QUADAS Score (0–14)
Dervin (Medial)	κ = .21	NT	NT	NT	NT	NT	NA
(Lateral)	κ = .25	NT	NT	NT	NT	NT	NA
Barry et al.[11] (Combined)	NT	86	43	1.5	.33	4.5	7
Noble & Erat[74] (Combined)	NT	72	13	.83	2.2	.38	9
Pookarnjanamorakot et al.[79]	NT	27	96	6.8	.76	8.9	11

Comments: The study by Eren[23] had 104 subjects, all of whom were male military recruits, which limits the applicability of these findings. Furthermore, the Karachalios et al.[45] study employs a case-control design, which dramatically overstates the diagnostic accuracy of the test and the .95 is an estimate of agreement. Therefore, almost without exception, the research shows that joint-line tenderness is of little value in diagnosing a meniscus tear. Furthermore, the interobserver agreement of joint-line tenderness is fair at best.

Forced Extension/Extension Block/Bounce Home Test

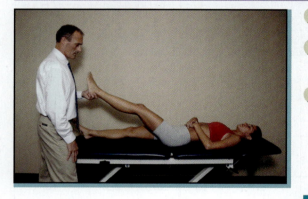

1. The patient is supine.

2. The examiner extends the affected knee to end range.

3. A positive test for meniscus tear is indicated by a block preventing full extension or pain at end-range extension.

UTILITY SCORE 3

Study	Reliability	Sensitivity	Specificity	LR+	LR−	DOR	QUADAS Score (0–14)
Kurosaka et al.[50] (Combined)	NT	47	67	1.4	.79	1.8	10
Dervin et al.[21] Combined	κ = .07	NT	NT	NA	NA	NA	NA
Noble & Erat[74] (Combined)	NT	38	67	1.2	.93	1.3	9
Fowler & Lubliner[28] (Combined)	κ =.29	44	85	2.9	.66	4.4	10

Comments: Neither pain at full extension nor an extension block seems to indicate a torn meniscus. No data is specifically available for the Bounce Home Test.

TESTS FOR A TORN TIBIAL MENISCUS

Squat/Duck Waddle/Childress Test

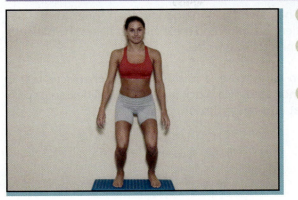

1. The patient is standing and then squats.

2. If no pain is reproduced, the patient is asked to "duck walk" in the squatting position.

3. A positive test for meniscus tear is indicated by a block preventing full flexion or pain at end-range flexion.

UTILITY SCORE 3

Study	Reliability	Sensitivity	Specificity	LR+	LR−	DOR	QUADAS Score (0–14)
Noble & Erat[74] (Combined)	NT	55	67	1.7	.67	2.5	9
Pookarnjanamorakot et al.[79] (Combined)	NT	68	60	1.7	.53	3.2	11
Comments: Neither pain with squatting nor with a "duck waddle" seems to indicate a torn meniscus.							

TESTS FOR A TORN TIBIAL MENISCUS

Flexion Block/Forced Flexion

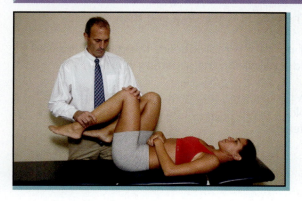

1 The patient is standing and then squats or the patient is supine and the examiner flexes the patient's knee to end-range.

2 In either case, a positive test for meniscus tear is indicated by a block preventing full flexion or pain at end-range flexion.

UTILITY SCORE 3

Study	Reliability	Sensitivity	Specificity	LR+	LR−	DOR	QUADAS Score (0–14)
Noble & Erat[74] (Combined)	NT	44	57	1.0	.98	1.0	9
Fowler & Lubliner[28] (Combined)	κ =.18	50	68	1.6	.74	2.2	10
Comments: A flexion block does not appear to indicate a torn meniscus.							

TESTS FOR A TORN TIBIAL MENISCUS

Effusion

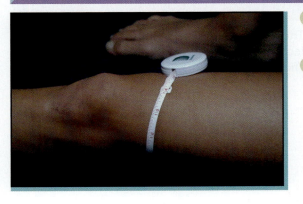

1. The examiner looks for or measures swelling about the knee.

2. A positive test for meniscus tear is indicated by more swelling/girth on the affected knee than the unaffected knee.

UTILITY SCORE 3

Study	Reliability	Sensitivity	Specificity	LR+	LR−	DOR	QUADAS Score (0–14)
Noble & Erat[74] (Combined)	NT	53	54	1.2	.87	1.4	9
Comments: Effusion does not appear to differentiate a torn meniscus.							

TESTS FOR A TORN TIBIAL MENISCUS

Figure 4 Test (Popliteomeniscal Fascicle Tears of the Lateral Meniscus)

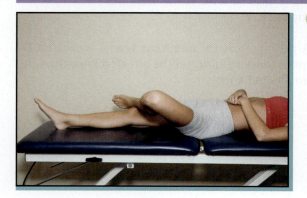

① The patient lies supine and places the foot of the affected knee on the contralateral knee, forming a "figure 4."

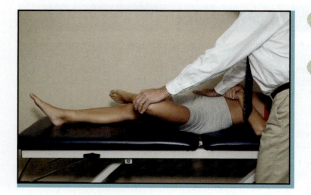

② The examiner pushes the affected knee toward the examining table.

③ A positive test is indicated by concordant pain over the lateral joint-line at the popliteal hiatus.

UTILITY SCORE   3

Study	Reliability	Sensitivity	Specificity	LR+	LR−	DOR	QUADAS Score (0–14)
Laprade & Konowalchuk[51]	NT	100	0	NA	NA	NA	9

Comments: The Figure 4 Test was developed to detect popliteomeniscal fascicle tears, which create instability of the lateral meniscus. This original article, while provocative, had only six patients with prolonged lateral knee pain and therefore indicates only the need for more research with this test.

TESTS FOR A TORN TIBIAL MENISCUS

Payr Sign

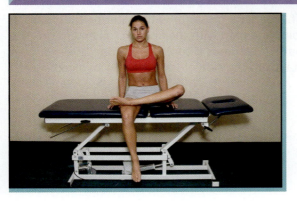

1 The patient sits and places the foot of the affected knee on the contralateral knee, forming a "figure 4."

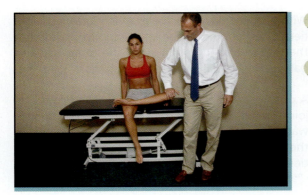

2 The examiner pushes the affected knee toward the floor.

3 A positive test for a posterior horn lesion of the medial meniscus is indicated by concordant pain over the medial joint-line.

UTILITY SCORE **3**

Study	Reliability	Sensitivity	Specificity	LR+	LR−	DOR	QUADAS Score (0–14)
Jerosch & Riemer[43]	NT	54	44	.96	1.05	.91	11
Comments: This test has as much effect on the posttest probability of detecting a torn tibial meniscus as a coin flip.							

TESTS FOR A TORN TIBIAL MENISCUS

Steinmann II Sign

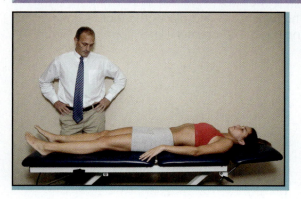

1 The patient presents with anterior tibiofemoral joint-line pain with the knee in full extension. The patient assumes a supine position. The examiner stands to the side of the patient's involved knee.

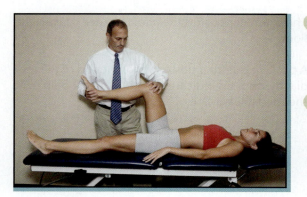

2 With the patient supine, the examiner grasps the patient's heel and flexes the knee and hip while using the thumb and index finger of the other hand to palpate the medial and lateral tibiofemoral joint-line.

3 A positive test for a meniscus tear is indicated by joint-line pain that moves in a posterior direction toward the collateral ligaments with knee flexion. If the pain doesn't move with knee flexion, the patient supposedly has a ligamentous issue.

UTILITY SCORE ?

Study	Reliability	Sensitivity	Specificity	LR+	LR−	DOR	QUADAS Score (0–14)
Not tested	NT	NT	NT	NA	NA	NA	NA

Comments: There have been no English-language studies that report the reliability or diagnostic accuracy of the Steinmann II Sign.

TESTS FOR TORN ANTERIOR CRUCIATE LIGAMENT (ACL) AND ANTERIOR ROTARY INSTABILITY

Composite Physical Exam (ACL Tear)

UTILITY SCORE   1

Study	Reliability	Sensitivity	Specificity	LR+	LR−	DOR	QUADAS Score (0–14)
O'Shea et al.[77]	NT	97	100	NA	NA	NA	9
Rose & Gold[82]	NT	100	100	NA	NA	NA	10
Simonsen et al.[93]	NT	62	75	2.5	.51	4.9	12
Kocabey et al.[47]	NT	100	100	NA	NA	NA	10
Kocher et al.[48]	NT	81	91	9.0	.21	42.9	11
Jackson et al.[41]	NT	74	95	15	.27	NT	NA

Comments: The composite physical examination for a torn ACL is highly accurate in adults with three of four studies showing sensitivities and specificities either at or near 100. The Kocher et al.[48] study would seem to indicate similar diagnostic accuracy for ACL tears in athletic children. Apparently, none of the physical examinations were performed in the acute stage of injury. The Jackson et al.[41] study is a meta-analysis and combines the data of 18 studies for ACL tear.

TESTS FOR TORN ANTERIOR CRUCIATE LIGAMENT (ACL) AND ANTERIOR ROTARY INSTABILITY

Lachman's Test (ACL Tear)

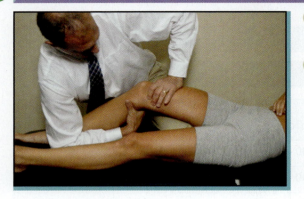

1 The patient is supine with the knee flexed to 15 degrees.

2 The examiner stabilizes the distal femur with one hand and grasps behind the proximal tibia with the other hand.

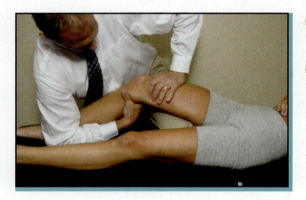

3 The examiner then applies an anterior tibial force to the proximal tibia.

4 A positive test for a torn ACL is indicated by greater anterior tibial displacement on the affected side when compared to the unaffected side.

TESTS FOR TORN ANTERIOR CRUCIATE LIGAMENT (ACL) AND ANTERIOR ROTARY INSTABILITY

UTILITY SCORE 1

Study	Reliability	Sensitivity	Specificity	LR+	LR−	DOR	QUADAS Score (0–14)
Bomberg[14]	NT	86	60	2.15	.23	9.3	9
Hardaker[34]	NT	74	NT	NA	NA	NA	8
Torg[103]	NT	96	100	NA	NA	NA	7
Learmonth[54]	NT	68	94	11.3	.38	37.7	6
Rubinstein[83]	NT	96*	100*	NA	NA	NA	9
Boeree[13]	NT	63	90	6.3	.41	15.2	8
Donaldson[22]	NT	99	NT	NA	NA	NA	8
Lee[55]	NT	91	100	NA	NA	NA	8
Liu[56]	NT	95	NT	NA	NA	NA	8
Cooperman[17]	κ = .38	65***	42***	NA	NA	NA	12
	κ = .35	77**	50**	NA	NA	NA	12

Comments: The Lachman Test improves the posttest probability of detecting a torn ACL by a moderate to large amount. However, the weighted kappa coefficient reported in the Cooperman et al.[17] study indicates that the test is performed with only fair interobserver agreement by both orthopedic surgeons and physical therapists when grading the amount of translation.

*Data are the mean result of five orthopedic surgeons.

**Data are the sum of the results from two physical therapists.

***Data are the sum of the results from two orthopedic surgeons.

TESTS FOR TORN ANTERIOR CRUCIATE LIGAMENT (ACL) AND ANTERIOR ROTARY INSTABILITY

Anterior Drawer Test (ACL Tear)

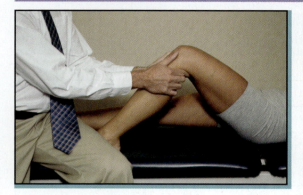

1 The patient is supine with the knee flexed to 90 degrees so that the foot is flat.

2 The examiner sits on the patient's foot and grasps behind the proximal tibia with thumbs palpating the tibial plateau and index fingers palpating the tendons of the hamstring muscle group medially and laterally.

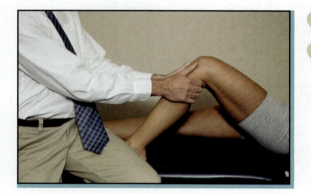

3 An anterior tibial force is applied by the examiner.

4 A positive test for a torn ACL is indicated by greater anterior tibial displacement on the affected side when compared to the unaffected side.

TESTS FOR TORN ANTERIOR CRUCIATE LIGAMENT (ACL) AND ANTERIOR ROTARY INSTABILITY

UTILITY SCORE 2

Study	Reliability	Sensitivity	Specificity	LR+	LR−	DOR	QUADAS Score (0–14)
Hardaker[34]	NT	18	NT	NA	NA	NA	8
Bomberg[14]	NT	41	100	NA	NA	NA	9
Rubinstein[83]	NT	76*	86*	NA	NA	NA	9
Jonsson[44] (Acute [A])	NT	33	NT	NA	NA	NA	8
(Chronic [C])	NT	95	NT	NA	NA	NA	8
Boeree[13]	NT	56	92	7.0	.48	14.6	8
Torg[103]	NT	52	100	NA	NA	NA	7
Donaldson[22]	NT	70	NT	NA	NA	NA	8
Lee[55]	NR	78	100	NA	NA	NA	8
Sandberg[85]	NT	39	78	1.8	.78	2.3	10
Noyes[76]	NT	25	96	6.2	.78	7.9	10
Liu[56]	NT	63	NT	NA	NA	NA	8
Anderson[7]	NT	27	NT	NA	NA	NA	12
Braunstein[15]	NT	91	89	8.3	.10	83	10
Warren[104,105]	NT	71	77	3.1	.38	8.2	7

Comments: The Anterior Drawer Test appears to be a specific test helpful at ruling in a torn ACL when the test is positive. The Anterior Drawer Test may become more sensitive in nonacute patients.

*Data is the mean result of five orthopedic surgeons.

TESTS FOR TORN ANTERIOR CRUCIATE LIGAMENT (ACL) AND ANTERIOR ROTARY INSTABILITY

Pivot-Shift Test (ACL Tear, Anterolateral Instability, Rotational Instability)

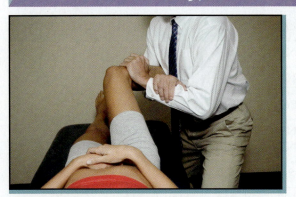

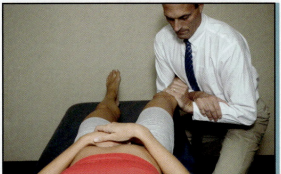

1 The patient assumes a supine position. The examiner stands to the side of the patient's involved knee.

2 The examiner grasps the patient's heel and flexes the knee to 90 degrees with one hand while using the palm of the other hand to medially rotate the tibia, effectively subluxing the lateral tibial plateau.

3 The examiner slowly extends the knee, maintaining rotation of the tibia.

4 As the patient's knee reaches full extension, the tibial plateau will relocate.

5 A positive test traditionally is indicated by an audible or palpable "thud" or "click."

UTILITY SCORE **2**

Study	Reliability	Sensitivity	Specificity	LR+	LR−	DOR	QUADAS Score (0–14)
Anderson[7]	NT	42	NT	NA	NA	NA	12
Bomberg[14]	NT	9	100	NA	NA	NA	9
Hardaker[34]	NT	29	NT	NA	NA	NA	8
Rubenstein[83]	NT	93*	89*	NA	NA	NA	9
Torg[103]	NT	9	100	NA	NA	NA	7
Sandberg[85]	NT	6	100	NA	NA	NA	10
Boeree[13]	NT	31	97	10.3	.71	14.5	8
Liu[56]	NT	71	NT	NA	NA	NA	8

Comments: The Pivot Shift Test appears to be a specific test helpful at ruling in a torn ACL when the test is positive.

*Data are the mean of five orthopedic surgeons. MacIntosh & Galway,[30] Hughston et al.,[39] Losee,[60] Slocum et al.,[94] Noyes et al.,[75] Bach et al.,[9] Martens and Mulier,[65] and Anderson and Lipscomb[6]—all have versions of the pivot-shift maneuver.

TESTS FOR TORN ANTERIOR CRUCIATE LIGAMENT (ACL) AND ANTERIOR ROTARY INSTABILITY

Anterior Drawer Test in External Rotation (ACL Tear, Anteromedial Instability)

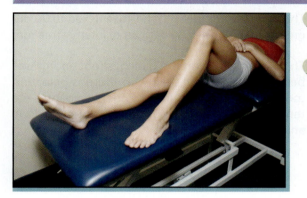

1. The patient is supine with the knee flexed to 90 degrees and the tibia in 15 degrees of external rotation.

2. The examiner sits on the patient's foot and grasps behind the proximal tibia with thumbs palpating the tibial plateau and index fingers palpating the tendons of the hamstring muscle group medially and laterally.

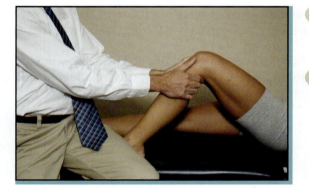

3. An anterior tibial force is applied by the examiner and more movement on the medial side will be detected.

4. A positive test for a torn ACL is indicated by greater anterior tibial displacement on the affected side when compared to the unaffected side.

UTILITY SCORE ?

Study	Reliability	Sensitivity	Specificity	LR+	LR−	DOR	QUADAS Score (0–14)
Larson[53]	NT	NT	NT	NA	NA	NA	NA
Comments: No data regarding the reliability or diagnostic accuracy of the Anterior Drawer in External Rotation is available.							

TESTS FOR TORN ANTERIOR CRUCIATE LIGAMENT (ACL) AND ANTERIOR ROTARY INSTABILITY

Anterior Drawer Test in Internal Rotation (ACL Tear, Anterolateral Instability)

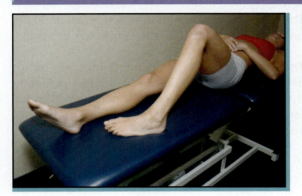

① The patient is supine with the knee flexed to 90 degrees and the tibia in 30 degrees of internal rotation.

② The examiner sits on the patient's foot and grasps behind the proximal tibia with thumbs palpating the tibial plateau and index fingers palpating the tendons of the hamstring muscle group medially and laterally.

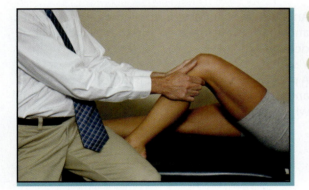

③ An anterior tibial force is applied by the examiner and greater movement of the lateral tibia is detected.

④ A positive test for a torn ACL is indicated by greater anterior tibial displacement on the affected side when compared to the unaffected side.

UTILITY SCORE ?

Study	Reliability	Sensitivity	Specificity	LR+	LR−	DOR	QUADAS Score (0–14)
Larson[53]	NT	NT	NT	NA	NA	NA	NA
Comments: No data regarding the reliability or diagnostic accuracy of the Anterior Drawer in Internal Rotation is available.							

TESTS FOR TORN ANTERIOR CRUCIATE LIGAMENT (ACL) AND ANTERIOR ROTARY INSTABILITY

▶ Active Lachman's Test (ACL Tear)

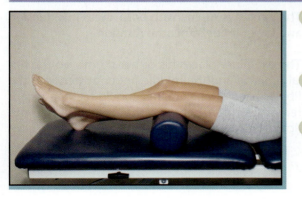

1 The patient assumes a supine position with a bolster under the distal femur so that the knee is flexed to 30–40 degrees.

2 The patient is asked to actively extend the involved knee and then to relax back to the starting position.

3 A positive test for a torn ACL is indicated by anterior glide of the proximal tibia.

UTILITY SCORE ?

Study	Reliability	Sensitivity	Specificity	LR+	LR−	DOR	QUADAS Score (0–14)
Cross et al.[19]	NT	NT	NT	NA	NA	NA	NA
Comments: The one study to examine the Active Lachman's[19] Test did not report reliability or diagnostic accuracy.							

TESTS FOR TORN ANTERIOR CRUCIATE LIGAMENT (ACL) AND ANTERIOR ROTARY INSTABILITY

Fibular Head Sign (ACL Tear, Anterolateral Instability)

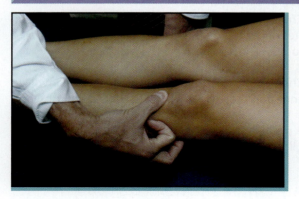

1 The patient is supine with both knees in extension and lower limbs in neutral rotation.

2 The examiner places his or her thumb on the tibial tubercle and the middle finger posterior to the fibular head. The examiner should feel the biceps femoris tendon between the middle finger and fibular head.

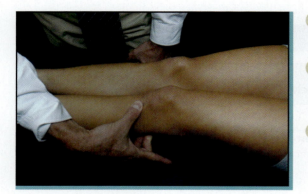

3 The examiner then extends his or her fingers to further palpate the fibular head.

4 A positive test for ACL tear is the inability to feel the biceps tendon between the middle finger and the fibular head.

5 Compare with the uninvolved knee.

UTILITY SCORE **?**

Study	Reliability	Sensitivity	Specificity	LR+	LR−	DOR	QUADAS Score (0–14)
Al-Duri[3]	NT	NT	NT	NA	NA	NA	NA

Comments: The one study to examine the Fibular Head Sign[3] did not report reliability or diagnostic accuracy and the test description was less than clear.

TESTS FOR TORN POSTERIOR CRUCIATE LIGAMENT (PCL) AND POSTERIOR ROTARY INSTABILITY

Composite Physical Exam

UTILITY SCORE 2

Study	Reliability	Sensitivity	Specificity	LR+	LR−	DOR	QUADAS Score (0–14)
O'Shea et al.[77]	NT	100	99	NA	NA	NA	9
Simonsen et al.[93]	NT	91	80	4.6	.11	41.8	12
Jackson et al.[41]	NT	81	95	16.2	.20	NT	NA

Comments: The higher numbers in the O'Shea et al.[77] article may be due to limited sample size (only 4 of 156 patients with a torn PCL) and patient population (male military personnel). The composite physical examination for a torn PCL is highly accurate, according to the Jackson et al.[41] meta-analysis, which combined the data from the Simonsen et al.[93] and O'Shea et al.[77] studies. The utility score of 2 reflects the weakness of the O'Shea et al.[77] article and the fact that only two articles have studied the composite exam for the PCL.

TESTS FOR TORN POSTERIOR CRUCIATE LIGAMENT (PCL) AND POSTERIOR ROTARY INSTABILITY

Posterior Drawer Test (PCL Tear)

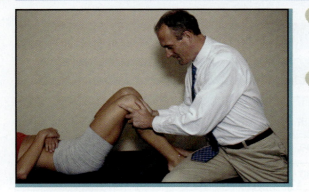

1. The patient is supine with the knee flexed to 90 degrees, the hip flexed at 45 degrees, and a neutral foot angle.

2. The examiner sits on the patient's foot to stabilize the extremity.

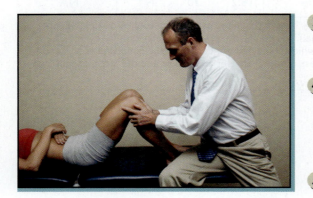

3. The examiner places both hands on the proximal anterior tibia with the thumbs on the medial and lateral joint-lines.

4. The proximal tibia is translated in a posterior direction and the amount of motion is estimated. This test is then repeated with the foot internally and then externally rotated and compared to the contralateral side.

5. A positive test for PCL tear is dependent on the amount of posterior motion of the tibia, Grade 1+ (0–5mm), grade 2+ (6–10mm), and grade 3+ (11mm+).

TESTS FOR TORN POSTERIOR CRUCIATE LIGAMENT (PCL) AND POSTERIOR ROTARY INSTABILITY

UTILITY SCORE **2**

Study	Reliability	Sensitivity	Specificity	LR+	LR−	DOR	QUADAS Score (0–14)
Clendenin et al.[16]	NT	100	NT	NA	NA	NA	9
Harilainen [36]	NT	33	NT	NA	NA	NA	6
Harilainen et al.[37]	NT	25	NT	NA	NA	NA	8
Fowler & Messieh[29]	NT	100	NT	NA	NA	NA	10
Hughston et al.[38]	NT	22	NT	NA	NA	NA	6
Moore & Larson[70]	NT	67	NT	NA	NA	NA	8
Loos et al.[59]	NT	51	NT	NA	NA	NA	6
Rubinstein[83]	NT	90	99	90	.10	NA	9

Comments: In the higher-quality studies, the Posterior Drawer Test[25] appears to have value as a sensitive test where a negative result would rule out a PCL tear. However, some studies show that detection of the drawer sign can be difficult in the acute injury secondary to muscle guarding. Hughston et al.[38] reports that a PCL injury can occur without stress on the arcuate complex, thus preventing a positive posterior drawer sign in the acute injury. Several of the studies were done retrospectively, were not blinded, and included very small sample sizes (<10).

TESTS FOR TORN POSTERIOR CRUCIATE LIGAMENT (PCL) AND POSTERIOR ROTARY INSTABILITY

Posterior Sag Sign or Godfrey's Test (PCL Tear)

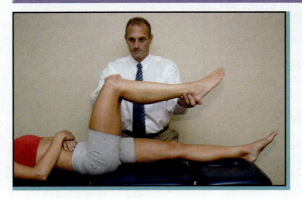

1 The patient is supine with the knee flexed to 90 degrees and the hip placed in 90 degrees of flexion.

2 The examiner supports the leg under the lower calf/heel, suspending the leg in the air.

3 A positive test for a PCL tear is posterior sagging of the tibia secondary to gravitational pull.

UTILITY SCORE   **2**

Study	Reliability	Sensitivity	Specificity	LR+	LR−	DOR	QUADAS Score (0–14)
Clendenin et al.[16]	NT	90	NT	NA	NA	NA	9
Fowler & Messieh[29]	NT	100	NT	NA	NA	NA	10
Staubli & Jakob[96]	NT	83	NT	NA	NA	NA	10
Loos et al.[59]	NT	46	NT	NA	NA	NA	6
Rubinstein[83]	NT	79	100	NA	NA	NA	9

Comments: The Sag Sign can be dependent upon the examiner's ability to detect a posterior shift of the tibia, which may or may not be obvious and may also be unreliable in the cases of multiple injures. The Godfrey's Test[25] differs from the Posterior Sag Sign because it includes a further step where the patient is asked to raise the foot and the anterior translation of the proximal tibia indicates a positive result. The Posterior Sag may have some value as a screening test when negative due to its high sensitivity.

TESTS FOR TORN POSTERIOR CRUCIATE LIGAMENT (PCL) AND POSTERIOR ROTARY INSTABILITY

Quadriceps Active Test (PCL Tear)

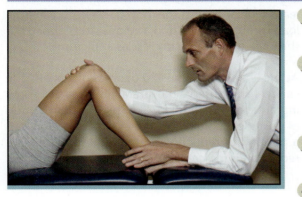

1 The patient is supine with the knee flexed to 90 degrees.

2 Keeping the eyes at the level of the subject's flexed knee, the examiner supports the subject's thigh and confirms the thigh muscles are relaxed while the foot is stabilized by the examiner's other hand.

3 The subject is asked to slide the foot gently down the table.

4 A positive test for PCL tear is anterior tibial displacement resulting from the quadriceps contraction.

UTILITY SCORE 2

Study	Reliability	Sensitivity	Specificity	LR+	LR−	DOR	QUADAS Score (0–14)
Daniel et al.[20]	NT	98	100	NA	NA	NA	8
Staubli & Jakob[96]	NT	75	NT	NA	NA	NA	10
Rubinstein[83]	NT	54	97	18	.47	38.3	9

Comments: This test appears to have some value as a specific test to detect a torn PCL when positive. However, the studies are of a quality that makes any conclusions about diagnostic accuracy tentative.

Reverse Pivot-Shift Test (PCL Tear, Posterolateral Rotary Instability [PLRI] Tear)

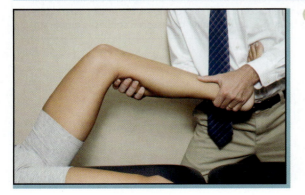

1 The patient lies supine with the knee flexed to 70–80 degrees. External rotation of the foot and leg is applied.

(continued)

TESTS FOR TORN POSTERIOR CRUCIATE LIGAMENT (PCL) AND POSTERIOR ROTARY INSTABILITY

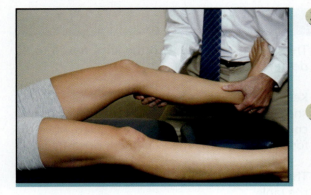

2 The knee is now allowed to straighten using nothing more than the weight of the leg. The examiner leans slightly against the foot, transmitting an axial load through the leg and a valgus stress applied to the knee using the iliac crest as a fulcrum.

3 As the knee approaches 20 degrees of flexion, one can feel and observe the lateral tibial plateau moving anteriorly with a jerk-like shift from a position of posterior subluxation and external rotation into a position of reduction and neutral rotation. This reduction is indicative of a positive test.

UTILITY SCORE 2

Study	Reliability	Sensitivity	Specificity	LR+	LR−	DOR	QUADAS Score (0–14)
Jakob et al[42]	NT	NT	NT	NA	NA	NA	NA
Fowler & Messieh[29]	NT	23	NT	NA	NA	NA	10
LaPrade & Wentorf[52]	NT	NT	NT	NA	NA	NA	NA
Shelbourne et al.[89]	NT	NT	NT	NA	NA	NA	NA
Rubinstein et al.[83] (Dynamic Posterior Shift)	NT	58	94	9.67	.47	20.6	9
Rubinstein et al.[83] (Reverse Pivot Shift)	NT	26	95	5.2	.78	6.7	9

Comments: Fowler and Messieh[29] report the Reverse Pivot-Shift Test as an occasional finding for an isolated tear of the PCL. Shelbourne et al.[89] and Rubinstein[83] describe a modification of the Reverse Pivot-Shift and call the test the Dynamic Posterior Shift Test. Rubinstein[83] differentiates between the Dynamic Posterior Shift and the Reverse Pivot-Shift representing the two sets of data, the first being the Dynamic Posterior Shift and the second the Reverse Pivot-Shift. The main difference between the two tests is that the Dynamic Posterior Shift Test controls rotation of the femur and tightens the hamstrings, providing axial loading across the knee joint. The Dynamic Posterior Shift accentuates the "clunk" as the knee nears extension. The test appears specific for ruling in a torn PCL if the test is positive but the quality of research studies is moderate.

TESTS FOR TORN POSTERIOR CRUCIATE LIGAMENT (PCL) AND POSTERIOR ROTARY INSTABILITY

Reverse Lachman's Test or Trillat's Test (PCL Tear)

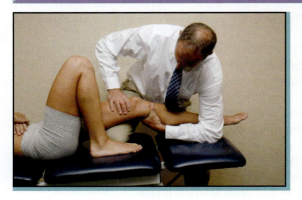

1 The patient is supine with the knee flexed to 20–30 degrees.

2 The examiner stabilizes the distal femur with one hand and grasps behind the proximal tibia with the other hand.

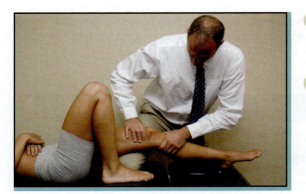

3 The examiner then applies an anterior tibial force followed by a posterior tibial force to the proximal tibia.

4 A positive test for a PCL tear is a soft or absent end-point in the posterior direction compared to the contralateral side.

UTILITY SCORE 3

Study	Reliability	Sensitivity	Specificity	LR+	LR−	DOR	QUADAS Score (0–14)
Rubinstein[83]	NT	62	89	5.64	.43	13.1	9

Comments: The Reverse Lachman's Test[25] is not a true reverse Lachman and examines both anterior and posterior translation of the tibia. Rubinstein[83] also reports sensitivity and specificity values for the Reverse Lachmans End-Point Test, although no description of the test could be found.

TESTS FOR TORN POSTERIOR CRUCIATE LIGAMENT (PCL) AND POSTERIOR ROTARY INSTABILITY

▶ Varus/Valgus Instability at 0 Degrees (PCL Tear)

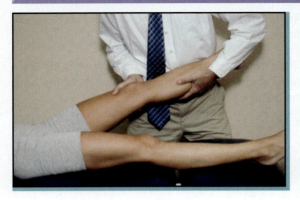

1 The patient is supine with the knee in full extension.

2 The examiner stands lateral to the patient's leg and cradling the lower leg in one hand, places the other hand over the lateral tibiofemoral joint-line.

3 The examiner applies a lateral to medial force at the tibiofemoral joint-line.

4 The test is repeated from the medial side of the patient's leg, providing a medial to lateral force wherein varus laxity is tested.

5 A positive test for a PCL tear is increased valgus and varus laxity when compared to the unaffected extremity.

UTILITY SCORE | **3**

Study	Reliability	Sensitivity	Specificity	LR+	LR−	DOR	QUADAS Score (0–14)
Hughston et al.[38]	NT	94	100	NA	NA	NA	6
Loos et al.[59]	NT	59	NT	NA	NA	NA	6

Comments: Typically the valgus/varus instability tests are used to detect tears of the medial and lateral collateral ligaments if performed at 20–30 degrees of knee flexion. However, a conclusion regarding the valgus test performed at 0 degrees detecting an associated rupture of the PCL cannot be made due to the low quality of the studies.

TESTS FOR TORN POSTERIOR CRUCIATE LIGAMENT (PCL) AND POSTERIOR ROTARY INSTABILITY

External Rotation Recurvatum Test

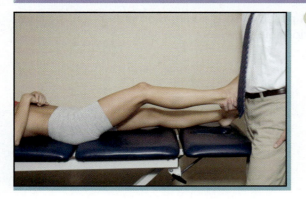

1 The patient lies supine with the examiner holding the heel of the leg in 30 degrees of knee flexion.

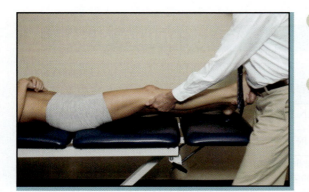

2 The examiner gradually extends the knee from 30 degrees of flexion while the opposite hand gently grasps the posterolateral aspect of the knee joint.

3 A positive test is the relative hyperextension and external rotation felt by the examiner compared to the opposite knee.

UTILITY SCORE 3

Study	Reliability	Sensitivity	Specificity	LR+	LR−	DOR	QUADAS Score (0–14)
Hughston et al.[38]	NT	39	NT	NA	NA	NA	6
Hughston & Norwood[40]	NT	NT	NT	NA	NA	NA	NA
LaPrade & Wentorf[52]	NT	NT	NT	NA	NA	NA	NA
Loos et al.[59]	NT	22	NT	NA	NA	NA	6
Rubinstein[83]	NT	3	99	3.0	.98	3.1	9

Comments: The low utility score reflects the poor quality of the articles. In the Hughston[38] article, the majority of the patients had tears of both the ACL and PCL. The value of a positive test to rule in PLRI needs to be confirmed by more than one study.

TESTS FOR TORN POSTERIOR CRUCIATE LIGAMENT (PCL) AND POSTERIOR ROTARY INSTABILITY

Anterior Abrasion Sign (PCL Tear)

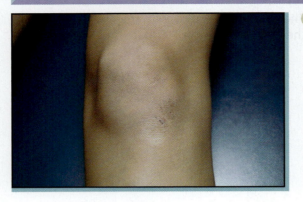

1 A positive test is an abrasion present on the anterior tibia.

UTILITY SCORE 3

Study	Reliability	Sensitivity	Specificity	LR+	LR−	DOR	QUADAS Score (0–14)
Loos et al.[59]	NT	14	NT	NA	NA	NA	6
Fowler & Messieh[29]	NT	7	NT	NA	NA	NA	10

Comments: Fowler and Messieh[29] report their data as occasional findings for the positive skin abrasion test as they were primarily looking at the posterior drawer and sag sign. This is a poor sign to detect a torn PCL.

TESTS FOR TORN POSTERIOR CRUCIATE LIGAMENT (PCL) AND POSTERIOR ROTARY INSTABILITY

Fixed Posterior Subluxation (PCL Tear)

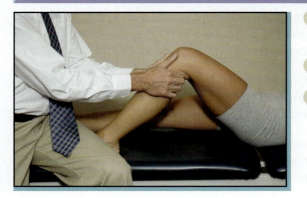

1 The patient lies supine with the knee flexed to 90 degrees.

2 The patient shows obvious posterior sagging.

3 A positive test is the inability to reduce the tibia to a neutral position during anterior tibial translation.

UTILITY SCORE ?

Study	Reliability	Sensitivity	Specificity	LR+	LR−	DOR	QUADAS Score (0–14)
Strobel et al.[101]	NT	NT	NT	NA	NA	NA	NA
Comments: The one study to examine the Fixed Posterior Subluxation[101] sign did not report reliability or diagnostic accuracy.							

TESTS FOR TORN POSTERIOR CRUCIATE LIGAMENT (PCL) AND POSTERIOR ROTARY INSTABILITY

Proximal Tibial Percussion Test (PCL Tear)

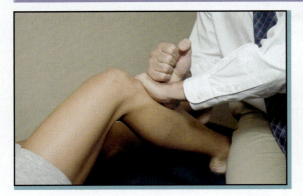

1 The patient lies supine with the hip flexed to 45 degrees and the knee in 90 degrees flexion and the examiner sitting on the patient's foot to stabilize it.

2 One of the examiner's hands is placed over the anterior-proximal tibia at the level of the tibial tubercle.

3 While the patient is relaxed, the examiner's other hand provides a blunt force to the back of the prepositioned hand.

4 A positive test is significant posterior joint pain similar to that of original injury.

UTILITY SCORE ?

Study	Reliability	Sensitivity	Specificity	LR+	LR−	DOR	QUADAS Score (0–14)
Feltham & Albright[25]	NT	NT	NT	NA	NA	NA	NA

Comments: The one study to examine the Proximal Tibial Percussion Test[25] did not report reliability or diagnostic accuracy. Due to the significant pain generated during this test, and the lack of evidence behind it, a clinician should question whether this test has any value.

TESTS FOR TORN POSTERIOR CRUCIATE LIGAMENT (PCL) AND POSTERIOR ROTARY INSTABILITY

Posterior Functional Drawer Test (PCL Tear)

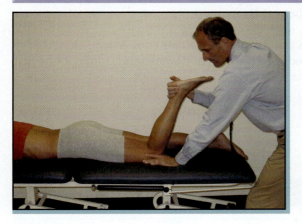

Prone

1 The patient lies prone with the knee flexed to 90 degrees, hip at 0 degrees flexion at the edge of the examining table.

2 The examiner maximally resists knee flexion and compares posterior pain and strength to the contralateral side.

3 Resistance is repeated at 20–30 degrees of knee flexion and compared to contralateral side.

4 A positive test is posterior pain and significant hamstring weakness at 90 degrees that is eliminated or reduced at 20–30 degrees when compared to the contralateral side.

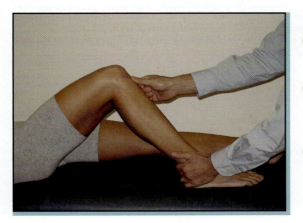

Supine

1 The patient is placed at 45 degrees hip flexion and 90 degrees knee flexion.

2 The examiner uses one hand to resist knee flexion at the heel and the other to palpate the anterior tibial plateau.

3 The examiner compares the strength of the hamstrings and patient report of posterior pain to the contralateral side.

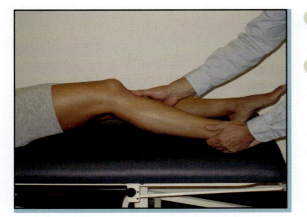

4 The test is repeated with the knee in 20–30 degrees flexion.

5 The examiner compares the strength of the hamstrings and patient report of posterior pain to the contralateral side and to exam finding at 90 degrees knee flexion.

(continued)

TESTS FOR TORN POSTERIOR CRUCIATE LIGAMENT (PCL) AND POSTERIOR ROTARY INSTABILITY

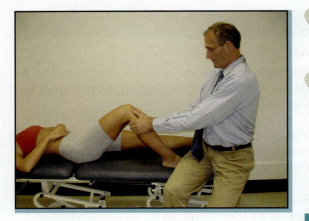

6 The examiner then applies an anterior drawer to the proximal tibia at 90 degrees knee flexion and the test is repeated.

7 A positive test is if an anterior drawer significantly reduced the pain and weakness is found in the first part of the exam.

UTILITY SCORE   **?**

Study	Reliability	Sensitivity	Specificity	LR+	LR−	DOR	QUADAS Score (0–14)
Feltham & Albright[25]	NT	NT	NT	NA	NA	NA	NA

Comments: The one study to examine the Posterior Functional Drawer[25] test did not report reliability or diagnostic accuracy. This test can reportedly be used in cases with partial tears or isolated PCL tears with minimal laxity for acute injuries. Post-rehabilitation, a positive test was associated with failure to return to high-level sports.

TESTS FOR TORN POSTERIOR CRUCIATE LIGAMENT (PCL) AND POSTERIOR ROTARY INSTABILITY

Modified Posterolateral Drawer Test or Loomer's Test (PCL Tear/PLRI)

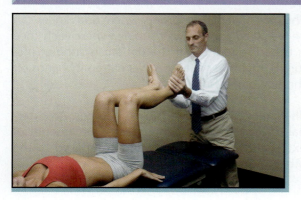

1. The patient lies supine with the hips and knees flexed to 90 degrees.

2. The examiner grasps the patient's feet and maximally externally rotates both feet.

3. A positive test has three interpretations:
   - Posterior sag of the tibia in neutral + no excessive rotation = isolated PCL tear
   - No posterior sag in neutral but excessive external rotation and posterior sag at the end of rotation = isolated PLRI
   - Posterior sag in neutral + excessive external rotation = PLRI and PCL tear.

UTILITY SCORE ?

Study	Reliability	Sensitivity	Specificity	LR+	LR−	DOR	QUADAS Score (0–14)
Loomer[57]	NT	NT	NT	NA	NA	NA	NA

Comments: The original research of this test[32] was in cadavers. The value of this test in diagnosis of PCL injury or PLRI is unknown.

TESTS FOR TORN POSTERIOR CRUCIATE LIGAMENT (PCL) AND POSTERIOR ROTARY INSTABILITY

Posterolateral Rotation Test or Dial Test (PCL Tear/PLRI)

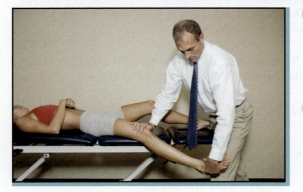

1 The patient lies either prone, where both knees can be tested concurrently, or supine, where each knee is tested separately. If the patient is supine (pictured), then the patient's lower extremity hangs off the side of the bed.

2 The knee(s) is/are flexed to 30 degrees. An external rotation force is then applied. The amount of external rotation is noted and compared to the other lower leg.

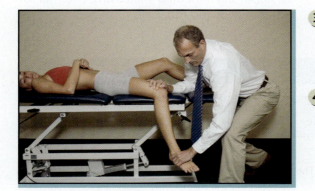

3 The knee(s) is/are now flexed to 90 degrees and again, an external rotation force is applied. The amount of external rotation is noted and compared to the other lower leg.

4 A positive test has three interpretations:
- More external rotation at 30 degrees than 90 degrees on the same leg = posterolateral corner injury
- More external rotation at 90 degrees than 30 = PCL tear
- Excessive external rotation in both positions when compared to the uninvolved leg = PCL and/or posterolateral corner tear.

UTILITY SCORE ?

	Reliability	Sensitivity	Specificity	LR+	LR−	DOR	QUADAS Score (0–14)
LaPrade & Wentorf[52]	NT	NT	NT	NA	NA	NA	NA
Allen[4]	NT	NT	NT	NA	NA	NA	NA

Comments: LaPrade and Wentorf,[52] Allen,[4] and Quarles[80] report on modifications of the dial test. No study reports on the diagnostic accuracy or reliability of this test.

TESTS FOR TORN POSTERIOR CRUCIATE LIGAMENT (PCL) AND POSTERIOR ROTARY INSTABILITY

Posterolateral Drawer Test (PLRI)

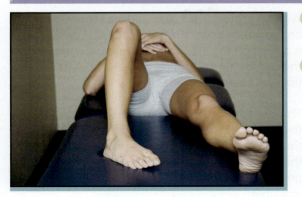

1 The patient lies supine with the hip flexed at 45 degrees and the knee flexed to 90 degrees.

2 The Posterior Drawer Test of the knee is now performed in neutral, external, and internal tibial rotation of 15 degrees.

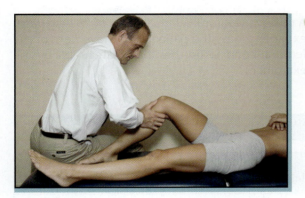

3 A positive test for PLRI is indicated by a relative posterior appearance of the lateral tibial condyle during the push phase of the drawer test when compared with the medial tibial condyle.

UTILITY SCORE ?

Study	Reliability	Sensitivity	Specificity	LR+	LR−	DOR	QUADAS Score (0–14)
Hughston & Norwood[40]	NT	NT	NT	NA	NA	NA	NA

Comments: Hughston and Norwood[40] suggest that internal rotation of the knee tightens the intact fibers of the PCL, which will not allow for anterior-posterior motion on the Posterior Drawer Test. If there is any posterior motion in complete internal rotation, then there must be an injury to the PCL. If the PCL is torn, the tibial rotation of the PLRI will not be present because the PCL pivot for rotation is absent. Shino et al.,[91] LaPrade and Wentorf,[52] and Quarles[80] all report modifications of the Posterolateral Drawer Test, none of which present any data on the test.

TESTS FOR TORN POSTERIOR CRUCIATE LIGAMENT (PCL) AND POSTERIOR ROTARY INSTABILITY

Standing Apprehension Test (PLRI)

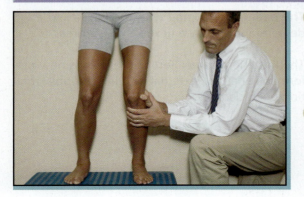

1. With the patient standing and and bearing weight on the affected leg, the tip of the examiner's thumb is placed on the anteriolateral femoral condyle with the rest of the thumb resting on the anterolateral tibia and joint line.

2. The patient is asked to flex the knee slightly while the examiner pushes the femoral condyle with the thumb. Increased rotation is felt as the tip of the thumb moves with the femur and the proximal portion of the thumb remained in contact with the lateral tibia.

3. A positive test for PLRI is a feeling of "giving way" experienced by the patient and movement of the femoral condyle on the tibial plateau felt by the examiner.

UTILITY SCORE | **?**

Study	Reliability	Sensitivity	Specificity	LR+	LR−	DOR	QUADAS Score (0–14)
Ferrari et al.[26]	NT	NT	NT	NA	NA	NA	NA
Comments: The one article describing the standing apprehension test did not report on any diagnostic accuracy or reliability values.							

TESTS FOR TORN POSTERIOR CRUCIATE LIGAMENT (PCL) AND POSTERIOR ROTARY INSTABILITY

Posterior Medial Displacement of the Medial Tibial Plateau with Valgus Stress (Posteromedial Rotatory Instability [PMRI])

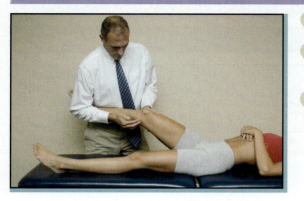

1 The patient lies supine with the knee extended.

2 The examiner produces hyperextension at the knee with a valgus force.

3 A positive test for isolated PMRI is sagging of the medial aspect of the tibia in the posteromedial corner. If the PCL is torn, the entire tibia will displace posteriorly.

UTILITY SCORE ?

Study	Reliability	Sensitivity	Specificity	LR+	LR−	DOR	QUADAS Score (0–14)
Larson[53]	NT	NT	NT	NA	NA	NA	NA

Comments: The one study[53] to examine the Posterior Medial Displacement of Medial Tibial Plateau with Valgus Stress Test did not report reliability or diagnostic accuracy.

TESTS FOR TORN COLLATERAL LIGAMENT

Composite Physical Exam (Medial Collateral Ligament [MCL] Tear)

UTILITY SCORE 2

Study	Reliability	Sensitivity	Specificity	LR+	LR−	DOR	QUADAS Score (0–14)
Simonsen et al.[93]	NT	88	73	3.3	.16	20.6	12

Comments: The composite physical examination for a torn MCL is fairly accurate according to Simonsen et al.[93] However, the utility score reflects the fact that only one article has examined the composite exam for the MCL.

Valgus Stress Test (MCL Tear)

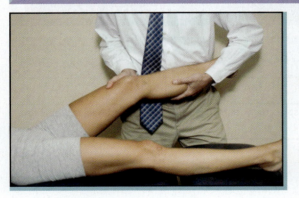

1 The patient is supine with hip slightly abducted and extended so the thigh is resting on the surface of the table.

2 The knee is flexed 30 degrees over the side of the table and the examiner places one hand about the lateral aspect of the knee while the other hand grasps the foot/ankle.

3 Gently apply a lateral to medial force to the knee, while the hand at the ankle externally rotates the leg slightly.

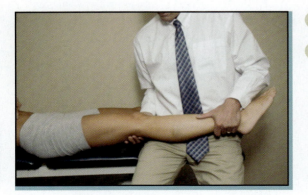

4 Repeat test with knee in full extension.

5 A positive test is excessive medial opening and concordant pain when compared to the uninvolved knee. If the test is positive at 30 degrees, the MCL is implicated. If the test is positive at 0 degrees, then the PCL and/or the joint capsule is implicated.

TESTS FOR TORN COLLATERAL LIGAMENT

UTILITY SCORE 2

Study	Reliability	Sensitivity	Specificity	LR+	LR−	DOR	QUADAS Score (0–14)
Harilainen[36]	NT	86	NT	NA	NA	NA	6
Harilainen[37]	NT	100	NT	NA	NA	NA	8
McClure et al.[66] (Extension)	κ = .06	NT	NT	NA	NA	NA	NA
(30° Flexion)	κ = .16	NT	NT	NA	NA	NA	NA
Sandberg et al.[85]	NT	80	NT	NA	NA	NA	8
Hughston et al.[38]	NT	94	100	NA	NA	NA	6

Comments: In both studies by Harilainen,[36,37] valgus testing was performed in 20 degrees of knee flexion. Since testing in extension was not done in these studies, a tear of the PCL could not be ruled out. In general, the Valgus Stress Test appears somewhat sensitive in ruling out a tear of the MCL when the test is negative but the quality of research makes this conclusion tenuous. More research is needed on the diagnostic accuracy and reliability of clinical tests with regard to the collateral ligaments.

Composite Physical Exam (Lateral Collateral Ligament [LCL] Tear)

UTILITY SCORE 3

Study	Reliability	Sensitivity	Specificity	LR+	LR−	DOR	QUADAS Score (0–14)
Simonsen et al.[93]	NT	100	20	NA	NA	NA	12

Comments: Only one article has examined the composite exam for the LCL and the low utility score reflects the limited sample size of the Simonsen et al.[93] article (only one LCL lesion).

TESTS FOR TORN COLLATERAL LIGAMENT

Varus Stress Test (LCL Tear)

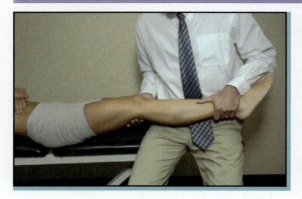

1 The patient is supine with hip slightly abducted and extended so the thigh is resting on the surface of the table.

2 The knee is flexed 30 degrees over the side of the table and the examiner places one hand about the medial aspect of the knee while the other hand grasps the foot/ankle.

3 Gently apply a medial to lateral force to the knee, while the hand at the ankle externally rotates the leg slightly.

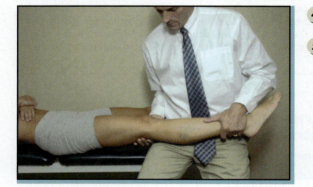

4 Repeat test with knee in full extension.

5 A positive test is excessive medial opening and concordant pain when compared to the uninvolved knee. If the test is positive at 30 degrees, the MCL is implicated. If the test is positive at 0 degrees, then the PCL and/or the joint capsule is implicated.

UTILITY SCORE 3

Study	Reliability	Sensitivity	Specificity	LR+	LR−	DOR	QUADAS Score (0–14)
Harilainen[36]	NT	25	NT	NA	NA	NA	6
Harilainen[37]	NT	0	NT	NA	NA	NA	8

Comments: In the Harilainen[36,37] studies, only four and one patient, respectively, were diagnosed with LCL tears confirmed by arthroscopy. Varus testing was performed in 20 degrees of knee flexion and testing in extension was not done, thus a tear of the PCL could not be ruled out. More research is needed to evaluate the diagnostic accuracy and reliability of the Varus Stress Test.

TESTS FOR PATELLOFEMORAL DYSFUNCTION

Patellar Apprehension Test or Fairbank's Apprehension Test

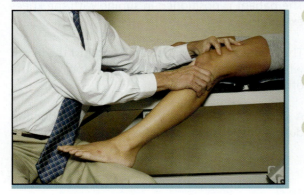

1 The patient is positioned in supine with a relaxed knee passively flexed to 30 degrees over the side of the examining table, foot resting on the examiner.

2 The examiner presses both thumbs on the medial aspect of the patella to exert a lateral force.

3 A positive test occurs when the patient shows signs of apprehension (resists the lateral force and attempts to extend the knee) or pain is reproduced.

UTILITY SCORE   2

Study	Reliability	Sensitivity	Specificity	LR+	LR−	DOR	QUADAS Score (0–14)
Nijs et al.[71]	NT	32	86	2.3	0.79	2.9	9
Haim et al.[33]	NT	7	92	0.87	1.0	.87	8
Niskanen et al.[72]	NT	37	70	1.2	0.90	1.3	9

Comments: This test, as used for patellar dislocation, appears to be more specific than sensitive, meaning a positive test would help rule in patellofemoral instability.

TESTS FOR PATELLOFEMORAL DYSFUNCTION

Waldron Test (Patellofemoral Joint Pathology)

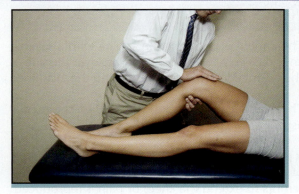

Phase I

1. The patient is positioned in supine with the knees extended.

2. The examiner presses the patella against the femur while performing passive knee flexion with the other hand.

3. A positive test is crepitus and pain reproduction during part of the range of motion.

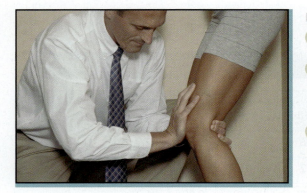

Phase II

1. The patient is positioned in standing.

2. The examiner places his hand on the patella and applies gentle compression of the patella against the femur as the patient performs a slow, full squat.

3. A positive test is crepitus and pain reproduction during the test.

UTILITY SCORE 3

Study	Reliability	Sensitivity	Specificity	LR+	LR−	DOR	QUADAS Score (0–14)
Nijs et al.[71]—Phase I	NT	45	68	1.41	0.81	1.7	9
Nijs et al.[71]—Phase II	NT	18	83	1.05	0.99	1.1	9
Comments: Nijs et al.[71] reported unimpressive positive and negative likelihood ratios for both Phase I and II.							

TESTS FOR PATELLOFEMORAL DYSFUNCTION

Passive Patellar Tilt Test (Patellofemoral Joint Instability)

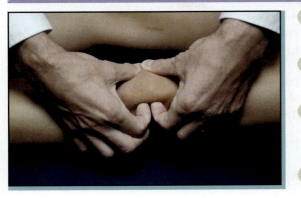

(1) The patient is positioned in supine with knees extended and quadriceps relaxed.

(2) The examiner stabilizes the extremity at the ankle in neutral rotation.

(3) The examiner lifts the lateral edge of the patella from the lateral femoral condyle using the thumb and index finger on both hands.

(4) A positive test occurs if the patella moves out of the trochlear groove and laterally subluxes.

UTILITY SCORE 3

Study	Reliability	Sensitivity	Specificity	LR+	LR−	DOR	QUADAS Score (0–14)
Watson et al.[106]	κ = 0.2–0.35*	NT	NT	NA	NA	NA	NA
Nissen et al.[73]	NT	NT	NT	NA	NA	NA	NA
Haim et al.[33]	NT	43	92	5.4	0.62	8.7	8
Watson et al.[107]	κ = 0.19**	NT	NT	NA	NA	NA	NA

Comments: The Watson et al.[106] article categorized subjects' patellae as having positive, negative, or neutral angle with respect to the horizon. Nissen et al.[73] described the Patellar Tilt Test as elevating the lateral patellar border while depressing the medial patellar border. Haim et al.[33] reported data on military recruits in which the examiner who conducted both clinical and radiological evaluations was not masked to the group's assignments.

*Three senior physical therapy students were included in the interobserver agreement. Intraobserver agreement varied from 0.44–0.50 for this test.

**Watson et al.[107] reports on two senior physical therapy students who performed medial/lateral patellar tilts in coordinates with McConnell's Test. Intraobserver agreement varied between 0.28 and 0.33.

TESTS FOR PATELLOFEMORAL DYSFUNCTION

Clarke's Sign/Patellar Grind/Patellar Tracking with Compression (Patellofemoral Joint Pathology)

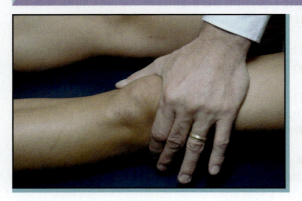

1 The patient is positioned in supine with both knees supported by a knee pad or bolster.

2 The examiner places a hand on the superior border of the patella and presses the patella distally while the patient is relaxed.

3 The patient is then asked to contract the quadriceps.

4 A positive test is pain and reproduction of symptoms.

UTILITY SCORE **3**

Study	Reliability	Sensitivity	Specificity	LR+	LR−	DOR	QUADAS Score (0–14)
Nijs et al.[71]	NT	49	75	1.94	0.69	2.8	9
Niskanen et al.[72]	NT	29	67	0.88	1.06	.83	9
Solomon et al.[95]	NT	NT	NT	NA	NA	NA	NA
Malanga et al.[63]	NT	NT	NT	NA	NA	NA	NA

Comments: Nijs et al.[71] do not clearly describe the angle of knee flexion for this test. Niskanen et al.[72] described a variation of Clarke's[71] sign, which was called the Patellar Inhibition Test. Variations of this test have also been described by Solomon et al.[95] and Malanga et al.[63] This test does not appear to be useful in diagnosing patellofemoral joint pathology.

TESTS FOR PATELLOFEMORAL DYSFUNCTION

Lateral Pull Test (Patellofemoral Tracking/Instability)

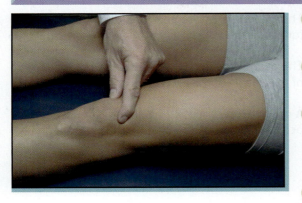

1 The patient is positioned in supine with knees extended and quadriceps relaxed.

2 The examiner stabilizes the extremity in neutral rotation at the ankle.

3 The patient was instructed to perform an isometric quadriceps femoris contraction, while the examiner observed the tracking of the patella with and without light palpation at the superior patellar pole.

4 A positive test was given when the patella tracked more laterally than superiorly.

UTILITY SCORE 3

Study	Reliability	Sensitivity	Specificity	LR+	LR−	DOR	QUADAS Score (0–14)
Watson et al.[106]	κ = 0.31*	NT	NT	NA	NA	NA	NA
Haim et al.[33]	NT	25	100	NA	NA	NA	8

Comments: Watson et al.[106] described a negative finding as superior or equidistant superior and lateral patellar tracking. The Lateral Pull Test conducted by Haim et al.[33] was labeled the active instability test and placed the patients supine with the knee flexed to 15 degrees prior to observing the tracking of the patella with an isometric quadriceps contraction. Haim et al.[33] described a positive test if the patella moved more than 3mm laterally.

*Two senior physical therapy students were included in the calculation of interobserver agreement. Intraobserver agreement varied from 0.39–0.47.

TESTS FOR PATELLOFEMORAL DYSFUNCTION

Patella Alta Test

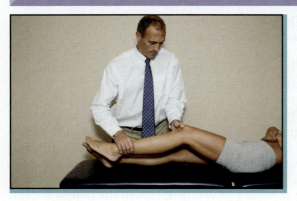

1 The patient is positioned in supine with the knee fully extended.

2 The examiner applies pressure over the lower pole of the patella of the extended knee and then flexes.

3 A positive test for patella alta is indicated when pain occurs during flexion.

UTILITY SCORE 3

Study	Reliability	Sensitivity	Specificity	LR+	LR−	DOR	QUADAS Score (0–14)
Haim et al.[33]	NT	49	72	1.75	0.71	2.5	8

Comments: Ironically, the likelihood ratios indicate that the Patella Alta Test[33] does not improve the posttest probability of detecting patella alta.

TESTS FOR PATELLOFEMORAL DYSFUNCTION

Vastus Medialis Coordination Test (Patellofemoral Tracking)

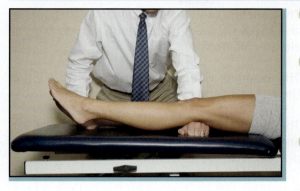

1. The patient is positioned in supine with the knee extended.

2. The examiner places his or her fist under the subject's knee and asks the patient to slowly extend the knee to full extension without pressing down or lifting away from the examiner's fist.

3. A positive test occurs when the patient has difficulty extending, does not extend the knee smoothly, or substitutes hip flexors to reach terminal extension.

UTILITY SCORE 3

Study	Reliability	Sensitivity	Specificity	LR+	LR−	DOR	QUADAS Score (0–14)
Nijs et al.[71]	ND	17	93	2.26	0.90	2.5	9

Comments: Although this test has a high reported specificity, which would make a positive finding valuable in ruling in vastus medialis incoordination, one study does not a physical exam test make.

TESTS FOR PATELLOFEMORAL DYSFUNCTION

▶ Eccentric Step Test (Patellofemoral Joint Dysfunction)

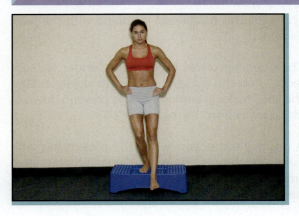

1 The patient is positioned in standing with bare feet and knees exposed, hands on hips, and up on an elevated platform.

2 The examiner gives a standard demonstration of the test and verbal instructions.*

3 The patient then preforms the test with one leg, and then repeats it on the other leg (no warmup or practice trials are allowed).

4 A positive test occurs when the patient reports knee pain during the test.

UTILITY SCORE 3

Study	Reliability	Sensitivity	Specificity	LR+	LR−	DOR	QUADAS Score (0–14)
Nijs et al.[71]	NT	42	82	2.34	0.71	3.3	9
Loudon et al.[62]	ICC = .94*	NT	NT	NA	NA	NA	NA

Comments: *The verbal instructions given to the patient included: "Stand on the step, put your hands on your hips, and step down from the step as slowly and as smoothly as you can" (Nijs et al.[71]).

**Loudon et al.[62] reported intratester reliability. Selfe et al.[88] have described a similar test utilizing a video analysis to determine the critical knee angle and angular velocity.

TESTS FOR PATELLOFEMORAL DYSFUNCTION

McConnell Test for Patellar Orientation (Patellofemoral Joint)

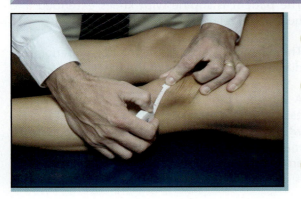

Medial/Lateral Glide

1 The patient is supine with knees extended and quadriceps relaxed.

2 The examiner determines the mid-point of the patella and then measures the distance from mid-patella to lateral femoral epicondyle and mid-patella to medial femoral epicondyle using a tape measure.

3 A positive test (score of 1) is given when distance from mid-patella to medial femoral epicondyle is >0.5 cm from lateral measurement. A score of 0 is equal medial and lateral distances.

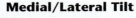

Medial/Lateral Tilt

1 The patient is supine with knees extended and quadriceps relaxed.

2 The examiner attempts to palpate the underside of the patellar borders.

3 A score of 0 is recorded when both the medial and lateral borders can be palpated. A score of 1 is given when >50% of lateral border, but not the posterior surface, can be palpated. A score of 2 is given when <50% of lateral border can be palpated.

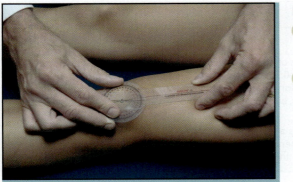

Patellar Rotation

1 The patient is supine with knees extended and quadriceps relaxed.

2 The examiner marks the superior and inferior aspects of the patella and draws a line between the two points and marks the medial and lateral aspects of the patella and creates a line. The long axis of the femur is also visualized and marked. A goniometer is used to evaluate the relationship of the two lines.

3 A score of 0 is given if two lines are parallel. A score of 1 is given if the inferior pole is lateral to femoral axis (obtuse angle of med/lat to femur). A score of −1 is given if inferior pole is medial to femoral axis (acute angle of med/lat to femur).

(continued)

TESTS FOR PATELLOFEMORAL DYSFUNCTION

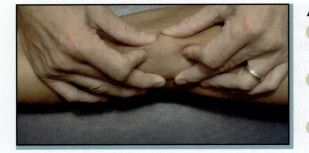

Anterior/Posterior Tilt

1 The patient is supine with knees extended and quadriceps relaxed.

2 The examiner palpates the inferior, superior, medial, and lateral aspects of the patella.

3 A score of 0 is given when distal 1/3 of patella is as easily palpated as proximal 1/3. A score of 1 is given when distal 1/3 is not as clearly palpable as proximal 1/3. A score of 2 is given when the distal 1/3 are not clearly palpable compared to proximal 1/3.

UTILITY SCORE ?

Study	Reliability	Sensitivity	Specificity	LR+	LR−	DOR	QUADAS Score (0–14)
Watson et al.[107] (M/L Glide)	κ = 0.02*	NT	NT	NA	NA	NA	NA
Tomsich et al.[102] (M/L Glide)	κ = 0.03**	NT	NT	NA	NA	NA	NA
Watson et al.[107] (M/L Tilt)	κ = 0.19*	NT	NT	NA	NA	NA	NA
Tomsich et al.[102] (M/L Tilt)	κ = 0.18**	NT	NT	NA	NA	NA	NA
Watson et al.[107] (Rotation)	κ = −0.03*	NT	NT	NA	NA	NA	NA
Tomsich et al.[102] (Rotation)	κ = −0.03**	NT	NT	NA	NA	NA	NA
Watson et al.[107] (A/P Tilt)	κ = 0.04*	NT	NT	NA	NA	NA	NA
Tomsich et al.[102] (S/I Tilt)	κ = 0.30**	NT	NT	NA	NA	NA	NA

Comments: *Watson et al.[107] reported interobserver agreement of two senior physical therapy students. The interobserver agreement ranged from 0.11–0.35 for med/lat glide, 0.28–0.33 for med/lat tilt, −0.06–0.00 for rotation, and 0.03–0.23 for ant/post tilt. McConnell[67] also reported on a test for chondromalacia patellae involving quadriceps contraction at varying degrees of knee flexion and medial patellar glides, but there has been no research regarding that tests's diagnostic accuracy either.

**Tomsich et al.[102] described slight variations in testing protocols and names for the McConnell measurements. Additionally, they reported interobserver agreement for three physical therapists and intraobserver agreement of medio/lateral glide (κ = 0.40), medio/lateral tilt (κ = 0.57), rotation (κ = 0.41), and superior/inferior tilt (κ = 0.50).

TESTS FOR PATELLOFEMORAL DYSFUNCTION

Zohler's Sign (Patellofemoral Joint Dysfunction)

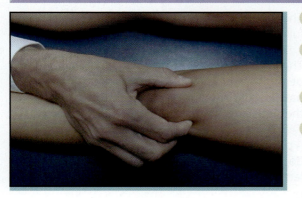

1 The patient lies supine with the knees extended.

2 The examiner pulls the patella distally and holds it in this position.

3 The patient is asked to contract the quadriceps.

4 A positive sign is pain.

UTILITY SCORE ?

Study	Reliability	Sensitivity	Specificity	LR+	LR−	DOR	QUADAS Score (0–14)
Strobel & Stedtfeld[100]	NT	NT	NT	NA	NA	NA	NA
Comments: The one study to examine Zohler's sign[100] did not report reliability or diagnostic accuracy.							

Tubercle Sulcus Test (Patellofemoral Joint Alignment)

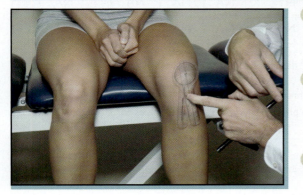

1 The patient is positioned in sitting with the knee flexed to 90 degrees and foot positioned in zero degrees of rotation.

2 The examiner draws a line from the center of the tibial tubercle to the inferior patellar pole. Another line is drawn from the femoral sulcus down the tibia perpendicular to the floor.

3 A positive test is an angle greater than 8 degrees.

UTILITY SCORE ?

Study	Reliability	Sensitivity	Specificity	LR+	LR−	DOR	QUADAS Score (0–14)
Nissen et al.[73]	NT	NT	NT	NA	NA	NA	NA
Comments: The study[73] that reported on this test did not report reliability or diagnostic accuracy.							

TESTS FOR PATELLOFEMORAL DYSFUNCTION

Q-Angle (Patellofemoral Joint Alignment)

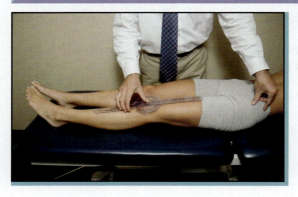

1 The patient is positioned in supine with the knee in full extension.

2 The examiner draws a line between the anterior superior iliac spine of the pelvis to the middle of the patella. Another line is drawn from the middle of the patella to the middle of the tibial tubercle.

3 A positive test is an angular value of greater than 10 degrees for males and greater than 15 degrees for females.

UTILITY SCORE ?

Study	Reliability	Sensitivity	Specificity	LR+	LR−	DOR	QUADAS Score (0–14)
Nissen et al.[73]	NT	NT	NT	NA	NA	NA	NA
Haim et al.[33]	NT	NT	NT	NA	NA	NA	NA
Haim et al.[33]	NT	NT	NT	NA	NA	NA	NA
Greene et al.[31]	ICC = .17–.29*	NT	NT	NA	NA	NA	NA
**Tomsich et al.[102]	ICC = .23	NT	NT	NA	NA	NA	NA

Comments: Nissen et al.[73] recommended the test be repeated in supine and in standing with 20 degrees of knee flexion and maximal internal, neutral, and external rotation. Haim et al.[33] described this test being performed at 90 degrees of knee flexion.

*Greene et al.[31] reported the interobserver measurements for three testers.

**Tomsich et al.[102] reported intertester measurements for three physical therapists and ICC values for intratester measurements of 0.63.

TESTS FOR PATELLOFEMORAL DYSFUNCTION

Q-Angle at 90 Degrees (Patellofemoral Joint Alignment)

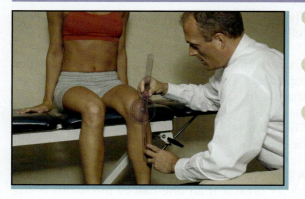

1 The patient is positioned in sitting with the knees extended.

2 A vertical line is drawn from the center of the patella to the center of the tibial tubercle.

3 A second horizontal line is drawn through the femoral epicondyle.
  • Angles greater than 10 degrees from the perpendicular are considered abnormal.

UTILITY SCORE **?**

Study	Reliability	Sensitivity	Specificity	LR+	LR−	DOR	QUADAS Score (0–14)
Haim et al.[33]	NT	NT	NT	NA	NA	NA	NA

Comments: The one study[100] to examine Q-angle at 90 degrees did not report reliability or diagnostic accuracy.

TESTS FOR PATELLOFEMORAL DYSFUNCTION

Lateral Patellar Glide (Patellofemoral Joint Instability)

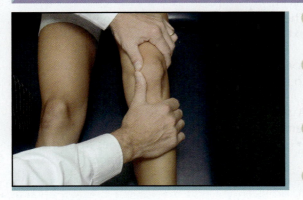

1 The patient is positioned in supine with the knee in full extension.

2 The examiner's thumbs are placed on the medial aspect of the patella, providing a lateral force on the patella.

3 The test is repeated at 20 and 45 degrees of knee flexion.

4 A positive test occurs when the patella laterally glides greater than one-half of the width of the patella.

UTILITY SCORE ?

Study	Reliability	Sensitivity	Specificity	LR+	LR−	DOR	QUADAS Score (0–14)
Nissen et al.[73]	NT	NT	NT	NA	NA	NA	NA
Haim et al.[33]	NT	NT	NT	NA	NA	NA	NA
Watson et al.[107]	κ = 0.02*	NT	NT	NA	NA	NA	NA

Comments: Nissen et al.[73] describe the positive test is indicative of laxity in the medial restraints.

*Watson et al.[107] reports on two senior physical therapy students. No information on the diagnostic accuracy of this test is available.

TESTS FOR PATELLOFEMORAL DYSFUNCTION

Medial Patellar Glide (Patellofemoral Joint Instability)

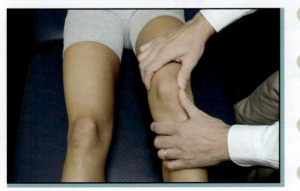

1 The patient is positioned in supine with the knee in full extension.

2 The examiner's thumbs are placed on the lateral aspect of the patella, providing a medial force on the patella.

3 The test is repeated at 20 and 45 degrees of knee flexion.

4 A positive test occurs when the patella medially glides greater than 30–40% of the width of the patella or greater than 10mm.

UTILITY SCORE ?

Study	Reliability	Sensitivity	Specificity	LR+	LR−	DOR	QUADAS Score (0–14)
Nissen et al.[73]	NT	NT	NT	NA	NA	NA	NA
Haim et al.[33]	NT	NT	NT	NA	NA	NA	NA
Watson et al.[107]	κ = 0.02*	NT	NT	NA	NA	NA	NA

Comments: In this study, Nissen et al.[73] report that the Medial Glide Test is reported in either percentages or millimeters, where 30–40% the width of the patella or 6–10mm of medial glide is considered normal. A glide of less than 6mm indicates a tight lateral retinaculum and a medial glide greater than 10mm most commonly indicated a hypermobile patella.

*Watson et al.[107] reports on two senior physical therapy students who performed medial/lateral glides.

TESTS FOR PLICA SYNDROME

MPP Test (Medial Patellar Plica Syndrome)

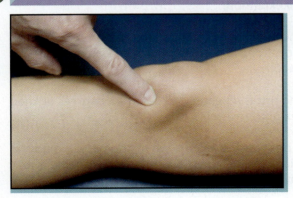

1. The patient assumes a supine position with knee in full extension. The examiner stands to the side of the patient's involved knee.

2. The examiner applies manual pressure to the plica at the inferomedial patellar border to force the plica between the medial femoral condyle and the joint-line.

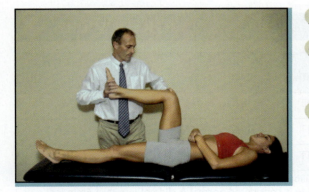

3. The examiner flexes the patient's knee to 90 degrees.

4. A positive test for a symptomatic medial patellar plica is indicated by more pain in extension than at 90 degrees flexion.

5. The painful knee is compared to the opposite side.

UTILITY SCORE ?

Study	Reliability	Sensitivity	Specificity	LR+	LR−	DOR	QUADAS Score (0–14)
Kim et al.[46]	NT	NT	NT	NA	NA	NA	NA

Comments: The one study to examine the MPP Test[46] did not report reliability or diagnostic accuracy. This diagnosis and a torn medial meniscus are often confused with each other but the symptomatic plica is thought to be a greater issue in active teenage individuals. A similar-sounding test was described by Flanagan et al.[27] in 1994.

Medial Plica Shelf Test (Medial Patellar Plica Syndrome)

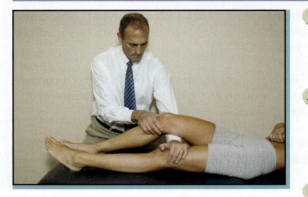

1 The patient assumes a supine position with knee flexed to 30 degrees. The examiner stands to the side of the patient's involved knee and reaches under that knee grasping the opposite thigh.

2 With the examiner's forearm acting as a bolster to maintain 30 degrees knee flexion, the examiner applies manual pressure to the lateral border of the patella with the opposite hand, causing a medial patellar glide.

3 A positive test for a symptomatic medial patellar plica is indicated by pain with the medial patellar glide.

UTILITY SCORE ?

Study	Reliability	Sensitivity	Specificity	LR+	LR−	DOR	QUADAS Score (0–14)
Mital & Hayden[69]	NT	NT	NT	NA	NA	NA	NA

Comments: The one study to examine the Medial Plica Shelf Test[69] did not report reliability or diagnostic accuracy. This diagnosis and a torn medial meniscus are often confused with each other but the symptomatic plica is thought to be a greater issue in active teenage individuals.

TESTS FOR PLICA SYNDROME

Medial Plica Test (Medial Patellar Plica Syndrome)

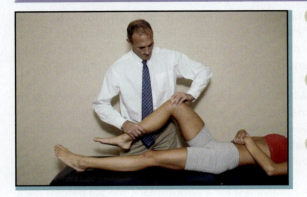

1. The patient assumes a supine position. The examiner stands to the side of the patient's involved knee.

2. The examiner palpates the medial femoral condyle while moving the patient's knee through flexion and extension.

3. A positive test for a symptomatic medial patellar plica is indicated by palpable crepitation.

UTILITY SCORE   ?

Study	Reliability	Sensitivity	Specificity	LR+	LR−	DOR	QUADAS Score (0–14)
Hardaker et al.[35]	NT	NT	NT	NA	NA	NA	NA

Comments: The one study to examine the Medial Plica Test[35] did not report reliability or diagnostic accuracy. This diagnosis and a torn medial meniscus are often confused with each other but the symptomatic plica is thought to be a greater issue in active teenage individuals.

TESTS FOR PLICA SYNDROME

Rotation Valgus Test (Medial Patellar Plica Syndrome)

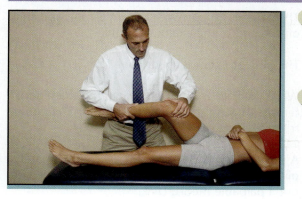

1. The examiner flexes the patient's knee while concurrently providing a valgus force, a medial patellar glide, and either internal or external tibial rotation.

2. A positive test for a symptomatic medial patellar plica is indicated by more pain either with or without a palpable medial click.

UTILITY SCORE ?

Study	Reliability	Sensitivity	Specificity	LR+	LR−	DOR	QUADAS Score (0–14)
Koshino & Okamoto[49]	NT	NT	NT	NA	NA	NA	NA

Comments: The one study to examine the Rotation Valgus Test[49] did not report reliability or diagnostic accuracy. This diagnosis and a torn medial meniscus are often confused with each other but the symptomatic plica is thought to be a greater issue in active teenage individuals.

TESTS FOR PLICA SYNDROME

Holding Test (Medial Patellar Plica Syndrome)

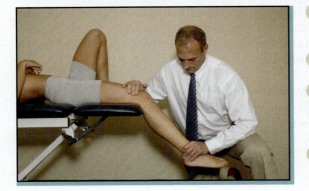

1. The patient is supine with the knee, foot, and ankle off the end of the examining table.

2. The patient extends his or knee fully.

3. While the knee is in full extension, the examiner attempts to push the knee into flexion. The patient resists the force.

4. A positive test for a symptomatic medial patellar plica is indicated by medial pain either with or without a palpable medial click.

UTILITY SCORE ?

Study	Reliability	Sensitivity	Specificity	LR+	LR−	DOR	QUADAS Score (0–14)
Koshino & Okamoto[49]	NT	NT	NT	NA	NA	NA	NA

Comments: The one study to examine the Holding Test[49] did not report reliability or diagnostic accuracy. Medial patellar plica syndrome and a torn medial meniscus are often confused with each other but the symptomatic plica is thought to be a greater issue in active teenage individuals. A combination of the Holding Test and the Rotation Valgus Test was reported by Amatuzzi et al.[5] in 1990 but no reliability or accuracy data were reported.

TESTS FOR PLICA SYNDROME

Patellar Stutter Test (Suprapatellar Plica Syndrome)

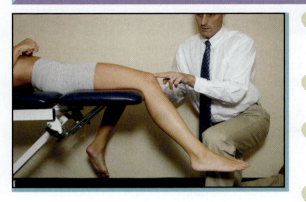

1) The patient is sitting with the knee flexed to 90 degrees, with foot and ankle off the end of the examining table.

2) The examiner places one finger on the patella while the patient slowly extends his or her knee.

3) Somewhere between 60 and 45 degrees of flexion, the patella stutters or jumps. This stutter is a positive test.

4) The author describes this test as best performed in the morning.

UTILITY SCORE ?

Study	Reliability	Sensitivity	Specificity	LR+	LR−	DOR	QUADAS Score (0–14)
Pipkin[78]	NT	NT	NT	NA	NA	NA	NA

Comments: The one study to examine the Patellar Stutter Test[78] did not report reliability or diagnostic accuracy. This diagnosis and anterior knee pain from chondromalacia patella are often confused with each other.

TESTS FOR PROXIMAL TIBIOFIBULAR JOINT INSTABILITY

Fibular Head Translation Test

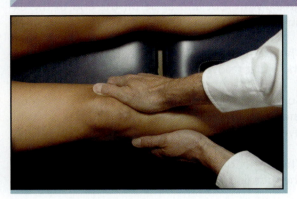

1 The examiner grasps the fibular head and provides a translatory force both in the anterior and the posterior directions.

2 A positive test is reproduction of the patient's pain and/or apprehension.

UTILITY SCORE ?

Study	Reliability	Sensitivity	Specificity	LR+	LR−	DOR	QUADAS Score (0–14)
Sijbrandij[92]	NT	NT	NT	NA	NA	NA	NA

Comments: The one study to examine the Fibular Head Translation Test[92] did not report reliability or diagnostic accuracy.

TESTS FOR PROXIMAL TIBIOFIBULAR JOINT INSTABILITY

Radulescu Sign

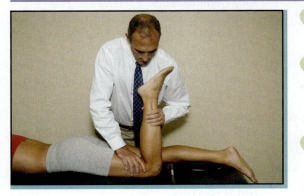

1 The patient lies prone with the knee flexed to 90 degrees.

2 The examiner stabilizes the patient's thigh with one hand while internally rotating the tibia with the other hand in an attempt to sublux the fibular head in an anterior direction.

3 A positive test is reproduction of the patient's pain, subluxation, and/or apprehension.

UTILITY SCORE   ?

Study	Reliability	Sensitivity	Specificity	LR+	LR−	DOR	QUADAS Score (0–14)
Baciu et al.[10]	NT	NT	NT	NA	NA	NA	NA
Comments: The one study to examine the Radulescu sign[10] did not report reliability or diagnostic accuracy.							

Key Points

1. Both the Ottawa Rules and the Pittsburgh Rules appear to be strong tools to screen for a knee fracture because a negative test would rule out a fracture and a positive test would lead to referral for an x-ray.

2. For meniscus tears:
   - The composite physical exam modifies posttest probability of detecting a lateral tear by a large amount.
   - The composite physical exam modifies posttest probability of detecting a medial tear by a small amount.
   - There is no single clear physical sign or test that is accurate in dianosing a meniscus tear, although some of the newer weight-bearing tests are intriguing.

3. For the ACL:
   - The composite physical examination has strong diagnostic accuracy in the nonacute patient.
   - The Lachman Test has the best diagnostic accuracy or any single physical exam test.
   - Both the pivot shift and anterior drawer are specific tests valuable at ruling in a torn ACL when positive.

4. There are no substantiated tests for symptomatic plica or proximal tibiofibular joint instability.

5. For the PCL:
   - The composite physical exam has potential for high diagnostic predictive values in detecting PCL tears. However, more studies need to be conducted to make the accuracy generalizable.
   - There is no all or none sign or test that is consistently accurate in diagnosing a torn PCL.
   - A positive Valgus or Varus Stress Test performed at 0 degrees may be indicative of a torn PCL.

6. For the MCL:
   - The value of the composite physical exam for a tom MCL is unknown.
   - The Valgus Stress Test is sensitive and has value in ruling out a torn MCL when the test is negative.
   - The Valgus Stress Test can be performed at both 0 degrees and 30 degrees of knee flexion to determine an isolated MCL tear (30 degrees) versus a combined PCL/MCL tear (0 degrees).

7. For the LCL:
   - The accuracy of the composite exam cannot be determined as only one article has been examined and the sample size only included one PCL lesion.
   - There are no proven tests to diagnose a torn LCL.

8. For the patellofemoral joint:
   - Although many tests have been described to clinically diagnose patellofemoral symptoms, the diagnostic accuracy and reliability are questionable.

References

1. Abdon P, Lindstrand A, Thorngren KG. Statistical evaluation of the diagnostic criteria for meniscal tears. *Int Orthop.* 1990;14:341–345.

2. Akseki D, Ozcan O, Boya H, Pinar H. A new weight-bearing meniscal test and a comparison with McMurray's test and joint line tenderness. *Arthroscopy.* 2004;20:951–958.

3. al-Duri Z. Relation of the fibular head sign to other signs of anterior cruciate ligament insufficiency: a follow-up letter to the editor. *Clin Orthop Relat Res.* 1992:220–225.

4. Allen CR, Kaplan LD, Fluhme DJ, Harner CD. Posterior cruciate ligament injuries. *Curr Opin Rheumatol.* 2002;14:142–149.

5. Amatuzzi MM, Fazzi A, Varella MH. Pathologic synovial plica of the knee: results of conservative treatment. *Am J Sports Med.* 1990;18: 466–469.

6. Anderson AF, Lipscomb AB. Clinical diagnosis of meniscal tears: description of a new manipulative test: *Am J Sports Med.* 1986;14: 291–293.

7. Anderson AF, Lipscomb AB. Preoperative instrumented testing of anterior and posterior knee laxity. *Am J Sports Med.* 1989;17: 387–392.

8. Apley, AG. The diagnosis of meniscus injuries. *JBJS.* 1947;29:78–84.

9. Bach BR, Jr., Warren RF, Wickiewicz TL. The pivot shift phenomenon: results and description of a modified clinical test for anterior cruciate ligament insufficiency. *Am J Sports Med.* 1988;16:571–576.

10. Baciu CC, Tudor A, Olaru I. Recurrent luxation of the superior tibio-fibular joint in the adult. *Acta Orthop Scand.* 1974;45:772–777.

11. Barry OC, Smith H, McManus F, MacAuley P. Clinical assessment of suspected meniscal tears. *Ir J Med Sci.* 1983;152:149–151.

12. Bauer SJ, Hollander JE, Fuchs SH, Thode HC, Jr. A clinical decision rule in the evaluation of acute knee injuries. *J Emerg Med.* 1995;13: 611–615.

13. Boeree NR, Ackroyd CE. Assessment of the menisci and cruciate ligaments: an audit of clinical practice. *Injury.* 1991;22:291–294.

14. Bomberg BC, McGinty JB. Acute hemarthrosis of the knee: indications for diagnostic arthroscopy. *Arthroscopy.* 1990;6:221–225.

15. Braunstein EM. Anterior cruciate ligament injuries: a comparison of arthrographic and physical diagnosis. *AJR Am J Roentgenol.* 1982; 138:423–425.

16. Clendenin MB, DeLee JC, Heckman JD. Interstitial tears of the posterior cruciate ligament of the knee. *Orthopedics.* 1980;3:764–772.

17. Cooperman JM, Riddle DL, Rothstein JM. Reliability and validity of judgments of the integrity of the anterior cruciate ligament of the knee using the Lachman's test. *Phys Ther.* 1990;70:225–233.

18. Corea JR, Moussa M, al Othman A. McMurray's test tested. *Knee Surg Sports Traumatol Arthrosc.* 1994;2:70–72.

19. Cross MJ, Schmidt DR, Mackie IG. A no-touch test for the anterior cruciate ligament. *J Bone Joint Surg Br.* 1987;69:300.

20. Daniel DM, Stone ML, Barnett P, Sachs R. Use of the quadriceps active test to diagnose posterior cruciate-ligament disruption and measure posterior laxity of the knee. *J Bone Joint Surg Am.* 1988;70–A:386–391.

21. Dervin GF, Stiell IG, Wells GA, Rody K, Grabowski J. Physicians' accuracy and interrater reliability for the diagnosis of unstable meniscal tears in patients having osteoarthritis of the knee. *Can J Surg.* 2001;44:267–274.

22. Donaldson WF, 3rd, Warren RF, Wickiewicz T. A comparison of acute anterior cruciate ligament examinations: initial versus examination under anesthesia. *Am J Sports Med.* 1985;13:5–10.

23. Eren OT. The accuracy of joint line tenderness by physical examination in the diagnosis of meniscal tears. *Arthroscopy.* 2003;19:850–854.

24. Evans PJ, Bell GD, Frank C. Prospective evaluation of the McMurray test. *Am J Sports Med.* 1993;21:604–608.

25. Feltham GT, Albright JP. The diagnosis of PCL injury: literature review and introduction of two novel tests. *Iowa Orthop J.* 2001;21:36–42.

26. Ferrari DA, Ferrari JD, Coumas J. Posterolateral instability of the knee. *J Bone Joint Surg Br.* 1994;76:187–192.

27. Flanagan JP, Trakru S, Meyer M, Mullaji AB, Krappel F. Arthroscopic excision of symptomatic medial plica: a study of 118 knees with 1–4 year follow-up. *Acta Orthop Scand.* 1994; 65:408–411.

28. Fowler PJ, Lubliner JA. The predictive value of five clinical signs in the evaluation of meniscal pathology. *Arthroscopy.* 1989;5:184–186.

29. Fowler PJ, Messieh SS. Isolated posterior cruciate ligament injuries in athletes. *Am J Sports Med.* 1987;15:553–557.

30. Galway HR, MacIntosh DL. The lateral pivot shift: a symptom and sign of anterior cruciate ligament insufficiency. *Clin Orthop Relat Res.* 1980:45–50.

31. Greene CC, Edwards TB, Wade MR, Carson EW. Reliability of the quadriceps angle measurement. *Am J Knee Surg.* 2001;14:97–103.

32. Grood ES, Stowers SF, Noyes FR. Limits of movement in the human knee: effect of sectioning the posterior cruciate ligament and posterolateral structures. *J Bone Joint Surg Am.* 1988;70:88–97.

33. Haim A, Yaniv M, Dekel S, Amir H. Patellofemoral pain syndrome: validity of clinical and radiological features. *Clin Orthop.* 2006.

34. Hardaker WT, Jr., Garrett WE, Jr., Bassett FH, 3rd. Evaluation of acute traumatic hemarthrosis of the knee joint. *South Med J.* 1990;83: 640–644.

35. Hardaker WT, Whipple TL, Bassett FH, 3rd. Diagnosis and treatment of the plica syndrome of the knee. *J Bone Joint Surg Am.* 1980;62: 221–225.

36. Harilainen A. Evaluation of knee instability in acute ligamentous injuries. *Ann Chir Gynaecol.* 1987;76:269–273.

37. Harilainen A, Myllynen P, Rauste J, Silvennoinen E. Diagnosis of acute knee ligament injuries: the value of stress radiography compared with clinical examination, stability, under anaesthesia and arthroscopic or operative findings. *Ann Chir Gynaecol.* 1986;75:37–43.

38. Hughston JC, Andrews JR, Cross MJ, Moschi A. Classification of knee ligament instabilities: Part I. The medial compartment and cruciate ligaments. *J Bone Joint Surg Am.* 1976;58: 159–172.

39. Hughston JC, Andrews JR, Cross MJ, Moschi A. Classification of knee ligament instabilities. Part II. The lateral compartment. *J Bone Joint Surg Am.* 1976;58:173–179.

40. Hughston JC, Norwood LA. The posterolateral drawer test and external rotational recurvatum test for posterolateral rotatory instability of the knee. *Clin Orthop.* 1980;147:82–87.

41. Jackson JL, O'Malley PG, Kroenke K. Evaluation of acute knee pain in primary care. *Ann Intern Med.* 2003;139:575–588.

42. Jakob RP, Hassler H, Staubli H-U. Observations on rotatory instability of the lateral compartment of the knee: experimental studies on the functional anatomy and pathomechanism of the true and reversed pivot shift sign. *Acta Orthop Scand.* 1981;52:1–32.

43. Jerosch J, Riemer S. [How good are clinical investigative procedures for diagnosing meniscus lesions?]. *Sportverletz Sportschaden.* 2004; 18:59–67.

44. Jonsson T, Althoff B, Peterson L, Renstrom P. Clinical diagnosis of ruptures of the anterior cruciate ligament: a comparative study of the Lachman test and the anterior drawer sign. *Am J Sports Med.* 1982;10:100–102.

45. Karachalios T, Hantes M, Zibis AH, Zachos V, Karantanas AH, Malizos KN. Diagnostic accuracy of a new clinical test (the Thessaly test) for early detection of meniscal tears. *J Bone Joint Surg Am.* 2005;87:955–962.

46. Kim SJ, Jeong JH, Cheon YM, Ryu SW. MPP test in the diagnosis of medial patellar plica syndrome. *Arthroscopy.* 2004;20:1101–1103.

47. Kocabey Y, Tetik O, Isbell WM, Atay OA, Johnson DL. The value of clinical examination versus magnetic resonance imaging in the diagnosis of meniscal tears and anterior cruciate ligament rupture. *Arthroscopy.* 2004;20:696–700.

48. Kocher MS, DiCanzio J, Zurakowski D, Micheli LJ. Diagnostic performance of clinical examination and selective magnetic resonance imaging in the evaluation of intraarticular knee disorders in children and adolescents. *Am J Sports Med.* 2001;29:292–296.

49. Koshino T, Okamoto R. Resection of painful shelf (plica synovialis mediopatellaris) under arthroscopy. *Arthroscopy.* 1985;1:136–141.

50. Kurosaka M, Yagi M, Yoshiya S, Muratsu H, Mizuno K. Efficacy of the axially loaded pivot shift test for the diagnosis of a meniscal tear. *Int Orthop.* 1999;23:271–274.

51. LaPrade RF, Konowalchuk BK. Popliteomeniscal fascicle tears causing symptomatic lateral

compartment knee pain: diagnosis by the figure-4 test and treatment by open repair. *Am J Sports Med.* 2005;33:1231–1236.

52. LaPrade RF, Wentorf F. Diagnosis and treatment of posterolateral knee injuries. *Clin Orthop.* 2002;402:110–121.

53. Larson RL. Physical examination in the diagnosis of rotatory instability. *Clin Orthop Relat Res.* 1983:38–44.

54. Learmonth DJ. Incidence and diagnosis of anterior cruciate injuries in the accident and emergency department. *Injury.* 1991;22:287–290.

55. Lee JK, Yao L, Phelps CT, Wirth CR, Czajka J, Lozman J. Anterior cruciate ligament tears: MR imaging compared with arthroscopy and clinical tests. *Radiology.* 1988;166:861–864.

56. Liu SH, Osti L, Henry M, Bocchi L. The diagnosis of acute complete tears of the anterior cruciate ligament: comparison of MRI, arthrometry and clinical examination. *J Bone Joint Surg Br.* 1995;77:586–588.

57. Loomer RL. A test for knee posterolateral rotatory instability. *Clin Orthop Relat Res.* 1991:235–238.

58. Loomer RL. A test for knee posterolateral rotatory instability. *Clin Orthop.* 1991;264:235–238.

59. Loos WC, Fox JM, Blazina ME, Del Pizzo W, Friedman MJ. Acute posterior cruciate ligament injuries. *Am J Sports Med.* 1981;9:86–92.

60. Losee RE. Concepts of the pivot shift. *Clin Orthop Relat Res.* 1983:45–51.

61. Losee RE. Diagnosis of chronic injury to the anterior cruciate ligament. *Orthop Clin North Am.* 1985;16:83–97.

62. Loudon JK, Wiesner D, Goist-Foley HL, Asjes C, Loudon KL. Intrarater reliability of functional performance tests for subjects with patellofemoral pain syndrome. *J Athl Train.* 2002;37:256–261.

63. Malanga GA, Andrus S, Nadler SF, McLean J. Physical examination of the knee: a review of the original test description and scientific validity of common orthopedic tests. *Arch Phys Med Rehabil.* 2003;84:592–603.

64. Mariani PP, Adriani E, Maresca G, Mazzola CG. A prospective evaluation of a test for lateral meniscus tears. *Knee Surg Sports Traumatol Arthrosc.* 1996;4:22–26.

65. Martens MA, Mulier JC. Anterior subluxation of the lateral tibial plateau: a new clinical test and the morbidity of this type of knee instability. *Arch Orthop Trauma Surg.* 1981;98:109–111.

66. McClure PW, Rothstein JM, Riddle DL. Intertester reliability of clinical judgments of medial knee ligament integrity. *Phys Ther.* 1989;69:268–275.

67. McConnell J. The management of chondromalacia patella. *Aust J Physiother.* 1986;32:215–223.

68. McMurray, TP. The semilunar cartilages. *Br J Surg.* 1942;29:407–414.

69. Mital MA, Hayden J. Pain in the knee in children: the medial plica shelf syndrome. *Orthop Clin North Am.* 1979;10:713–722.

70. Moore HA, Larson RL. Posterior cruciate ligament injuries: results of early surgical repair. *Am J Sports Med.* 1980;8:68–78.

71. Nijs J, Van Geel C, Van der auwera D, Van de Velde B. Diagnostic value of five clinical tests in patellofemoral pain syndrome. *Man Ther.* 2006;11:69–77.

72. Niskanen RO, Paavilainen PJ, Jaakkola M, Korkala OL. Poor correlation of clinical signs with patellar cartilaginous changes. *Arthroscopy.* 2001;17:307–310.

73. Nissen CW, Cullen MC, Hewett TE, Noyes FR. Physical and arthroscopic examination techniques of the patellofemoral joint. *J Orthop Sports Phys Ther.* 1998;28:227–285.

74. Noble J, Erat K. In defence of the meniscus: a prospective study of 200 meniscectomy patients. *J Bone Joint Surg Br.* 1980;62-B:7–11.

75. Noyes FR, Grood ES, Cummings JF, Wroble RR. An analysis of the pivot shift phenomenon: the knee motions and subluxations induced by different examiners. *Am J Sports Med.* 1991;19:148–155.

76. Noyes FR, Paulos L, Mooar LA, Signer B. Knee sprains and acute knee hemarthrosis: misdiag-

nosis of anterior cruciate ligament tears. *Phys Ther.* 1980;60:1596–1601.

77. O'Shea KJ, Murphy KP, Heekin RD, Herzwurm PJ. The diagnostic accuracy of history, physical examination, and radiographs in the evaluation of traumatic knee disorders. *Am J Sports Med.* 1996;24:164–167.

78. Pipkin G. Knee injuries: the role of the suprapatellar plica and suprapatellar bursa in simulating internal derangements. *Clin Orthop Relat Res.* 1971;74:161–176.

79. Pookarnjanamorakot C, Korsantirat T, Woratanarat P. Meniscal lesions in the anterior cruciate insufficient knee: the accuracy of clinical evaluation. *J Med Assoc Thai.* 2004;87: 618–623.

80. Quarles JD, Hosey RG. Medial and lateral collateral injuries: prognosis and treatment. *Prim Care Clin Office Pract.* 2004;31:957–975.

81. Richman PB, McCuskey CF, Nashed A, et al. Performance of two clinical decision rules for knee radiography. *J Emerg Med.* 1997;15: 459–463.

82. Rose NE, Gold SM. A comparison of accuracy between clinical examination and magnetic resonance imaging in the diagnosis of meniscal and anterior cruciate ligament tears. *Arthroscopy.* 1996;12:398–405.

83. Rubinstein RA, Jr., Shelbourne KD, McCarroll JR, VanMeter CD, Rettig AC. The accuracy of the clinical examination in the setting of posterior cruciate ligament injuries. *Am J Sports Med.* 1994;22:550–557.

84. Saengnipanthkul S, Sirichativapee W, Kowsuwon W, Rojviroj S. The effects of medial patellar plica on clinical diagnosis of medial meniscal lesion. *J Med Assoc Thai.* 1992;75:704–708.

85. Sandberg R, Balkfors B, Henricson A, Westlin N. Stability tests in knee ligament injuries. *Arch Orthop Trauma Surg.* 1986;106:5–7.

86. Seaberg DC, Jackson R. Clinical decision rule for knee radiographs. *Am J Emerg Med.* 1994; 12:541–543.

87. Seaberg DC, Yealy DM, Lukens T, Auble T, Mathias S. Multicenter comparison of two clin-

ical decision rules for the use of radiography in acute, high-risk knee injuries. *Ann Emerg Med.* 1998;32:8–13.

88. Selfe J, Harper L, Pederson I, Breen-Turner J, Waring J. Four outcome measures for patellofemoral joint problems. Part I. Development and validity. *Physiotherapy.* 2001;87:507–515.

89. Shelbourne KD, Benedict F, McCarroll JR, Rettig AC. Dynamic posterior shift test: an adjuvant in evaluation of posterior tibial subluxation. *Am J Sports Med.* 1989;17:275–277.

90. Shelbourne KD, Martini DJ, McCarroll JR, VanMeter CD. Correlation of joint line tenderness and meniscal lesions in patients with acute anterior cruciate ligament tears. *Am J Sports Med.* 1995;23:166–169.

91. Shino K, Horibe S, Ono K. The voluntarily evoked posterolateral drawer sign in the knee with posterolateral instability. *Clin Orthop.* 1987;215:179–186.

92. Sijbrandij S. Instability of the proximal tibio-fibular joint. *Acta Orthop Scand.* 1978;49:621–626.

93. Simonsen O, Jensen J, Mouritsen P, Lauritzen J. The accuracy of clinical examination of injury of the knee joint. *Injury.* 1984;16:96–101.

94. Slocum DB, James SL, Larson RL, Singer KM. Clinical test for anterolateral rotary instability of the knee. *Clin Orthop Relat Res.* 1976:63–69.

95. Solomon DH, Simel DL, Bates DW, Katz JN, Schaffer JL. Does this patient have a torn meniscus or the ligament of the knee? Value of the physical examination. *JAMA.* 2001;286: 1610–1620.

96. Staubli H-U, Jakob RP. Posterior instability of the knee near extension. *J Bone Joint Surg Br.* 1990;72-B:225–230.

97. Stiell IG, Greenberg GH, Wells GA, et al. Prospective validation of a decision rule for the use of radiography in acute knee injuries. *Jama.* 1996;275:611–615.

98. Stiell IG, Greenberg GH, Wells GA, et al. Derivation of a decision rule for the use of radiography in acute knee injuries. *Ann Emerg Med.* 1995;26:405–413.

99. Stiell IG, Wells GA, Hoag RH, et al. Implementation of the Ottawa Knee Rule for the use of radiography in acute knee injuries. *Jama.* 1997;278:2075–2079.

100. Strobel M, Stedtfeld HW. *Diagnostic evaluation of the knee.* Berlin: Springer-Verlag; 1990.

101. Strobel MJ, Weiler A, Schulz MS, Russe K, Eichhorn H-J. Fixed posterior subluxation in posterior cruciate ligament-deficient knees: diagnosis and treatment of a new clinical sign. *Am J Sports Med.* 2002;30:32–38.

102. Tomsich DA, Nitz AJ, Threlkeld AJ, Shapiro R. Patellofemoral alignment: reliability. *J Orthop Sports Phys Ther.* 1996;23:200–208.

103. Torg JS, Conrad W, Kalen V. Clinical diagnosis of anterior cruciate ligament instability in the athlete. *Am J Sports Med.* 1976;4:84–93.

104. Warren RF, Marshall JL. Injuries of the anterior cruciate and medial collateral ligaments of the knee: a long-term follow-up of 86 cases—part II. *Clin Orthop Relat Res.* 1978:198–211.

105. Warren RF, Marshall JL. Injuries of the anterior cruciate and medial collateral ligaments of the knee: a retrospective analysis of clinical records—part I. *Clin Orthop Relat Res.* 1978:191–197.

106. Watson CJ, Leddy HM, Dynjan TD, Parham JL. Reliability of the lateral pull test and tilt test to assess patellar alignment in subjects with symptomatic knees: student raters. *J Orthop Sports Phys Ther.* 2001;31:368–374.

107. Watson CJ, Propps M, Galt W, Redding A, Dobbs D. Reliability of McConnell's classification of patellar orientation in symptomatic and asymptomatic subjects. *J Orthop Sports Phys Ther.* 1999;29:378–385.

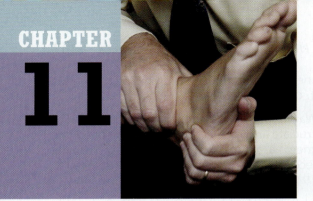

Physical Examination Tests for the Lower Leg, Ankle, and Foot

TEST FOR FIRST RAY MOBILITY

Manual Examination of the First Ray

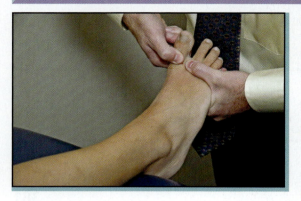

1. The patient lies in a supine position.

2. The second through fifth digits are stabilized by one hand of the examiner while the other hand stabilizes the first ray. The stabilization is held just distal to the metatarsal-phalangeal joint.

3. The examiner applies a dorsal and a plantar force to the first ray to determine first ray mobility. Typically, movement is considered normal or hypomobile.

4. A positive test is reduction of motion into dorsiflexion or plantarflexion.

UTILITY SCORE ?

Study	Reliability	Sensitivity	Specificity	LR+	LR−	DOR	QUADAS Score (0–14)
Glasoe et al.[7]	.16 kappa	NT	NT	NA	NA	NA	NA
Glasoe et al.[8] (Use of a Ruler)	0.05 ICC	NT	NT	NA	NA	NA	NA
Comments: This test demonstrates poor agreement and unknown diagnostic accuracy.							

TESTS FOR SYNDESMOTIC ANKLE SPRAINS

Fibular Translation Test

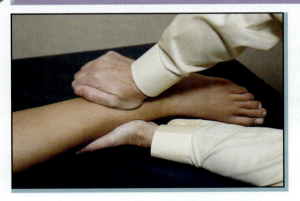

1. The patient lies in a sidelying position.

2. The examiner applies anterior and posterior forces on the fibula at the level of the syndesmosis.

3. A positive test is pain during translation and more displacement to the fibula than the compared side.

UTILITY SCORE 2

Study	Reliability	Sensitivity	Specificity	LR+	LR−	DOR	QUADAS Score (0–14)
Beumer et al.[3]	NT	82	88	6.8	0.2	33.4	8
Comments: Beumer et al.[3] only found increased translation when all ligaments were removed in cadavers.							

TESTS FOR SYNDESMOTIC ANKLE SPRAINS

External Rotation Test

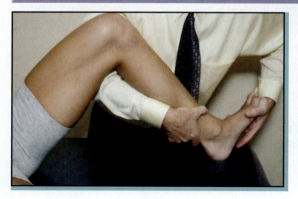

1. The patient lies in a supine position; the knee of the patient is flexed to 90 degrees.

2. The examiner holds the ankle in a neutral position then applies an externally rotated movement to the ankle.

3. A positive test is reproduction of concordant symptoms during movement.

UTILITY SCORE 2

Study	Reliability	Sensitivity	Specificity	LR+	LR−	DOR	QUADAS Score (0–14)
Alonso et al.[1]	.75 kappa	NT	NT	NA	NA	NA	NA
Beumer et al.[3]	NT	NT	95	NA	NA	NA	8

Comments: Beumer et al.[3] found significant displacement with this test in cadavers with ligaments individually sectioned.

TESTS FOR SYNDESMOTIC ANKLE SPRAINS

Cotton Test

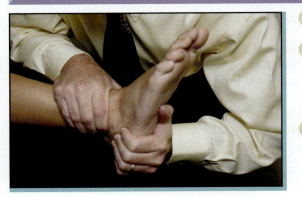

1 The patient lies in a supine position.

2 The examiner stabilizes the tibia with one hand and applies a lateral force to the ankle with the other. Occasionally, dorsiflexion is added to improve the sensitivity of the test.

3 A positive test is lateral translation of the ankle.

UTILITY SCORE **3**

Study	Reliability	Sensitivity	Specificity	LR+	LR−	DOR	QUADAS Score (0–14)
Beumer et al.[4]	NT	NT	NT	NA	NA	NA	NA
Beumer et al.[3]	NT	46	NT	NA	NA	NA	8

Comments: To translate the foot on the tibia effectively, the tibia requires appropriate stabilization. Consider stabilizing the tibia on the plinth.

TESTS FOR SYNDESMOTIC ANKLE SPRAINS

Syndesmosis Squeeze Test

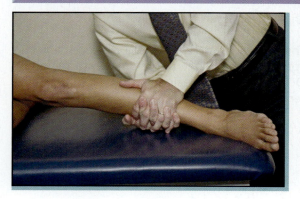

1. The patient lies in a supine or sidelying position.

2. The examiner applies a manual squeeze, pushing the fibula into the tibia, applying a force at the midpoint of the calf.

3. The test is considered positive if the proximal force causes distal pain near the syndesmosis.

UTILITY SCORE   ?

Study	Reliability	Sensitivity	Specificity	LR+	LR−	DOR	QUADAS Score (0–14)
Alonso et al.[1]	.50 kappa	NT	NT	NA	NA	NA	NA

Comments: This test is also described as the squeeze test of the leg and occasionally the distal tibiofibular compression test, if performed distal to the mid-point of the lower leg. Some describe a positive finding as pain when the squeeze is released.

TEST FOR ANTERIOR TALUS DISPLACEMENT RELATIVE TO THE TIBIA

Anterior Drawer Test

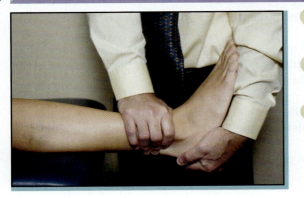

1 The patient lies in a supine position. The ankle is prepositioned into slight plantarflexion.

2 The examiner provides an anterior glide of the calcaneus and talus on the stabilized tibia.

3 A positive test is excessive translation of one side in comparison to the opposite extremity.

UTILITY SCORE   2

Study	Reliability	Sensitivity	Specificity	LR+	LR−	DOR	QUADAS Score (0–14)
Hertel et al.[9]	NT	78	75	3.1	0.29	10.6	8

Comments: The test is designed to measure damage to the anterior talofibular ligament. The examiner should observe the presence of a dimple or sulcus sign near the region of the anterior talofibular ligament.

TEST FOR SUBTALAR JOINT STABILITY

Medial Subtalar Glide Test

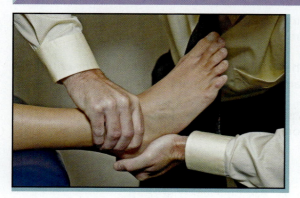

1. The patient lies in a supine position.

2. The examiner stabilizes the talus superiorly while gripping the calcaneus at the plantar aspect of the foot.

3. The examiner applies a medial glide of the calcaneus on the fixed talus.

4. A positive test is gross laxity during the procedure.

UTILITY SCORE 2

Study	Reliability	Sensitivity	Specificity	LR+	LR−	DOR	QUADAS Score (0–14)
Hertel et al.[9]	NT	78	75	3.1	0.29	10.6	8

Comments: Actual subtalar movement is minimal, subsequently gross laxity during assessment should be indicative of instability.

TEST FOR SUBTALAR JOINT PRONATION

Subtalar Joint Neutral (Open and Closed Chain)

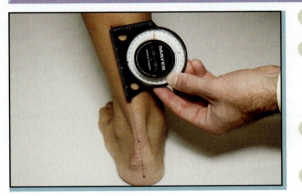

1 The patient stands.

2 The examiner places the patient in a subtalar neutral position. Subtalar neutral is found by palpation of the patient's tali in which both medial and lateral aspects are felt equally by the examiner.

3 Often, subtalar neutral is examined by measuring the position of the calcaneus using an inclinometer.

4 A positive test is excessive pronation or supination during obtained subtalar neutral.

UTILITY SCORE ?

Study	Reliability	Sensitivity	Specificity	LR+	LR−	DOR	QUADAS Score (0–14)
Picciano et al.[16] (Open Chain)	0.00 ICC	NT	NT	NA	NA	NA	NA
Picciano et al.[16] (Closed Chain)	0.15 ICC	NT	NT	NA	NA	NA	NA

Comments: Many question the benefit of finding subtalar neutral. Note the exceptionally poor reliability in detecting subtalar joint neutral.

TESTS FOR MIDTARSAL JOINT PRONATION

Navicular Drop Test

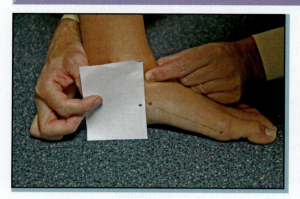

1. The patient stands. The examiner places the patient in a subtalar neutral position. Subtalar neutral is found by palpation of the patient's tali in which both medial and lateral aspects are felt equally by the examiner.

2. The most prominent aspect of the navicular bone is palpated and marked with a pen.

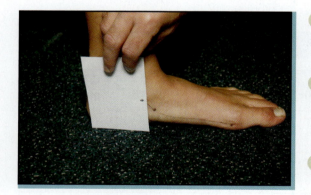

3. The examiner marks the height of the "neutral" position on a 3 × 5 note card. The patient is then instructed to stand normally.

4. Once the patient stands normally, the navicular height is again measured using the 3 × 5 card. The difference of the two measures is taken. The process is repeated for the opposite foot.

5. A significant difference of one side in comparison to the opposite is considered a positive finding.

TESTS FOR MIDTARSAL JOINT PRONATION

UTILITY SCORE ?

Study	Reliability	Sensitivity	Specificity	LR+	LR−	DOR	QUADAS Score (0–14)
Smith et al.[19] (Left Foot)	.72 ICC	NT	NT	NA	NA	NA	NA
Smith et al.[19] (Right Foot)	.82 ICC	NT	NT	NA	NA	NA	NA
Loudon et al.[12] (Right Foot)	.87 kappa	NT	NT	NA	NA	NA	NA
Picciano et al.[16]	0.57 ICC	NT	NT	NA	NA	NA	NA
Sell et al.[17] (Resting)	0.95 ICC	NT	NT	NA	NA	NA	NA
Sell et al.[17] (Neutral)	0.92 ICC	NT	NT	NA	NA	NA	NA
Sell et al.[17] (Measurement of Difference)	0.83 ICC	NT	NT	NA	NA	NA	NA
Vinicombe et al.[22]	0.33 ICC	NT	NT	NA	NA	NA	NA

Comments: It is questionable whether a significant drop is also indicative of dysfunction. The measurement does appear to be somewhat consistent.

Feiss Line

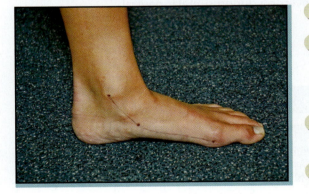

1 The patient is placed in a standing position.

2 Three marks are made on the patient's foot. One mark is made on the medial aspect of the malleolus, another at the navicular tubercle, and another at the medial aspect of the first metatarsal head.

3 The examiner places the patient in subtalar weight-bearing neutral.

4 The patient is instructed to weight-bear normally. A positive test is a dramatic drop (increased angle) of the Feiss line.

UTILITY SCORE ?

Study	Reliability	Sensitivity	Specificity	LR+	LR−	DOR	QUADAS Score (0–14)
Not tested	NT	NT	NT	NA	NA	NA	NA

Comments: It is likely that one will see a high amount of false positives with this test.

TEST FOR REARFOOT VARUS AND VALGUS

Calcaneal Position Technique

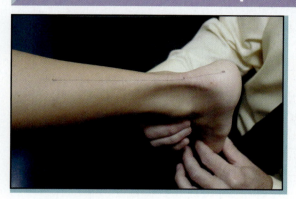

1. The patient lies in a prone position with both legs hanging over the plinth.

2. The calcaneus is palpated medially and laterally and bisected by placing dots in the inferior aspect and middle aspect of the calcaneus. A line is drawn to connect the dots.

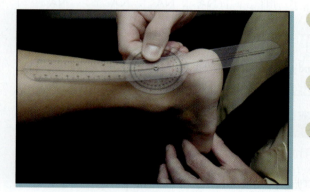

3. The examiner then finds subtalar neutral by palpating the patient's tali in which both medial and lateral aspects are felt equally by the examiner.

4. A goniometer is used to measure the varus or valgus of the calcanei.

5. A positive test is substantial rearfoot inversion or eversion during subtalar neutral.

UTILITY SCORE   3

Study	Reliability	Sensitivity	Specificity	LR+	LR−	DOR	QUADAS Score (0–14)
Sell et al.[17] (Neutral)	.85 ICC	NT	NT	NA	NA	NA	NA
Sell et al.[17] (Resting)	.85 ICC	NT	NT	NA	NA	NA	NA
Comments: This test differs from the subtalar joint neutral assessment in that it is performed in non-weight-bearing versus standing.							

TEST FOR MEDIAL LIGAMENT INTEGRITY

Lateral Talar Tilt Stress Test

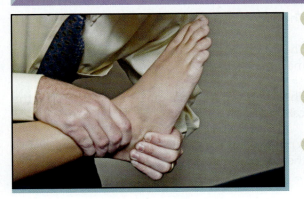

1 The patient is placed in a sitting or supine position.

2 The examiner grasps the ankle of the patient at the malleoli.

3 The examiner applies a quick lateral thrust to the calcaneus.

4 A positive test is excessive laxity when compared to the opposite side.

UTILITY SCORE ?

Study	Reliability	Sensitivity	Specificity	LR+	LR−	DOR	QUADAS Score (0–14)
Not tested	NT	NT	NT	NA	NA	NA	NA
Comments: The test remains unstudied.							

TEST FOR LATERAL LIGAMENT INTEGRITY

Medial Talar Tilt Stress Test

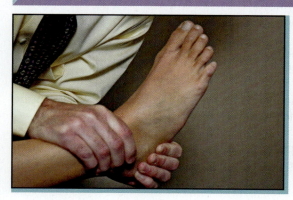

1 The patient is placed in a sitting or supine position.

2 The examiner grasps the ankle of the patient at the malleoli.

3 The examiner applies a quick medial thrust to the calcaneus.

4 A positive test is excessive laxity when compared to the opposite side.

UTILITY SCORE **3**

Study	Reliability	Sensitivity	Specificity	LR+	LR−	DOR	QUADAS Score (0–14)
Hertel et al.[9]	NT	67	75	2.7	0.44	6.1	8
Comments: Expect positive findings after inversion sprains.							

TEST FOR ACHILLES TENDON INTEGRITY

Thompson Test

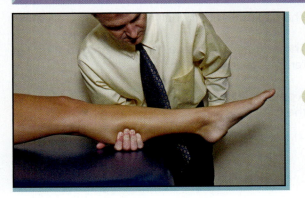

1. The patient lies in a supine position.

2. The examiner applies a squeeze to the calf of the patient's affected leg.

3. A positive test is a nonresponse during the squeeze test.

UTILITY SCORE 3

Study	Reliability	Sensitivity	Specificity	LR+	LR−	DOR	QUADAS Score (0–14)
Thompson & Doherty[21]	NT	40	NT	NA	NA	NA	7
Comments: The test has surprisingly low sensitivity. Patient history is essential concurrently when performing this test.							

TEST FOR TARSAL TUNNEL SYNDROME

Tinel's Sign

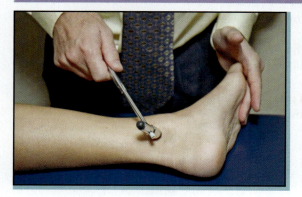

1. The patient lies in a sidelying position.

2. The examiner applies a tapping force to the posteromedial aspect of the ankle.

3. A positive finding is reproduction of tingling during the test.

UTILITY SCORE 3

Study	Reliability	Sensitivity	Specificity	LR+	LR−	DOR	QUADAS Score (0–14)
Oloff & Schulhofer[14]	NT	58	NT	NA	NA	NA	5
Comments: Like all Tinel's tests, throughout the body, the test provides only marginal sensitivity.							

TESTS FOR ANTERIOR ANKLE IMPINGEMENT

Forced Dorsiflexion Test

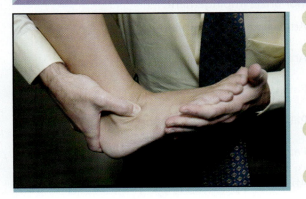

1. The patient assumes a sitting position.

2. The examiner stabilizes the distal aspect of the tibia and places his or her thumb on the anterolateral aspect of the talus near the lateral gutter. Pressure is applied.

3. The examiner applies a forceful dorsiflexion movement.

4. A positive test is reproduction of pain at the anterolateral aspect of the foot during forced dorsiflexion.

UTILITY SCORE 2

Study	Reliability	Sensitivity	Specificity	LR+	LR−	DOR	QUADAS Score (0–14)
Alonso et al.[1]	.36 kappa	NT	NT	NA	NA	NA	NA
Molloy et al.[13]	NT	95	88	7.9	0.06	133.7	8

Comments: Alonso et al.[1] tested for a syndesmosis injury. Although the diagnostic values for the test are strong, the quality of the study and the reliability among examiners is poor.

TESTS FOR ANTERIOR ANKLE IMPINGEMENT

Clinical Prediction Rule of Impingement

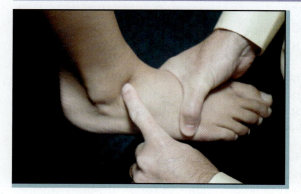

Five of six symptoms below are considered positive for anterior ankle impingement:

1 Anterolateral ankle joint tenderness.

2 Anterolateral ankle joint swelling.

3 Pain with forced dorsiflexion.

4 Pain with single-leg squat on the affected side.

5 Pain with activities.

6 Absence of ankle instability.

UTILITY SCORE | **2**

Study	Reliability	Sensitivity	Specificity	LR+	LR−	DOR	QUADAS Score (0–14)
Liu et al.[11]	NT	94	75	3.8	0.08	47	7

Comments: Some disagreement exists whether absence of ankle instability should be a rule for impingement. The quality of the single study is suspect.

TEST FOR ANKLE SWELLING

Figure-8 Test

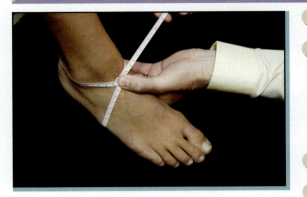

1. The patient lies in a supine or sitting position.

2. Using a flexible tape measure, and starting at the mid-point of the anterior aspect of the ankle, the examiner winds the tape measure around both the medial and lateral malleolus (but distal to each) and under the foot. The final winding should replicate a figure 8.

3. The examiner measures the distance of the excursion.

4. The test is a measurement of the girth of one limb to another. Substantial differences from one side to another is a positive finding.

UTILITY SCORE ?

Study	Reliability	Sensitivity	Specificity	LR+	LR−	DOR	QUADAS Score (0–14)
Petersen et al.[15]	.98 ICC	NT	NT	NA	NA	NA	NA
Tatro-Adams et al.[20]	.99 ICC	NT	NT	NA	NA	NA	NA
Comments: It is essential to identify the same landmarks to perform the figure-8 tests when comparing both sides.							

TEST FOR STRESS FRACTURE OR INTERDIGITAL NEUROMA

Morton's Test

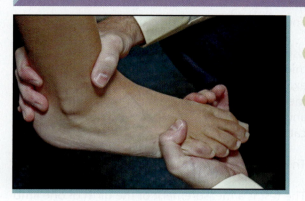

1 The patient lies in a supine or sitting position.

2 The examiner applies a squeeze to the metatarsal heads from lateral to medial toward mid-line.

3 A positive test is reproduction of patient symptoms.

UTILITY SCORE ?

Study	Reliability	Sensitivity	Specificity	LR+	LR−	DOR	QUADAS Score (0–14)
Not tested	NT	NT	NT	NA	NA	NA	NA
Comments: A false positive is possible in patients with metatarsalgia.							

TESTS FOR DEEP VEIN THROMBOSIS

Well's Clinical Prediction Rule for Deep Vein Thrombosis

1 Query or assess the patient for the following major criteria:
- Active cancer within the last 6 months
- Paralysis
- Recently bedridden
- Localized tenderness
- Thigh and calf are swollen
- Strong family history of DVT

2 Query or assess the patient for the following minor criteria:
- History of recent trauma
- Pitting edema
- Dilated superficial veins
- Hospitalized within last 6 months
- Erythema

3 A positive test is > 3 of the major criteria and > 2 of the minor criteria.

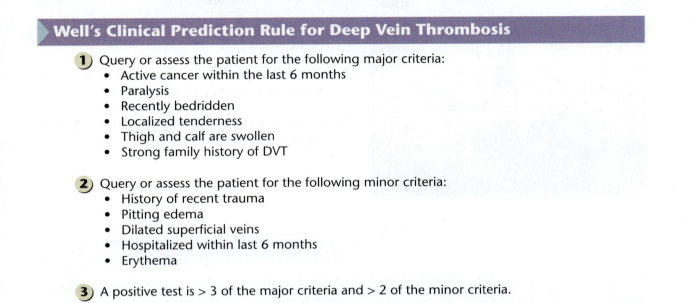

Study	Reliability	Sensitivity	Specificity	LR+	LR−	DOR	QUADAS Score (0–14)
Wells et al.[23]	NT	78	98	39	0.22	123.7	8

UTILITY SCORE **2**

Comments: At present, only one fairly designed study has examined these criteria; otherwise, the findings are promising.

TESTS FOR DEEP VEIN THROMBOSIS

Calf Swelling

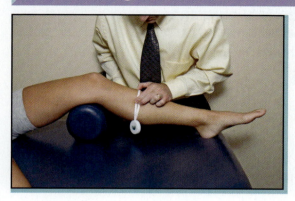

1. The patient lies in a supine position with the knee slightly flexed.

2. The examiner performs a circumferential measure of the calf and compares the size to the opposite side.

3. A positive test is a difference of 15 mm for men and 12 mm for women.

UTILITY SCORE   2

Study	Reliability	Sensitivity	Specificity	LR+	LR−	DOR	QUADAS Score (0–14)
Cranley et al.[5]	NT	90	92	11.3	0.11	103.5	7
Shafer & Duboff[18]	NT	NT	NT	NA	NA	NA	NA
Comments: This special test would benefit from further examination.							

TESTS FOR DEEP VEIN THROMBOSIS

Homan's Sign

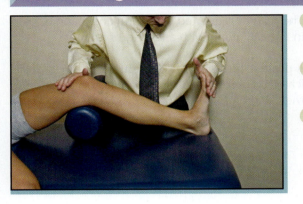

1 The patient lies in a supine position with the knee slightly flexed.

2 The examiner applies a forceful dorsiflexion maneuver.

3 A positive test is popliteal pain and calf pain.

UTILITY SCORE 3

Study	Reliability	Sensitivity	Specificity	LR+	LR−	DOR	QUADAS Score (0–14)
Cranley et al.[5]	NT	48	41	.81	1.27	0.64	7
Knox[10]	NT	35	NT	NA	NA	NA	4
Comments: A number of conditions may lead to false positives. The test does not appear to be diagnostic.							

TESTS FOR DEEP VEIN THROMBOSIS

Calf Tenderness

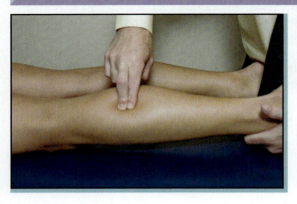

1 The patient is queried regarding an aching or pain in the calf along with a feeling of fullness.

2 A positive test is report of these symptoms, specifically if reproduced during manual compression of the calf.

UTILITY SCORE 3

Study	Reliability	Sensitivity	Specificity	LR+	LR−	DOR	QUADAS Score (0–14)
Cranley et al.[5]	NT	82	72	2.9	0.25	11.7	7
Shafer & Duboff[18]	NT	35	NT	NA	NA	NA	4
Comments: It is likely the fair to moderate diagnostic value from the Cranley et al.[5] study was associated with testing bias.							

TESTS FOR DEEP VEIN THROMBOSIS

Popkin's Sign

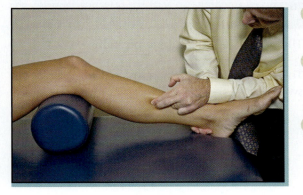

1 The patient lies in a supine position with the knee slightly flexed.

2 The examiner applies pressure with his or her index finger over the anterior medial aspect of the lower extremity.

3 A positive test is reproduction of pain or patient grimacing.

UTILITY SCORE ?

Study	Reliability	Sensitivity	Specificity	LR+	LR−	DOR	QUADAS Score (0–14)
Shafer & Duboff[18]	NT	NT	NT	NA	NA	NA	NA
Comments: Untested and somewhat unbelievable.							

TEST FOR SURGICAL STABILIZATION REQUIRED WITH FRACTURED FIBULA

Clinical Prediction Rule for Surgical Stabilization

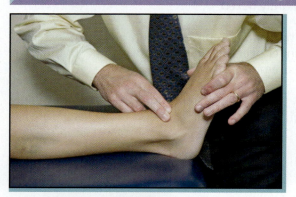

1 The patient lies in a supine position.

2 The examiner observes and palpates the ankle for swelling.

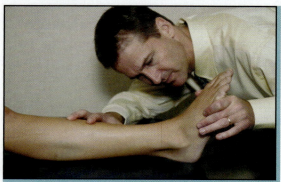

3 The examiner further observes the ankle for tenderness and ecchymosis.

4 A positive test is identified by positive stress x-rays in addition to clinical findings.

UTILITY SCORE **2**

Study	Reliability	Sensitivity	Specificity	LR+	LR−	DOR	QUADAS Score (0–14)
Egol et al.[6] (Medial Tenderness)	NT	56	80	2.8	0.55	5.1	8
Egol et al.[6] (Swelling)	NT	55	71	1.9	0.63	2.9	8
Egol et al.[6] (Ecchymosis)	NT	26	91	2.9	0.81	3.6	8
Egol et al.[6] (Tenderness and Swelling)	NT	39	91	4.3	0.67	6.5	8
Egol et al.[6] (Tenderness and Ecchymosis)	NT	20	97	6.7	0.82	8.1	8
Egol et al.[6] (Swelling and Ecchymosis)	NT	21	91	2.3	0.87	2.7	8
Comments: The test demonstrates strong specificity and is likely not a good screen.							

TEST FOR FOOT AND ANKLE FRACTURES

Ottawa Ankle Rules

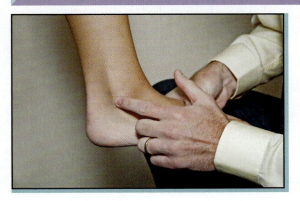

1 An ankle x-ray is required if there is any pain in the anterior aspect of the medial and lateral malleoli and anterior talar dome region, and any of the following findings:
- Bone tenderness at the posterior aspects of the medial malleolus
- Bone tenderness at the lateral malleolus
- Inability to weight-bear immediately after the injury and in the emergency room

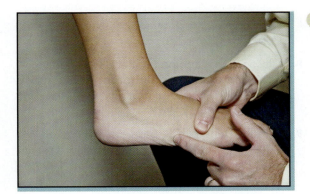

2 A foot x-ray series is required if there is any pain in the dorsal medial and lateral aspect of the mid-foot and any of the following findings:
- Bone tenderness at the base of the fifth metatarsal
- Bone tenderness at the navicular
- Inability to weight-bear immediately after the injury and in the emergency room

UTILITY SCORE 1

Study	Reliability	Sensitivity	Specificity	LR+	LR−	DOR	QUADAS Score (0–14)
Bachmann et al.[2]	NT	98	32	1.4	0.07	18.8	NA

Comments: A positive test requires radiographic assessment. Pooled results included studies that demonstrated QUADAS scores of 9 to 12. The test is an excellent screen.

Key Points

1. Clinical special tests of the lower leg, ankle, and foot are woefully understudied.

2. Most of the clinical special tests of the lower leg, ankle, and foot have been studied using poor designs and are hampered by internal bias.

3. Commonly used tests for deep vein thrombosis tend to be more specific than sensitive (occasionally) and lack proper study design.

4. The Ottawa rules include pooled analysis of 27 different studies with moderate to good methodology. The rules are excellent screens for ruling out the need for an x-ray among adults and children.

5. Although several syndesmosis tests exist, only a few have been studied for diagnostic accuracy.

6. The commonly used talar stress tests have been poorly tested. It is likely that results depend on the vigor of the stress used by the examiner.

7. The navicular drop test appears to be a moderately reliable test for pronation; however, the contribution of the findings of the test to pathology is untested.

References

1. Alonso A, Khoury L, Adams R. Clinical tests for ankle syndesmosis injury: reliability and prediction of return to function. *J Orthop Sports Phys Ther.* 1998;27(4):276–284.

2. Bachmann LM, Kolb E, Koller MT, Steurer J, ter Riet G. Accuracy of Ottawa ankle rules to exclude fractures of the ankle and mid-foot: systematic review. *BMJ.* 2003;326(7386):417.

3. Beumer A, Swierstra BA, Mulder PG. Clinical diagnosis of syndesmotic ankle instability: evaluation of stress tests behind the curtains. *Acta Orthop Scand.* 2002;73(6):667–669.

4. Beumer A, van Hemert WL, Swierstra BA, Jasper LE, Belkoff SM. A biomechanical evaluation of clinical stress tests for syndesmotic ankle instability. *Foot Ankle Int.* 2003;24(4):358–363.

5. Cranley JJ, Canos AJ, Sull WJ. The diagnosis of deep venous thrombosis: fallibility of clinical symptoms and signs. *Arch Surg.* 1976;111(1):34–36.

6. Egol KA, Amirtharajah M, Tejwani NC, Capla EL, Koval KJ. Ankle stress test for predicting the need for surgical fixation of isolated fibular fractures. *J Bone Joint Surg Am.* 2004;86-A(11):2393–2398.

7. Glasoe WM, Allen MK, Saltzman CL, Ludewig PM, Sublett SH. Comparison of two methods used to assess first-ray mobility. *Foot Ankle Int.* 2002;23(3):248–252.

8. Glasoe WM, Grebing BR, Beck S, Coughlin MJ, Saltzman CL. A comparison of device measures of dorsal first ray mobility. *Foot Ankle Int.* 2005;26(11):957–961.

9. Hertel J, Denegar CR, Monroe MM, Stokes WL. Talocrural and subtalar joint instability after lateral ankle sprain. *Med Sci Sports Exerc.* 1999;31(11):1501–1508.

10. Knox FW. The clinical diagnosis of deep vein thrombophelbitis. *Practitioner.* 1965;195:214–216.

11. Liu SH, Nuccion SL, Finerman G. Diagnosis of anterolateral ankle impingement: comparison between magnetic resonance imaging and clinical examination. *Am J Sports Med.* 1997;25(3):389–393.

12. Loudon JK, Bell SL. The foot and ankle: an overview of arthrokinematics and selected joint techniques. *J Athl Train.* 1996;31(2):173–178.

13. Molloy S, Solan MC, Bendall SP. Synovial impingement in the ankle: a new physical sign. *J Bone Joint Surg Br.* 2003;85(3):330–333.

14. Oloff LM, Schulhofer SD. Flexor hallucis longus dysfunction. *J Foot Ankle Surg.* 1998;37(2): 101–109.

15. Petersen EJ, Irish SM, Lyons CL, Miklaski SF, Bryan JM, Henderson NE, Masullo LN. Reliability of water volumetry and the figure eight method on patients with ankle joint swelling. *J Orthop Sports Phys Ther.* 1999;29(10):609–615.

16. Picciano AM, Rowlands MS, Worrell T. Reliability of open and closed kinetic chain subtalar joint neutral positions and navicular drop test. *J Orthop Sports Phys Ther.* 1993;18(4): 553–558.

17. Sell KE, Verity TM, Worrell TW, Pease BJ, Wigglesworth J. Two measurement techniques for assessing subtalar joint position: a reliability study. *J Orthop Sports Phys Ther.* 1994;19(3): 162–167.

18. Shafer N, Duboff S. Physical signs in the early diagnosis of thrombophlebitis. *Angiology.* 1971;22(1):18–30.

19. Smith J, Szczerba JE, Arnold BL, Perrin DH, Martin DE. Role of hyperpronation as a possible risk factor for anterior cruciate ligament injuries. *J Athl Train.* 1997;32(1):25–28.

20. Tatro-Adams D, McGann SF, Carbone W. Reliability of the figure-of-eight method of ankle measurement. *J Orthop Sports Phys Ther.* 1995; 22(4):161–163.

21. Thompson TC, Doherty JH. Spontaneous rupture of tendon of Achilles: a new clinical diagnostic test. *J Trauma.* 1962;2:126–129.

22. Vinicombe A, Raspovic A, Menz HB. Reliability of navicular displacement measurement as a clinical indicator of foot posture. *J Am Podiatr Med Assoc.* 2001;91(5):262–268.

23. Wells PS, Hirsh J, Anderson DR, Lensing AW, Foster G, Kearon C, Weitz J, D'Ovidio R, Cogo A, Prandoni P. Accuracy of clinical assessment of deep-vein thrombosis. *Lancet.* 1995;345 (8961):1326–1330.

Index